Topics in Down Syndrome

MEDICAL & SURGICAL CARE for CHILDREN with DOWN SYNDROME

A Guide for Parents

Edited by D.C. Van Dyke, M.D.,
Philip Mattheis, M.D., Susan Schoon Eberly, M.A.,
and Janet Williams, R.N., Ph.D.

WOODBINE HOUSE ✵ 1995

ABP-2615

Cover illustration & design: Lili Robins
Text illustrations: Richard Huber

Library of Congress Cataloging-in-Publication Data

Medical & surgical care for children with Down syndrome : a guide for parents / edited by D.C. Van Dyke . . . [et al.].

p.   cm. — (Topics in Down sydrome)
Includes bibliographical references and index.
ISBN 0–933149–54–9 : $14.95
1. Down's syndrome—Patients—Medical care. 2. Down's syndrome—Patients—Surgery. 3. Down's syndrome—Patients—Health and hygiene. I. Van Dyke, Don C. II. Series.
RJ506.D68M43 1995
618.92'858842–dc20   95–1177
                                                          CIP

Manufactured in the United States of America

10 9 8 7 6 5 4 3 2

APR 17 1997

Table of Contents

Note from the Editors

The strength and uniqueness of this book lies in the contributions of more than 25 authors representing numerous disciplines in the fields of medicine, nutrition, rehabilitation, and dentistry. The challenge of the book is to present a large volume of sometimes complex information in a way that is useful to parents and non-medical professionals. While all aspects of the vast body of medical knowledge about children with Down syndrome cannot be dealt with in a single book, we have made an effort to cover the key areas and issues.

Each chapter is written from the expertise and the experience of the contributors, who are established experts in their field as it pertains to Down syndrome. In addition, some of the editors and authors have personal knowledge of Down syndrome, whether learned from children of their own or from close friends who have children with Down syndrome.

Children with Down syndrome who have medical conditions are first and foremost children. To emphasize that this book is about children first, we have included photographs of children and adults with Down syndrome throughout the book.

Throughout this book, personal pronouns are alternated from chapter to chapter. We felt uncomfortable referring only to either males or females, and felt that using "he or she" or "she/he" would be unwieldy. Hopefully this arrangement is clear.

We hope the book will be useful to people with and without a medical background who need a practical and organized approach to planning for the care of their child with Down syndrome. And we hope that this book will be a helpful resource to parents and other individuals in meeting the needs of people with Down syndrome.

With all best wishes for your family and your child,

Don C. Van Dyke, M.D.   Susan Schoon Eberly, M.A.
Janet William, RN., Ph.D.   Philip Mattheis, M.D.

Acknowledgments

We wish to acknowledge the many individuals who graciously and without remuneration contributed their expertise to the development of this book. We are especially indebted to a number of individuals from the Division of Developmental Disabilities of the Department of Pediatrics, University of Iowa College of Medicine, and to the staff of University Hospital School, University of Iowa Hospitals and Clinics. In particular, we thank Ginny Miller of the Division of Developmental Disabilities for her editorial and technical expertise, as well as her patience and good humor during the preparation of this book.

Special thanks are extended to Dr. Lula Lubchenco for her Foreword, to Emily Perl Kingsley for her Preface, and to Dr. Allen C. Crocker for his Introduction. We are also grateful to Susan Stokes and the staff at Woodbine House.

In closing, we are deeply indebted to the individuals with Down syndrome and their families who provided information, insight, ideas, and support for this project. A special vote of thanks to Molly Mattheis, patient-parent representative at the Division of Developmental Disabilities, and Dr. Carlyn Christensen-Szalanski, for their careful and caring review of many of the chapters.

Editors

Don C. Van Dyke, M.D.
Division of Developmental Disabilities
The Univeristy of Iowa Hospitals and Clinics
Iowa City, Iowa 52242

Susan Schoon Eberly, M.A.
Division of Developmental Disabilities
The University of Iowa Hospitals and Clinics
Iowa City, Iowa 52242

Philip Mattheis, M.D.
Rural Institute on Disabilities
University of Montana
Missoula, Montana 59812

Janet Williams, R.N., M.A., Ph.D.
College of Nursing
The University of Iowa
Iowa City, Iowa 52242

Graphic Designer
Richard Huber
Division of Developmental Disabilities
The University of Iowa Hospitals and Clinics
Iowa City, Iowa 52242

Contributing Authors

Frederick A. Berry, M.D.
Professor of Anesthesia and Pediatrics
Department of Anesthesia
University of Virginia
Charlottesville, Virginia 22908

Timothy M. Buie, M.D.
Attending Pediatric Gastroenterologist
Wellesley Hospital, Newton Massachusetts
Framingham Union Hospital
Boston, Massachusetts 02115

W. Carl Cooley, M.D.
Assistant Professor of Pediatrics
Associate Director of Clinical Services
Dartmouth Center for Genetics and Child Development
Dartmouth-Hitchcock Medical Center
Hanover, New Hampshire 03756

Anthony J. Cousineau, M.D.
Fellow Associate
Pediatric Cardiology
Department of Pediatrics
The University of Iowa Hospitals and Clinics
Iowa City, Iowa 52242

Allen C. Crocker, M.D.
Associate Professor of Pediatrics
Harvard Medical School
Director, Developmental Evaluation Center
University Affiliated Program
The Children's Hospital
Boston, Massachusetts 02115

Pedro A. de Alarcon, M.D.
Division Head, Professor of Pediatrics
Hematology/Oncology

Children's Medical Center
University of Virginia
Charlottesville, Virginia 22908

Susan Schoon Eberly, M.A.
Publications Supervisor
Division of Developmental Disabilities
The University of Iowa Hospitals and Clinics
Iowa City, Iowa 52242

Thomas E. Elkins, M.D.
Abe Mickal Professor and Head
Department of Obstetrics and Gynecology
School of Medicine in New Orleans
Louisiana State University Medical Center
New Orleans, Louisiana 90112

Alejandro F. Flores Sandoval, M.D.
Clinical Instructor of Pediatrics
Harvard Medical School
Assistant Clinical Professor
Boston University School of Medicine
Consultant in Gastroenterology
Boston Children's Hospital
Assistant Physician
Boston City Hospital
Boston, Massachusetts 02165

Thomas P. Foley, Jr., M.D.
Professor of Pediatrics
Director, Division of Endocrinology, Metabolism, and Diabetes Mellitus
School of Medicine
University of Pittsburgh
Children's Hospital of Pittsburgh
Pittsburgh, Pennsylvania 15213

Kevin T. Kavanagh, M.D., M.S., F.A.C.S.
Department of Ear, Nose & Throat
LeBonheur Children's Hospital
The University of Tennessee
St. Jude's Children's Hospital

Memphis, Tennessee 38103

Emily Perl Kingsley
Writer, Children's Television Workshop (*Sesame Street*)
Chappaqua, New York 10514

Ronald M. Lauer, M.D.
Professor and Director
Pediatric Cardiology
Department of Pediatrics
The University of Iowa Hospitals and Clinics
Iowa City, Iowa 52242

S. Michael Lawhon, M.D.
Orthopedic Surgeon
Wellington Orthopedics and Sports Medicine
Cincinnati, Ohio 45219

David R. Leshtz, M.A.
Disabilities Educator
University Affiliated Program
The University of Iowa Hospitals and Clinics
Iowa City, Iowa 52242

Marta M. Little, M.D.
Clinical Assistant Professor
Department of Internal Medicine
The University of Iowa Hospitals and Clinics
Iowa City, Iowa 52242

Lula O. Lubchenco, M.D.
Professor of Pediatrics Emeritus
University of Colorado
Health Science Center
Denver, Colorado 80262

Philip Mattheis, M.D.
Division of Developmental Disabilities
The University of Iowa Hospitals and Clinics
Iowa City, Iowa 52242

Arthur J. Nowak, D.M.D.
Professor of Dentistry and Pediatrics
College of Dentistry and Medicine
The University of Iowa
Iowa City, Iowa 52242

Peggy L. Pipes, M.P.H., R.D.
Clinical Nutritionist
Child Development and Mental Retardation Center
University of Washington
Seattle, Washington 98815

Robert A. Sargent, M.D.
Associate Clinical Professor of Ophthalmology
University of Colorado Health Science Center
Denver, Colorado 80262

Elaine C. Siegfried, M.D.
Assistant Professor of Dermatology and Pediatrics
Department of Internal Medicine
Division of Dermatology
St. Louis University Medical Center
St. Louis, Missouri 63104

George H. S. Singer, Ph.D.
Associate Professor of Pediatrics
Director, Hood Center for Family Support
Dartmouth-Hitchcock Medical Center
Hanover, New Hampshire 03756

C. Steven Smith, M.D.
Private Practice
Clinical Allergy and Immunology
Louisville, Kentucky 40207

Don C. Van Dyke, M.D.
Associate Professor of Pediatrics
Department of Pediatrics
Division of Developmental Disabilities
The University of Iowa Hospitals and Clinics
Iowa City, Iowa 52242

Foreword
Lula O. Lubchenco, M.D.

Medical information for parents and friends at the birth of a child with Down syndrome child is readily available and usually covers those early important days, weeks, and years. As the child reaches school age or enters adolescence different types of information are needed.

This book is designed to provide a resource for parents of both infants and school-age children with Down syndrome. The editors and their associates at the University of Iowa Hospitals and Clinics have gathered an impressive group of contributors to write chapters in this book. Each author is a specialist in his or her field, and, in addition, has had considerable experience with persons who have Down syndrome. In-depth information is provided for those who wish "to know everything." And if the material in the chapter is not enough to quench this thirst, additional references are given at the end of each chapter.

The chapters cover everything a parent might wish to know, from immunizations to the latest treatment for leukemia. They describe how every part of the human body functions as well as how trisomy 21 alters these functions. The authors cross reference from one chapter to another, making it clear that the person with Down syndrome is more than just a collection of isolated symptoms. Consequently, the reader becomes aware of how the different parts and processes of the human body interact.

The goal of each of the writers is to help parents steer their child with Down syndrome toward a healthy, well-adjusted life. Guidelines are given from early childhood to prepare for the time—which comes sooner than you think—to "let go." This frightening thought is buffered by a description of the many opportunities available today to people with disabilities, but more importantly, it emphasizes the surprising abilities of the person with Down syndrome to live an independent or semi-independent life.

This book is tailor-made for parents, friends, and health care professionals to guide the child who has Down syndrome toward a healthy adulthood.

Preface
Emily Perl Kingsley

In mulling over what I might include in this preface, I thought that I would start by affixing a title... as follows:

War and Peace

I hasten to reassure you that the title does not mean that this preface will be 883 pages long. What I hope it will suggest, though, is the wide range, the gamut of experiences which we have endured in our interactions with medical professionals in the 20 years since the birth of our son who has Down syndrome.

War

Twenty years ago, when our son Jason was only a few hours old, our medical professional, our obstetrician, proceeded to commit every solecism possible in the way he presented the news to us that our son had been born with Down syndrome.

First of all, he spoke to my husband, Charles, *alone,* instead of giving the news to us together, thus leaving Charles with the difficult and painful job of breaking the news to me and attempting to answer my myriad questions.

Secondly, he used the hated "M-word." (This by itself should have tipped us off immediately as to the doctor's outdated attitude and obsolete information—but, sadly, we were not well-enough informed yet to recognize this giveaway clue!)

Thirdly, his assessment of the situation and recommendation were as follows:

"Your child is a mongoloid. He will never sit or stand, walk or talk. He will never be able to distinguish his parents from any other adults who are nice to him. He will never have a meaningful thought. I suggest that you institutionalize him immediately and tell your friends and family that your baby died in childbirth."

The only worse story I ever heard was the one in which the obstetrician, after delivering the same kind of speech, flipped the institutionalization papers onto the new mom's bed, turned on his heels, and walked out of the hospital room without another word.

Our doctor happened to have been an older man, educated in Europe, and, amazingly, in 41 years of obstetrical practice he had never delivered a baby with Down syndrome. I believe it threw him—professionally and personally. Clearly he had not kept up with any of the current literature about the considerable potential and capabilities of individuals with Down syndrome.

Even in those days, 1974, concepts like "infant stimulation" and "early intervention" were beginning to be discussed and programs were being developed to begin the essential early training of these children. But obviously, this unfortunate doctor had not done his homework in these matters and relied on the antiquated training he had received in a Scottish medical school decades earlier.

In addition, it is my personal belief that delivering "bad news" is a particularly difficult thing for obstetricians. I believe that physicians who choose a specialization in obstetrics do so because they enjoy an area of medicine in which, almost all the time, they are bringing joy and fulfillment to people. What nicer job than spending much of your life announcing "It's a girl! It's a boy! Congratulations!"

Contrast that with other areas of medical specialization in which physicians are dealing with death and disease on a much more constant basis. In oncology, for example, giving people bad news is an ever-present part of the job. Doctors who choose those areas of specialization must have the personality and develop the ability to discuss these difficult and painful topics on a daily basis.

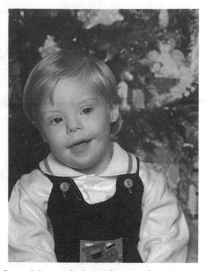

In obstetrics, on the other hand, you're *not* dealing with death and disease nearly so much—and I believe that physicians choose that specialization for exactly that reason. Having to inform people of a "problem" or a "disability" often makes them distinctly uncomfortable and they don't always handle it all that well! Certainly our case bears that out and this belief of mine has been confirmed by many other parents with whom I've spoken who have shared our unfortunate experience.

I should say that it was through the exposure to other parents and children, through a local support group for parents of children with Down syndrome, that we discovered just how misguided our original obstetrician had been in his assessment and prognosis.

I am happy to report that, not withstanding our unfortunate introduction to the "world of Down syndrome," our son is doing beautifully. He recently graduated from a regular high school with a regular full academic diploma. He is a capable and well-adjusted young man who is bright, imaginative, and creative. And he is the joy of our lives.

Peace

Happily, we have also experienced the "other side of the coin." We've encountered professionals (many more, thankfully, on this side of the coin than the other) who have de-

voted themselves to keeping up with all of the current literature, philosophies, and attitudes about children with Down
syndrome and who are sensitive, encouraging, and optimistic.

Fortunately too, the outreach network has improved enormously from the way it was 19 years ago. Our local parent support group frequently receives three separate phone calls
within the first 24 hours, informing us of a new baby's birth,
usually from the hospital nursing staff, the social worker, and
the genetic counselor who's been called in. In this way, we are
able to visit with new parents immediately and give them full
and accurate information, answer their questions, and demystify the situation.

With all respect to the most inspired and compassionate
of physicians, nothing is quite the same as talking to another
parent!

In that early conversation, we are always sure to give the
following, seemingly contradictory, advice to new parents:
Choose a pediatrician who is completely familiar with the "dif-
ferentness" of your child as well as the "sameness" of your
child.

What this means is this: On the one hand, you must feel
comfortable that a pediatrician is totally up to date with all of
the most current research and information regarding all of
the conditions that are unique to Down syndrome. In Jason's
early life, we frequently had the experience of having our pediatrician explain that, while he ordinarily prescribed a certain medication for a particular problem, his patients who had
Down syndrome reacted better to a *different* medication. The
fact that people with Down syndrome have narrow ear canals
and are particularly susceptible to ear infections led our pediatrician to check Jason's ears—no matter what else was the reason for our visit. We always felt that our pediatric team was on
top of anything specific to Down syndrome that could possibly
be present.

In this case, a doctor who tells you, "Oh, we'll just treat
your child exactly like any other child" is somewhat of a red

flag to me. You want
to feel confident that
your doctors are
reading all of the
newest literature
and keeping up with
all progress being
made in the medical
treatment of those
conditions which ac-
company Down syndrome.

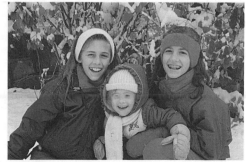

On the other hand, you also want to make sure that your
doctors will be treating your child with entirely as much dignity, respect, and caring as they would extend to any other
child. You must know—utterly—that your child will receive
that same quality of care, with the same immediacy and thor-
oughness of care, that the doctor would afford any child. In
that respect, your child *must* be seen as "just another child"
with the same integrity and worth as any child in that doctor's practice.

In our area we have come to know many of the doctors
who enjoy and believe in our children. We pass the word to
each other and when a new baby is born, we are able to recommend sympathetic and knowledgeable doctors. In that way,
those doctors tend to have large numbers of patients with
Down syndrome and it becomes more and more necessary for
them to keep themselves up to date. Needless to say, we are
also in a position to advise new parents about doctors to avoid
because of their outdated attitudes.

I am happy to say that in the 19 years of our involvement
with Down syndrome, and in the 19 years of exposure to the
professional community helping our new families as they continue to come along, I have observed a tremendous improvement in the attitudes of physicians, nurses and other medical
professionals dealing with our children. You almost never
hear of a doctor giving parents the kind of advice we received.

Unfortunately, I can't say "never." It still occurs from time to time—but, thankfully, it's extremely rare.

With better public awareness, people everywhere are seeing individuals with Down syndrome as just that—*individuals*—with individual profiles, capabilities, and personalities. There is a much more general recognition that people with Down syndrome are entitled to every human and civil right enjoyed by anyone else, to every legal protection, and to the availability of any medical or educational program necessary to help them to achieve their considerable potential and live full, active, and productive lives.

Introduction
Allen C. Crocker, M.D.

Understanding has grown substantially about the best ways to provide accurate and effective health care for children with Down syndrome. This real increase in knowledge now makes it possible to demystify many of the formerly puzzling differences seen in people with Down syndrome. A possible by-product, of course, of gathering all this modern information could be to overwhelm parents and families. Some might say that all these chapters may create a false impression of vulnerability. Many of the chapters discuss potentially alarming matters like orthopedic, respiratory, or neurologic problems. But surely the availability of current knowledge, put appropriately (and, even, lovingly) in context, is a true improvement over the amorphous impersonal care of children with Down syndrome just a decade or two ago.

It is remarkable that so much is known. When you consider that persons with Down syndrome represent less than one tenth of a percent of the population (1 in 1000 births) it is intriguing that so much advocacy and organization (and writing of books) exists about them. Clearly, many workers and families have been captured in a common effort, one characterized by appreciation and joining. The books on health care such as this one are produced in an attempt to get it right, to honor persons with trisomy 21, and to build for the best quality of life.

The Health Care Trip Begins

The baby with Down syndrome has already shown good survival capacity by the time of birth. In many other kinds of chromosomal change in human fetuses there is a high mortality rate early in pregnancy. Making it to birth, the new baby with Down syndrome is usually in good condition, and notably appealing. As the health care team examines the child, two items must be promptly considered. These will be described in much detail in the chapters that follow. The most compelling element, of course, is the possible presence of a significant malformation of the heart. The other is the chance that obstruction exists within the gastrointestinal tract. A forewarning about either of these may have been provided from ultrasound examinations in the last three months of pregnancy. Each of these phenomena is manageable with proper care.

All things considered, the newborn period usually proceeds well. Things may be quite tumultuous for the parents, but the baby is doing nicely. The surprise (usually) and challenge engendered by the arrival of this special new human may show itself in an unsettled environment, which can become part of the problem. Parent-to-parent encouragement is a priceless assistance in the adjustment. The importance of parent-to-parent contacts is emphasized throughout this book, particularly in Chapter 1, "Decision Making for Parents," and Chapter 19, "Resources for 'Resilient' Families."

As childhood proceeds, other health issues may present themselves. These are less pressing, and can be dealt with in turn. A helpful concept is to view these little people as "alike/unalike" other children. The "alike" parts are in the majority, of course. They are discussed well by Dr. Cooley in Chapter 2, which deals with preventive medical care, and include such usual components as immunization, treatment of acute infections and other upsets, safety guidance, and attention to principles of nutrition, growth, and behavioral concerns. The "unalike" elements are gentle but real, and are what this book is about. It is important to understand that children with Down syndrome have somewhat altered risks for various medically significant features. They are more likely to have certain conditions than are other children. The problems they may experience, however, are not different in nature from issues that also arise with typical children, and with children who have other developmental disorders. Children with Down syndrome get more notice because the rate of occurrence of these conditions and problems is different. Consequently, it is quite important for the care provider and the family to be aware of the elements of their child's biological specialness so that needed interventions can be timely and fitting. These elements are discussed in detail in the chapters that follow.

Access to Good Health Care

Families seek care from physicians and other health care workers that is well informed, resourceful, and empathetic. Numerous developments have occurred in the last 15 to 20 years to make high quality care a reasonable expectation for children with Down syndrome. There are a wide range of health care providers who practice in many different settings. All high quality doctors, including the family physician, should be able to help children with Down syndrome. The comments that follow describe some of the different types of pediatric practices.

The type of health care provider that we can call *Physician A* carries the major responsibility for your child's medical care. This is the general pediatrician providing primary care in the community, usually with a stable location and regular contact. General physicians commonly have not had extensive training in child development issues (or in the special features of children with "syndromes"), but their busy careers assist them in gaining useful information about human variation and special family dynamics. These physicians generally know their child patients well. Problem solving for complex issues may be more of a challenge, but this can be assisted by referring patients to specialists when needed. In addition, the opportunity exists for advocacy on behalf of the child and family,

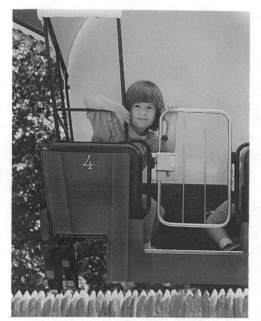

and the primary care pediatrician can be an important ally in the community and school.

Physician B also runs a primary care office, but for a variety of reasons has a particular interest in the care of children with special needs. A personal tie to children with disabilities, from community activities or from his or her family, may sometimes be an element in this interest. Usually this person has had conventional pediatric training, but becomes involved in continuing education courses and conferences regarding developmental disorders. Such physicians have something of a dilemma regarding office logistics, since deliberate review sessions for special children and their families take a longer time to be done right and there are many meetings to attend and reports to write. Somehow these warm persons make it work. There seem to be more of them now than a decade ago, perhaps because children with disabilities are a lively and growing force in the physician's patient population.

Finally there is another type of care provider whom we shall call *Physician C.* These people work in hospitals or child development centers. They have had fellowships or other postgraduate training in children's developmental disorders, and their practice is full-time in this area. In this setting it is expected that special knowledge about different conditions and possible complications will be available, plus state-of-the-art diagnostic and intervention techniques. These physicians can be particularly valuable when a child with Down syndrome needs to be admitted to a hospital. They commonly work as part of multi- or interdisciplinary teams, blending medical insight with insights from other child development professionals for evaluation and program planning.

Day to day health care for children with special needs inevitably (and appropriately) rests with the community practitioners, Physicians A and B. A survey of pediatricians in Massachusetts a few years ago showed that most saw about five children with Down syndrome in their practices. The use of developmental pediatricians (Physician C) for primary care is generally not feasible or really advantageous, but they should be liberally used for assessment or consultation as needed. Local parent groups are a good source of information regarding pediatricians in the area who are potential allies. Interestingly, there are now more than 20 specialized "Down syndrome clinics" in various child development centers around the country; they are listed at the end of Chapter 19. Chapter 19 also contains information on parent advocacy groups that can guide you to the most useful services in your area.

The Family Health Care Record System

Parents sometimes joke that a filing cabinet would be a beneficial baby gift for the family with an infant with special needs (including children with Down syndrome). There is so much to become familiar with, to explore, to record, and to remember. Inevitably the process will be more secure and effective if a good mechanism for storing information exists, though personal taste will dictate which method fits best.

First, families should keep a log or a journal, recording notes about health-related events. This can include names of physicians and other health care providers, dates of immunizations, measurements of growth, times of illness, medications and their responses, and, of course, the little person's developmental achievements.

Secondly, make good use of the numerous recent books available. You may want to loan them out later to other new parents, but keep a record of their authors, titles, and dates (note the many references in the resource sections at the end of each chapter in this book). Be sure to subscribe to *Exceptional Parent Magazine*, and save all the back issues. You can order from P. O. box 3000, Dept. EP, Denville, NJ 07845–9919. Health care matters are regularly discussed in this magazine. Information sheets and releases on many specific health topics can be obtained from the National Down Syndrome Congress (the phone number is 800/232–NDSC). These reports are periodically revised. Likewise, the *Down Syndrome News* (which is published by the NDSC) customarily has articles on guidance for good health care, with warm attention to the needs of parents. Other advocacy groups with a special focus on individuals with Down syndrome are described in Chapter 19.

Thirdly, it is of great value for you to maintain a permanent file of specific medical documents and reports of studies. If your child has received services from a variety of physicians or facilities for different aspects of care, your family records may constitute the most complete file and will have many uses. In hospitals or centers, records sometimes get misfiled or even lost; the family's notes can be a wonderful back-up. Work with your health care provider's office to obtain copies of key items—it is your right to have full access to these. Reasonable materials would be copies of assessments, letters between doctors or facilities, discharge summaries from hospitals, consultation reports, x-ray and laboratory reports, descriptions of the chromosome studies, and even bills and claim forms. If, on handling these, you note elements that puzzle you, or you think they may not be accurate, it is entirely appropriate to speak up and get explanations or corrections.

All of this collecting and filing may seem a little mechanistic at first, but it does assist you to become an "informed consumer." You can also anticipate that the material will serve as a comforting documentary of successes and gains.

A Philosophy for Medical Care

This book will show you that a great deal of current information supports appropriate health care for the child with Down syndrome. There is now effective treatment for many of the conditions that can affect children with Down syndrome. Treatment of many of the most pressing concerns, such as cardiac problems, ocular (eye) function, seizures if they occur, and endocrine difficulties, can now be handled well. On occasion, repeated infections may be bewildering, and certain gastrointestinal problems can be challenging. For some children preservation of optimal hearing requires considerable effort. Growth and personal adjustment can sometimes be elusive. And, in adult life, the prevention of early changes related to aging remains incompletely understood.

Considerable change is occurring in the circumstances of care for individual children with Down syndrome and other developmental disorders. Attitudes of health care providers and families have changed a lot in the last decade. Social evolution, the emphasis of children's rights, and professional development are all part of it. Families can now consider themselves full partners in health care diagnosis, decisions, and quality assurance. It is entirely reasonable for you to require your pediatrician to share your philosophy and attitude about your child with Down syndrome. These matters should be talked over, early on, and then later again if needed. Don't be shy about changing physicians if the fit is not good. Actually, you and your child have a lot to teach the doctor, as well as the other way around, and that can be a most fulfilling

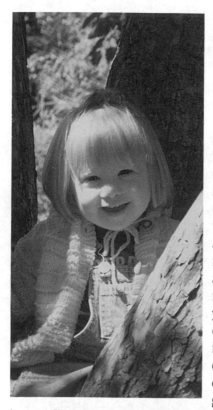

process. The medical visit often goes best if the parent(s) bring written questions to the session, and make direct notes about the conclusions.

Your pediatrician can and should be of much help in assuring effective use of early intervention, creative school programs, and physical therapy, occupational therapy, speech therapy, arts therapy, and so forth. In mutual problem-solving about health and development concerns, you and your physician may reach out together for other opinions. The response of "I don't know" is an honorable one, as long as it is earnestly given and followed through by an effort to gain the information needed. The use of a Physician C type, and of the resources of a developmental center, can be helpful for all parties. However, resort to unusual or alternative, sometimes extreme, therapies or manipulations is rarely a solution (see Chapter 15).

Finally, be of good faith! Regarding health matters, for children with Down syndrome as for all children, there may be discouraging moments, but appropriate assistance is at hand in the great majority of situations. The big stories in the life of a child with Down syndrome are usually not medically related. Rather they concern individual progress, accommodation, fulfillment, and happiness. After the visit to the doctor's office is over, you can move on to the "wellness" model, dealing with central stuff of life and its rewards. In our generation a true "cure" for Down syndrome is not in sight, but intelligent means exist for the achievement of good general health and excellent life opportunities.

1 | Making Decisions as the Parent of a Child with a Disability

George H.S. Singer, Ph.D.

All Parents Are Decision Makers

Parents make decisions about their children every day. They decide what to make for dinner and what time to pick up the baby from day care. They decide if a child should be scolded for a misbehavior or if it is better to let it go. They decide how much time they can put into helping a child with homework and how to balance one child's need for help with a brother or sister's wish to have them come to a little league game. For most of these decisions parents rely upon what they see other parents doing, they draw upon experiences from their own childhoods, and they rely on day-to-day routines to make many decisions automatically.

Parents of children with disabilities are also decision makers. Many of the decisions that a parent makes about a child with a disability are the same as the ones they need to make for their other children. "Do I send her to school today with that cough? How late should I let her stay up on a school night? Is she safe playing outside after dark?"

But there are also many unusual decisions. In some cases, parents must decide early in the pregnancy whether they want to become the parents of a child with Down syndrome. Soon after birth, some parents of children with Down syndrome will have to make difficult decisions about surgeries. Later they must decide how much they want to be involved in early intervention services or what degree of inclusion they want for their child in school. Parents of a child with Down syndrome may also have to make many more decisions about medical care than other parents. Many of these decisions cannot be made automatically, nor can they be made by looking to see what the neighbors do. There are few guidelines to go by. Parents usually cannot rely on their own childhood experiences because they did not grow up in a family where a child had a disability. As a result, these parents have to make a lot more decisions with no "rules of thumb" to draw upon.

When it comes to medical decisions, parents often have to deal with difficult technical issues and complex medical terms and procedures. Most parents are not prepared for this sudden immersion in the medical world. In the language of social science, there are few norms to follow. Consequently, parents of children with Down syndrome are exceptional decision makers. They have to make medical decisions with little guidance from their culture. What can be done so that decision making for a child with Down syndrome will be a process that leaves parents feeling that they are in charge and that they have made good decisions?

Two crucial kinds of support can help with medical decision making:

1) getting in touch with other parents of children with Down syndrome or other disabilities; and
2) forming an alliance with a supportive and knowledgeable medical professional.

Parent-to-Parent Support

The special help that parents can get from other parents is best summed up by a father who said, "You can't imagine unless you have been there yourself." Other parents of children with disabilities can provide you with a special kind of support. They are familiar with many of the feelings that you will have as you adjust to being the parent of a child with a disability. They are familiar with the day-to-day realities of living with a child with special needs. They are familiar with the special contributions that children with Down syndrome make to their families. Also, they are likely to "know the ropes" when it comes to getting the right kind of medical help. They may be able to tell you what their experience has been with different physicians and point you toward a doctor or a clinic that is particularly good with children with Down syndrome.

One of the reasons that parent-to-parent helping can be very effective is because you share common experiences with other parents. They know what it is like to be on the receiving end of the news that their child has an exceptional condition. They know what it is like to tell their relatives about the new baby. And they probably have had to make medical decisions similar to the ones you face. Parent-to-parent connections are likely to work best if the parent you contact is able not only to share feelings with you but also to help you take a positive view. If a parent-to-parent helper is too negative, or is so positive that it makes you feel that your own sad feelings aren't "right," then the match may not work out. You may have to try talking to more than one veteran parent before you find the right match. Sometimes parents report that they tried to talk to another parent and it didn't go well the first time. Keep trying—the rewards of connecting with a "kindred soul" can be great. It is not uncommon for parents to report that other parents changed their life by sharing their experiences.

When you talk to other parents of children with Down syndrome you can ask them about specific medical conditions that may effect your child. It is very likely that they have had similar experiences. They may be able to tell you what it is like, for example, to take care of an infant after surgery, or to treat a child at home for chronic ear infections. They will understand that these situations affect you and your family, as well as your child. They may be able to give you some suggestions about how to arrange for help while your child is in the hospital, or about ways to take care of yourself while caring for your child. In other words, they will understand how care

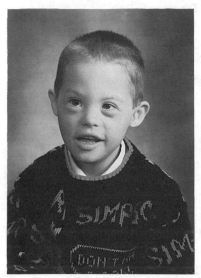

giving and decision making feels, and how it can have an impact on you and your family.

Often the diagnosis of a child with Down syndrome takes place in a way that makes parents feel powerless. For example, many children are identified in the hospital soon after birth. In this situation, parents usually have given a lot of control over to the medical staff. Having a baby in a hospital is treated as a medical event in which doctors and nurses make the big decisions. The medical workers have special expertise, and parents feel that they must rely upon this knowledge for their own health as well as their baby's.

This means that the world in which a baby with Down syndrome is first identified is a world that is run by technical experts who know many facts and many words that are not commonly part of the parents' day to day life. It is in this technical, "expert" world that parents first learn that their baby is different.

Parents of children with disabilities will often remark that they finally decided one day that their baby was a child first and a person with a disability second. Sometimes I ask parents, "Why did you ever start thinking your baby was a disability first and a child second?" They usually answer by saying that when they were given the baby's diagnosis, they thought it meant that this child was something *completely* different— a different kind of baby, one that they did not know anything about. This difference was linked to a need for experts, to the technical nature of a hospital, and to a strange world of medical terms and procedures. It is as if these parents unexpectedly got a baby from a different world—a technical, medical world.

Sometimes the nurses and doctors in the hospital communicate to parents that something very bad has happened when a baby with Down syndrome is born. Parents talk about the way the nurses got very quiet when their baby was born and the way no one would make eye contact with the mother. Or they will sometimes say that their doctor was difficult to hear and understand when he or she first told them about their baby. Sometimes the medical procedures are different when a baby with a disability is born. For example, instead of giving the baby to the mother and father to hold right away, the baby is taken away for observation or, sometimes, for intensive care. Sometimes the first sight that parents have of their new baby is in an incubator, surrounded by tubes and wires. All of these practices can make a parent think that this baby is something really different—a "child with a disability" first, and a baby second.

Parents often talk about a day when they decide, "This baby is my kid. She is a baby first, someone with a disability second." They feel as if they make this decision all at once, at the point when they begin to feel stronger and less intimidated by their baby's condition. A lot of experiences lead up to this decision. Many of these experiences come from simply getting to know the new baby. After holding her, feeding her, changing her, and watching her, parents start to see this baby as a unique person, someone who has a special place in their family and in their hearts. These experiences are part of a process that is often called *bonding*. Bonding is an important part of a new relationship with any baby. It can sometimes take longer to emerge with a baby with a disability.

Another part of deciding to see the baby as a member of the family first and as an exceptional child second has to do with grieving. Most parents have an idea in mind of what they expect their baby to be like when it is born. These ideas often include dreams such as "He'll be a great baseball player," or "She'll grow up to be a scientist." Sometimes the ideas about the baby can be a lot more concrete: "He'll be cute and have curly hair like his father." Every baby comes into a world in which her mom and dad have some expectations. This "ideal baby" has been growing in the parent's minds for at least nine months, and in some ways it is as real as the flesh and blood child who is born. When parents suddenly learn that their baby has Down syndrome, they may experience the sudden loss of their ideal child. This loss can feel as real and as painful as if their child had actually died. And so some parents (not all) go through a time of grief in which they feel as sad as if they have had a great loss. Many parents of children with disabilities have these feelings. It can be very reassuring to talk to other parents of children with disabilities in order to understand that these feelings are normal—and also that they fade and become less important with time.

So, the decision to view the new baby as your child first and a baby with a disability second can grow out of having:

- experiences that help you to bond with the baby;
- passing through a grieving process; and
- making contact with other people who have had similar experiences and have "come out the other end"

It can also make a tremendous difference if you can find a medical professional who can be your ally as you practice your new role as a parent.

Developing a Reliable Ally in the Medical Field

Another very important kind of support for making medical decisions can and should come from a relationship with a medical professional. Ideally, this support would come from your family doctor, although your special ally may also be a specialist, a physician's assistant, or a nurse. Parents who adapt well to having a child with special health care needs are able to develop a working partnership with a medical professional. This "reliable alliance" can make a tremendous difference as you deal with the necessity to make difficult choices.

Several ingredients make up a reliable alliance. First, the attitude that you carry into the relationship makes a difference. Many parents who have adjusted well to being "exceptional parents" talk about the way that they decided to take charge of their relationship with their doctor and hospital. They say things like, "I decided I was the customer and that I needed to be treated right." Or they will say, "I decided that I might not know all of the technical information about this baby, but I am her parent. I know what it's like to be the person who is most responsible for this baby in the whole world." Professionals who become reliable allies with parents treat the mother and father with respect. They listen to the parents' concerns and they also rely on the parents to give them important information about the baby. Reliable allies treat parents like partners.

Here is a list of phrases that parents have used when asked to describe the professional who is their reliable ally:

She listens to me.

He takes my observations seriously.

He treats me like I'm an important part of the team.

She values my opinion.

She will ask if the treatment plan will fit into our daily schedule.

He lets me know that he cares about how I am feeling, as well as about my baby's health.

She uses language that I can understand.

He takes the time to talk to me.

*I trust that she will call me back if I need to get * *in touch.*

He treats my child like a person.

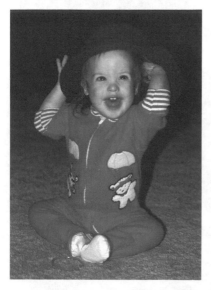

You can see from these statements that a reliable ally is not only competent in his or her profession, but also has some relationship skills that make a big difference to parents. One way to find a professional who can become your "reliable ally" is by talking with other parents to get the benefit of their experience.

Parents who have had a lot of medical experience also talk about two important roles that they play. One is to keep hope alive. The second is to keep reminding everyone that this baby is, first of all, a person.

Sometimes parents feel like they are the only ones who keep hope alive for their child. Often professionals seem to believe that they should tell parents all of the worst possible things that might happen to a baby with disabilities. Their motives for giving a lot of bad news can be very good. However, many parents feel that in order to keep going over the long haul, they have to remain hopeful. Sometimes it can feel like a battle against people who are negative. Deciding to keep hope alive can be as simple as reminding yourself of all the happy moments you have had, and will have, with your baby. Or remembering that your child may be different than other children, but will still have a good life. For example, the father of a child with a rare genetic condition recently explained that it was very helpful to attend a meeting of parents who have children with the same rare disorder. He saw some older children with the condition playing with their brothers and sisters at a swimming pool. He said, "All of a sudden I realized that these children can be happy and have good times. Nobody told me that. Because of all the problems my little girl has had, somehow I forgot that she might have a good life." For some parents a major decision is the decision to keep hope.

Another decision that some parents talk about is deciding to *insist* that other people recognize the personhood of their child. This decision is similar to deciding to view the child as a child first and a person with a disability second. For example, one mother talked about a time when her son was in intensive care in a hospital. He had been in a terrible car accident and was comatose because of a head injury. She said, "I couldn't stand the thought that the doctors and nurses would think of my son as just a thing with tubes going in and out of him." In order to keep the personhood of her child alive in their minds, she collected photographs of her son from different times in his life. She put these pictures all around his hospital room and next to his bed. They reminded staff that he was special person to his family, a real child with a real life.

Similarly, parents of children who must stay in an intensive care neonatal unit (ICNU) will often talk about how important it is that the doctors and nurses treat their baby like a person who has feelings. For example, one mother remembered a resident who was particularly sensitive to this. Whenever he gave a report to the mother and father, he always held the baby at the same time, rocked her, and talked to her gently and affectionately. Sometimes parents choose to begin to advocate for their child soon after birth by insisting that others treat the baby as a person with feelings.

Deciding to Advocate for Your Child

A related decision that many parents make is deciding to advocate for their child. Once again, parents report that this decision happens along with a kind of shift in their understanding. For example, one father said. "One day it really hit home for me. If I'm not out there fighting for my child, nobody is going to do it. I just realized that it is up to me." Parents have to make decisions about how much time and energy they want to commit to advocacy. Some parents join advocacy organizations and put a lot of time and effort into the work of these organizations. Other parents decide that they have to give priority to other parts of their lives. Again, there is no correct answer to the question of how committed you should be to advocacy for your child and others with disabilities.

Finding a Balance

Parents of children with Down syndrome have to decide about maintaining some important balances in their lives. Here are some of the parts of the family system that parents have to balance:

- Time for their child with Down syndrome with time for their other children;
- Time for their child with time for each other; and
- Time for their child with time for oneself.

There is no magic formula that will tell what the right balance is. Generally, you can tell if things get way out of balance. Brothers and sisters will let you know through what they say or what they do if they are feeling neglected. You can tell whether your marriage is getting too little attention if it has been a long time since you and your spouse had fun together, or if you feel you are drifting apart. And you can tell if you need to be giving more to yourself if you are often feeling exhausted, discouraged, or just plain resentful.

In thinking about these balances, it can be helpful to remember that you will have the job of parent for a long time. This is a marathon race, not a sprint. And so you have to pace yourself. Talking to other parents can sometimes provide you with information about how they balance these competing priorities. Sometimes you have to decide to get some extra help in order to keep a balance in the family. For example, many parents make use of special child care services so that they can have time for themselves or for their other children.

Finding a Balance between *Habilitation* and *Acceptance*

Here is another set of decisions that parents of children with Down syndrome must deal with over time. They have to decide how much time, effort, and expense should go into giving their child special training. Often children with Down syndrome will work with more than one professional at a time. For example, a child might be getting habilitation services from a physical therapist, an occupational therapist, and a speech therapist. These professionals often give homework assignments for the child and their parents.

Parents have to decide how much time they want to devote to habilitation work with their child. Some balance is necessary between helping the child to develop to the fullest (habilitation), and allowing the child to simply be herself as she is (acceptance). Again, there is no recipe book that can tell you what the ideal balance is, but it can be helpful to talk to others about these decisions. Also, it is important to note that these choices are not "one time only decisions." In reality, they often have to be adapted to fit changing family circumstances. In some years you may decide that it is very important to spend a lot of time teaching your child self-help skills. In other years, you may decide that you want to let your child have as much free time as possible.

Realistic Expectations

Mothers and fathers have to decide many times a day how much to expect of a child with a Down syndrome. For example, if you tell your child, "Be sure to take your medicine at lunch time," what should you do at the end of the day if the pills are still in her lunch pail? Several questions come to mind. Is it fair to ask a child with mental retardation to remember for so long? Is it forgetfulness or does the child not like the medicine? Once again, there is no easy answer.

When I work with parents of children with disabilities, I tell them that the safest assumption when a child does not follow directions is to assume that the task is too hard for her or she did not understand, rather than to assume that she is refusing to cooperate. These judgments have to be made over and over again, and they can change from one circumstance to the next. For example, a child who rides the bus at the end of the school day may need to be supervised closely until she gets on board, while a second child might do well with just a reminder from the teacher. A third child may be very capable of managing completely independently. Or, your child's ability to cope may vary from day to day, depending upon what is happening at the end of the school day, before and while she is waiting for the bus. It may become necessary to look closely at each day's schedule to identify things that make Monday harder than Thursday, for example.

Sometimes other parents or teachers can give you useful information about what kinds of expectations are fair to have for your child. For example, a teacher might know that your child can do a task at school, so that you know it will be fair to ask her to do it at home.

Deciding what is fair often involves thinking about the values that matter for your child. For example, many parents decide that they want their child to live as normal a life as possible. They try to see that she participates in as many family and community activities as possible. A value that is important to many parents is the concept of "the dignity of risk."

That is, they decide to let their child experience many different situations in order to learn to be as independent as possible.

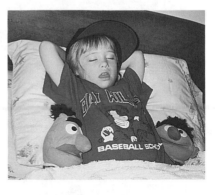

Summary

In summary, there are many kinds of decisions that parents have to make in living with a child with Down syndrome. All parents have to make judgments about raising their children. They often get guidance by watching what other parents do or by remembering their own childhoods. But when a child with a disability joins the family, there are fewer guidelines. Many decisions are the small choices that make up the flow of daily life. But other decisions represent major shifts in thinking. To help with both kinds of decisions, it can make a big difference to have reliable allies—your spouse, your extended family, other parents, friends, and professionals. Talking about these choices with others can generate a vital kind of support that will help you to make the best decisions you can for your child.

Resources

Exceptional Parent Magazine, P.O. Box 3000, Denville, NJ 07834; 800/247-8080.

2 | Preventive Health Care for Children with Down Syndrome

W. Carl Cooley, M.D.

Introduction—Prevention and Health Promotion

Pediatric health care has a long history of emphasizing the value of prevention. Prevention means avoiding illness, injury, or disability by taking action before a problem develops. Prevention can also mean reducing the severity of a problem when it cannot be entirely prevented. Typical examples of prevention include immunizing for infections like measles and polio, wearing seat belts to prevent death or serious injury in automobile accidents, and brushing teeth and using fluoride to prevent cavities. Prevention is actually part of a larger idea called *health promotion* in which a healthy, fulfilling life is the goal, rather than simply preventing bad things from happening along the way.

Your child with Down syndrome needs the same preventive or health-promoting care as any other child. This care is usually provided through a series of visits to a pediatrician, family physician, nurse practitioner, child health associate, or maternal and child health clinic.

These "well child visits" involve a review of parental concerns and a discussion of your child's health, development, and daily habits (eating, sleep, play) since the previous visit. Measurements of height, weight, and head circumference are taken, and a physical examination is performed. Tests may be done to screen for lead poisoning, anemia, or problems with hearing and vision, and immunizations (shots) may be given according to a schedule. Counseling called "anticipatory guidance" is also provided about things to watch for, new foods to introduce, accidents to avoid, and changes in your child's behavior which may occur prior to the next visit. These health promotion visits are in contrast to visits which occur because a child is ill.

Preventive care may also be provided when your child is ill. This may take the form of information and counseling about your child's illness. For example, if your child is prone to repeated colds that become complicated by pneumonia, you can learn to spot the early signs and seek treatment. If your child has a skin infection, you can learn dry skin care that could prevent skin infections in the future.

All of these services should be the same for children with Down syndrome, and the health care provider should pay the same attention to "regular" concerns as he or she would for a child without Down syndrome. That means that nearly all children with Down syndrome should follow the same sequence of "well child visits," receive the same immunizations, and undergo the same measurements, physical examinations, and screening tests as all children. Parents of children with Down syndrome should expect to receive the same advice and counseling about accident prevention and safety, about eating and sleeping, and about behavior management as that offered to parents of other children.

In addition to the usual preventive health measures recommended for all children, there are some specific areas of care which may warrant more attention in the child with Down syndrome. Having Down syndrome does not mean that your child requires more health care, but it does increase the risk for certain kinds of problems. Some of these problems are serious and potentially life-threatening, such as congenital heart disease. Other problems are less serious and more like the health concerns of most children—but if these conditions are not discovered and treated, they may cause more serious illness or may slow down some areas of development. For example, the child with Down syndrome who has a hearing problem that is not identified and treated will have more problems with language development, more difficulty socializing, and may be at greater risk for additional learning problems later on.

This chapter provides an overview of some of the specific preventive health care that may benefit your child with Down syndrome and your family. Details about specific conditions or problems will be found in later chapters; for example, additional information about hearing problems is provided in Chapter 8 on ear, nose, throat, and sinus concerns. The references at the end of this chapter include more technical books and articles about the health care concerns of people with Down syndrome. These may interest some parents, and may also be recommended by parents to their doctors and other health care providers.

Preventive Health Care Plan

Most primary health care services are provided in or close to a child's own community by health care professionals (doctors, nurses, physician assistants) who are familiar with the child and his family. These services may occur in a doctor's office, health center, or clinic. Primary health care services include both well child visits ("check-ups") and the care of children when they are sick. Primary health care is the type of care that does not require consultation with a specialist or a visit to a specialized clinic. Developing and following a preventive health care plan is one of the most important roles of the primary health care provider.

Children with Down syndrome and their families usually receive preventive health care through their relationship with a knowledgeable and interested primary health care provider. Ideally, this professional is aware of the preventive care needs of children with Down syndrome and is able to include those needs in an overall plan for preventive health care. Figures 1

Figure 1—Pediatric Immunization

AGE	IMMUNIZATION
2 months	DPT, OPV, HIB
4 months	DPT, OPV, HIB
6 months	DPT, HIB
9 - 12 months	Tb Test
15 months	MMR, HIB
18 months	DPT, OPV
5 years	DPT, OPV

DPT = diptheria, pertussis, tetanus
OPV = oral polio vaccine
HIB = hemophilus b vaccine
MMR = measles, mumps, rubella (German measles)
Tb test = tuberculosis screening test

and 2 include elements of the preventative health care plan for your child. Your concerns, questions, and suggestions should play an important role in the development of this plan.

Just as parents have a right to take part in the planning of their child's education, you should also be supported as a partner in the process of planning for health care. For example, you may have information about issues like atlantoaxial instability (discussed in Chapter 10) or thyroid conditions (discussed in Chapter 5) that should help determine when and how your child will be monitored for these conditions. Your child's primary health care provider should seek and value your input.

The American Academy of Pediatrics provides pediatricians, family physicians, and other health care providers with guidelines and recommendations for preventive health care planning for all children. This outline of well child visits, immunizations, screening tests, and counseling should be the starting point for the preventive health care plan for your child with Down syndrome. This will ensure that routine preventive health care is never overlooked. Figure 1 lists the usual schedule of immunizations recommended for young children. Most children with Down syndrome should follow the same immunization schedule.

Experts on the health care of children with Down syndrome recognize that, in addition to routine preventive health care, children should be screened for certain conditions that are known to occur more frequently with Down syndrome. Not all experts agree on exactly what kind of screening is needed, exactly when or how often it should be done, or exactly who should do it. Some recommendations are based on careful, accurate research, and other recommendations are the "best guesses" of experienced professionals.

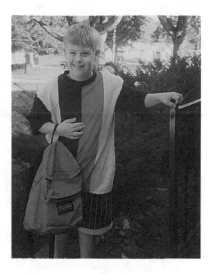

This situation can create confusion for parents about what is best for their child. It creates confusion, as well, for primary care physicians and nurses about what is needed.

Figure 2, Healthwatch for the Person with Down Syndrome, summarizes the preventive health care concerns that parents can share with their primary health care provider. In addition, the references at the end of this chapter provide a list of books and articles that contain more detailed information about preventive health care recommendations for the child with Down syndrome.

Newsletters for parents, such as the *Down Syndrome News* of the National Down Syndrome Congress (1605 Chantilly Drive, Atlanta, GA 30324; 1–800–232–6372), are also useful resources for up-to-date recommendations and information. Down syndrome clinics or programs are available at a number of medical centers around the country. These programs can be valuable resources for both parents and primary care professionals, but should not be regarded as a substitute for primary care. The National Down Syndrome Congress has a list of Down syndrome programs in each region of the United States.

Figure 2—Healthwatch for the Person with Down Syndrome

Adapted with permission from Crocker and Rubin (1989)

CONCERN	CLINICAL EXPRESSION	WHEN SEEN	PREVALENCE	MANAGEMENT
congenital heart disease	complete AV canal septal defects mitral prolapse	newborn or first six weeks; later for mitral prolapse	40 - 50%;	Pediatric cardiology consultation; echocardiogram; surgery; dental prophylaxis
hypotonia	reduced muscle tone; increased range of joint movement; motor function problems	throughout life; tends to improve with age	100%	guidance by physical therapy early intervention program
delayed growth	usually near or below third percentile of general population for height	throughout life	100%	nutritional support; DS growth charts check heart/thyroid; ?growth hormone in future
developmental delays	some global delay, degree varies; specific processing problems; specific language delay	first year; monitor throughout life	100%	early intervention individual educational plan language intervention
hearing problems	middle ear problems (fluid and infections) sensorineural hearing loss	screen in first six months; recheck annually	50-70%	audiology, tympanometry ENT consultation myringotomy tubes if needed
vision problems	refractive errors strabismus cataracts	eye exam in 1st month; then annually	50% 35% 15%	pediatric ophthalmologic consultation and appropriate treatment
cervical spine problems	atlanto-axial instability skeletal anomalies may cause spinal cord injury	initial x-ray screen at 3 years old	15%	orthopedic; neurology; neuro-surgery; avoid high risk activity; surgery if spinal cord compression
thyroid disease	hypothyroidism (rarely hyper-)	some congenital; check annually	15%	endocrinology consultation; replacement therapy
overweight	excessive weight gain	late preschool; adolescence/adult life	common	life style changes around food/exercise; check thyroid function; ?depression
seizure disorder	generalized or myoclonic; hypsarrhythmia	any time	5-10%	neurology consultation, EEG, medication
emotional problems	behavioral changes; depression	adolescence; young adult	common	inclusive education; counseling; support during transition from school to work

variable occurrence of: gastrointestinal anomalies; Hirschsprungs; leukemia; alopecia areata; diabetes; sleep apnea; hip dysplasia

Preventive Health Care before Birth

Down syndrome is sometimes diagnosed before birth. Several tests that can be done in the first half of a pregnancy allow chromosome testing of the unborn baby. Some couples do these tests in order to terminate the pregnancy through abortion if Down syndrome is found. However, more and more couples are choosing to continue the pregnancy. Knowing before birth that a baby has Down syndrome allows parents to prepare for the child's healthy arrival in a number of ways.

First, parents have time to prepare themselves, their families, and their friends. The birth itself can be the joyful, celebrated event it should be, since the shock and much of the emotional pain about the diagnosis of Down syndrome is in the past. Parents also have time to become more informed about Down syndrome and some of the issues they will need to confront. Parents may use the time during the pregnancy to meet other parents and individuals with Down syndrome, who can serve as a source of information and support.

Second, these parents will have time to learn about and make contacts with services and resources in the community, such as early intervention programs, family support services, and financial and medical assistance programs. Finally, tests can be done before the baby is born to check for heart or bowel defects. If a baby is known to have a bowel defect, plans could be made in advance for the medical care that might be needed soon after birth. This information might lead to a decision to give birth in a hospital whose staff includes a pediatric surgeon, and whose services include newborn intensive care, in case surgery will be needed.

Preventive Health Care for the Newborn

For most parents of newborns with Down syndrome the first awareness of the diagnosis comes soon after the child's birth. Though some parents recognize that their child has

Down syndrome at first sight, most are informed of this by their physician. How the news is conveyed can be an important first step in the preventive health care of a child with Down syndrome. The news is often a shocking surprise, and it may devastate parents for a period of time. However, the doctor who takes the time to be warm and supportive, who listens to parents' fears and questions, who finds positive ways to temper the negative news, and who models caring and acceptance of the baby by holding him and referring to him by name, will help to speed and strengthen a family's adjustment.

A physician like this will recognize and facilitate the parents' need for information and for contact with other parents of children with Down syndrome. This kind of doctor will respect each family's process of coping and coming to terms with an unfamiliar and, for some, overwhelming situation. Capable and thoughtful counseling about the diagnosis of Down syndrome can help prevent serious disruptions in family life and can foster a positive vision for the child as a family member and citizen.

Most newborns with Down syndrome appear healthy and require little or no extra medical care compared with other babies. They require the same careful assessment and initial observation as any new baby to be sure that they have arrived safely and in good health. Newborns are typically screened for uncommon and serious, but treatable, conditions such as *hypothyroidism* (low thyroid gland function) and *phenylketonuria* (PKU). The newborn with Down syndrome should also have these tests. Babies with Down syndrome have a somewhat higher risk of being born with low thyroid function, so this part of the "newborn screen" is particularly important.

In addition to the routine physical examination performed on all newborns, doctors will need to look carefully for any problems that may occur more frequently in a baby with Down syndrome. Heart and bowel problems are the most serious and are discussed below and in Chapters 3 and 9. Eye problems such as cataracts or glaucoma may also be present at birth (these are discussed in Chapter 6). These conditions must be identified and treated at an early age to prevent serious vision impairment.

Among the most important preventive practices for a baby with Down syndrome is screening to detect congenital heart defects. Children with Down syndrome have almost a 50% chance of being born with a heart defect. Many heart defects are serious enough to require surgery. If some heart defects are not discovered in the first few months, they may cause changes in the lungs which make corrective surgery impossible. In the past, doctors relied on listening with a stethoscope for a heart murmur to diagnose a heart defect. Now we know that serious defects can be present without a heart murmur. For this reason, all babies with Down syndrome should undergo careful screening for heart defects soon after birth. If possible this should include consultation with a pediatric cardiologist and should always include an echocardiogram, which provides a "picture" of the baby's heart without causing pain or harm to the baby.

One in every ten babies with Down syndrome is born with a defect in his intestinal tract which may cause obstruction (blockage). This may occur in any part from the esophagus (the tube from the mouth to stomach) to the rectum, but the most common blockage is called *duodenal atresia* and occurs in the small intestine just beyond the stomach. Babies with this sort of problem will not be able to keep down their food. Shortly after they are born, they will begin to vomit everything that they are fed. Babies who behave in this way will need x-rays to find the blockage. Most problems of this sort must be repaired by surgery.

Babies who are free of major heart or bowel defects are not likely to present any special problems as newborns. Parents' feeding plans (breast or bottle feeding) should be supported and encouraged. Though sometimes a baby with Down syndrome won't eat vigorously at first, good feeding habits usually become established in a day or two if properly supported.

Sometimes a hospital staff member will remark that babies with Down syndrome "can't breast feed." This may be the first occasion when parents will find themselves suspicious, and rightfully so, about an ill-informed professional who uses the word "can't" a little too freely.

For some babies, feeding will be challenging and may require further counseling with close follow-up of the baby's growth and nutritional status (nutrition concerns are discussed in Chapter 17). The LaLeche League of America publishes a pamphlet entitled "Breast Feeding the Baby with Down Syndrome," which is a good source of additional information for parents whose child is breast feeding. Your local hospital can tell you how to contact a branch of the LaLeche League in your area.

Preventive Health Care for the Young Child

As mentioned above, preventive health care for the child with Down syndrome begins with the same care that is provided to all children. This includes having a primary physician or other health care provider upon whom the child's family can depend as a resource not only for direct care, but for coordination of any other needed health care services, for information and counseling, and for advocacy and support. People with Down syndrome, and their families, have greatly benefited from society's belief in this more enlightened era that all children deserve the opportunity to grow up in a loving family environment. If children with Down syndrome benefit from living at home, then they benefit even more when families lead as natural and "normal" a lifestyle as possible. This kind of lifestyle includes the person with Down syndrome in family activities. Such a lifestyle is not turned upside down by the competing demands of professionals, but finds a balance between what is necessary or helpful and what is excessive. Physicians and other health care providers need to be sensitive to the demands faced by families and help prioritize them when necessary. Families should be encouraged to lead lives that feel natural to them and that are not driven by the fact that a child in the family has Down syndrome (see Chapter 19).

Early well child visits are occasions to monitor your infant's physical growth. This monitoring should be carried out both on regular growth charts used for all children and on growth charts especially developed for children with Down syndrome. This provides two ways of monitoring growth and may help to evaluate the causes of growth failure should it occur. In particular, children with Down syndrome are usually shorter than other children the same age. If a child is small even when measured on the Down syndrome growth charts, then further tests may be in order. On the other hand, the weight (as opposed to the height or length) charts for people with Down syndrome may allow the weight of an overweight child to appear "OK." In this case looking closely at the child's proportions (weight compared to height), and comparison with "regular" growth charts is needed.

Physical growth may also be different in its details. The head and facial features (eyes, nose, jaw, ears, etc.) of children with Down syndrome are smaller and may grow more slowly than in other children. As a result, facial structures such as tear ducts, sinus passages, and *eustachian tubes* (connecting the middle ear to the back of the throat) may be smaller in size and become blocked more easily. This contributes to an increased likelihood of tear duct, sinus, and ear infections in some children. Smaller jaw structures may contribute to incorrect alignment of teeth. Even the *trachea*, or airway to the lungs, may itself be smaller, which can contribute to respiratory infections like croup and to partial blockage of the airway during sleep *(obstructive sleep apnea),* placing some children with Down syndrome at increased risk. Awareness of and attention to these factors may help the primary health care provider prevent secondary problems. Parents who are aware

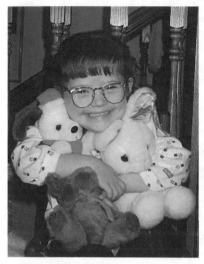

of and understand these issues will be better observers of their children at home.

Many children with Down syndrome have no more problems with infections than other children. However, for a variety of reasons, some children have more difficulty (Chapter 4 discusses immunity and infections in detail). The presence of congenital heart disease may contribute to respiratory infections in some children while the smaller size of the trachea (airway) may increase the likelihood of croup. Infections of the middle ear, sinuses, or nasal passages may be frequent enough to warrant the continuous use of antibiotics on a preventive basis, especially during the winter months. Some children who have frequent episodes of pneumonia or other respiratory problems may benefit from pneumococcal vaccine (to prevent certain types of bacterial pneumonia) and from annual doses of influenza (flu) vaccine.

Screening for problems with vision and hearing is a fundamental aspect of preventive health care in all children. However, the risk of problems with vision and hearing is higher among children with Down syndrome (Chapters 6 and 8 discuss vision and hearing problems). In addition, even mild impairments of these important senses may interfere with development more significantly in a child with Down syndrome. As a result, more active approaches are needed at an earlier age. As mentioned, newborns with Down syndrome should be carefully screened for birth defects affecting the eyes, such as cataracts or glaucoma. Over half of all children with Down syndrome may have problems with vision that require glasses or other treatment. After newborn screening, your child with Down syndrome should be seen at least annually by a pediatric ophthalmologist for continued monitoring of eye function.

Hearing is obviously crucial for language, social skills, and learning to develop to the highest potential. Half to three-quarters of people with Down syndrome may have some problem with hearing. The majority of these problems are treatable if identified. Therefore, screening of hearing should begin in infancy and include periodic assessment by a qualified audiologist skilled at testing infants and familiar with children with Down syndrome. Such testing should occur at six months and twelve months of age and annually thereafter unless circumstances require more frequent testing.

People with Down syndrome are also at higher risk for developing problems with thyroid gland function (discussed in detail in Chapter 5). Usually this results in *hypothyroidism*, or under-activity of the thyroid gland. Hypothyroidism may cause constipation, weight gain, slower growth in height, loss of stamina, decreased tolerance of heat or cold, and slowing of learning or development. Some of these characteristics may occur in people with Down syndrome who have normal thyroid gland activity. The only way to be certain that your child has normal thyroid activity is to have him tested to see if the levels of thyroid hormone in the blood are normal. Each child should be screened for hypothyroidism at birth as part of the "newborn screen" done on all children. After that, your child should be tested each year to see if the levels of thyroid hormone (called T4) and pituitary gland hormone (this hormone controls the thyroid gland, and is called TSH for *thyroid stimulating hormone*) are normal. If the test results are abnormal, an endocrinologist familiar with thyroid function in children with Down syndrome should be consulted about further tests or treatment.

Primary health care providers should also screen children with Down syndrome for *atlanto-axial instability* (discussed in detail in Chapter 10). Atlanto-axial instability refers to looseness of the joint between the first and second vertebrae (spine bones) in the neck. This looseness can be seen on the x-rays of about 15 percent of people with Down syndrome. It is believed that this looseness may lead to an increased risk of injury to the spinal cord and possible permanent harm. Only about 1 percent (1 in 100) of individuals actually develop problems with their spinal cord. Sometimes there are problems in other joints in the neck or with bones that are abnormally formed. Screening for these concerns is recommended when the child is 2½ to 3 years of age, at about 8 to 10 years of age when participation in organized athletics may begin, and every ten years thereafter. This screening consists of x-rays of the neck in several positions (with the neck bent, extended, and in the middle position). Children who have abnormal x-rays may need to be followed more closely and may need to be restricted from sports such as tumbling and competitive diving that can place excessive strain on the neck.

Dental care is another area that should be part of a preventive health care plan. Dental services should be obtained from a pediatric dentist or a general dentist who is comfortable with children and knowledgeable about Down syndrome. Prevention of cavities involves the same approaches as with all children. *Malocclusion* (teeth that are not properly aligned) occurs in nearly all children with Down syndrome, and may prompt earlier consultation with an orthodontist to plan a treatment program (discussed in detail in Chapter 12). When dental care is required, it is important to remember that children with congenital heart defects (even after surgery) may need to take an antibiotic just before and just after dental visits to prevent an infection of the heart called *endocarditis*.

Preventive Health Care Issues in the Older Child

Older children with Down syndrome should continue to be screened for problems with hearing, vision, thyroid function, atlanto-axial instability and teeth. Growth should be monitored with increasing attention to signs of being over weight. Problems with weight may be prevented or reduced by early attention to nutrition, exercise, eating habits and the role that food and meals play in family life.

During adolescence, psychological and emotional issues may begin to replace other health issues as areas of concern for children with Down syndrome. Withdrawal, sadness, anger, and depression may develop as a child's awareness of his disability or differences from other children grows more clear. Primary health care professionals should help parents advocate for fully inclusive school programs and for active strategies that encourage friendship and socialization, in order to prevent the child from feeling isolated from other children.

Emerging sexuality raises a host of worries and concerns for all children and their parents (discussed in Chapter 13). These concerns are often increased when they are not anticipated or are poorly understood. Beginning in the early grades, school programs should deal with the issues of health, hygiene, sexuality, and social skills. These subjects need to be presented clearly and thoughtfully, with the goal of enhancing behaviors that prevent exploitation and promote social competence and self-esteem.

Concerns about reproductive health need to be addressed for both males and females. Until recently it was believed that males with Down syndrome were infertile, but recent research has established that at least one male with Down syndrome has become a father. The development of primary and secondary sexual characteristics during puberty is not significantly different for boys with Down syndrome than for other boys. (*Primary sexual characteristics* are those characteristics of the male or female that are necessary for reproduction; *sec-*

ondary sexual characteristics are those characteristics that
are not necessary for reproduction.)

The age that puberty begins, and the age at which it is
completed, are the same for young men with Down syndrome
as for other young men. Appropriate counseling to meet the
emotional and cognitive needs of your child should be available. There are many unknowns regarding the fertility and
sexual function of young men with Down syndrome, and this
is an area that needs continuing research.

Like most young people, the child with Down syndrome
wants to be a part of his community, and to make plans for a
useful adult life beyond the school years. Reasonable preparation for work opportunities that do not remove a young person from the mainstream of school life can help make this a
reality.

Upon the completion of high school, many young people
with Down syndrome leave what has been a very active, struc-
tured, supportive, and full daily life. Some individuals go on to
post-secondary education or to productive employment in the
competitive work force. However, in some communities the
opportunities for young adults with disabilities to find work,
housing, and leisure activity and to engage in meaningful relationships are still very limited. In other instances, parents are
not ready to "let go" and encourage a transition to a more independent life in the community. The consequences of limited opportunities for a fulfilling life as an adult may be
despondency or demoralization. The symptoms of this may include withdrawal, anger, apparent loss of self-care and other
skills, and depression.

Preparations that will prevent this negative outcome must
begin in the early school years or sooner. Parents need to for-
mulate and nurture a clear vision of their child's future, and
to work for educational and vocational programs that will foster that vision. Your child is more likely to be prepared for
adult life if regular activities in regular settings, natural encounters with a network of friends, and preparation for in-

creasing independence have
been emphasized during his
formative years.

A Final Word

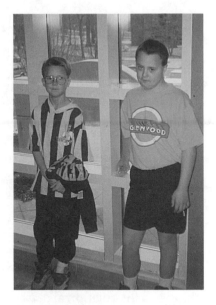

The best preventive
health care in the world is
useless if certain conditions
are not met. First, primary
preventive care must be ac-
cessible. This means that
the services are available in
or near a family's commu-
nity. The services must be
affordable for families. Usually being able to afford
health care means having some form of private or public insurance to pay for it. Families need help with identifying
sources of insurance and other financial support including
Medicaid, Supplemental Security Income through Social Security, and services through each state's program for children
with special health care needs. Sometimes insurance companies, or managed health care plans (HMOs) will refuse to pay
for necessary preventive services for a child with Down syndrome. Often this is due to a lack of understanding of the special reasons these services are necessary. Many times a letter
from the child's physician or a discussion with someone *in
authority* at the insurance company or HMO will result in a
decision to cover the needed services. The references at the
end of this chapter include an excellent booklet, "Paying the
Bills: Tips for Families on Financing Health Care for Children
with Special Needs," that will inform you about a range of
sources of financial aid. State offices of maternal and child
health and state developmental disabilities councils may also

have helpful information for families about financial resources.

Second, effective preventive health care must pay attention to family needs as well as the needs of the individual
child. It is clear that families that are overwhelmed with stress
have less success meeting the needs of family members, including those of the family member who has Down syndrome.
Many states are developing family support programs which
may provide respite care, help with the coordination of all the
services a child or family receives, information and advocacy,
and even cash or vouchers to help families purchase needed
services on their own.

Finally, families need information. They need to have up-
to-date information about Down syndrome in a format that is
easy to read and understand. They need information about
their rights and about the services to which they are entitled.
They need information about becoming capable advocates for
their child and information about where to get more information. The material contained in this book and access to health
care professionals who are willing to work as partners in
health promotion can provide an important source of support
for every family's natural expectation that their child with
Down syndrome will have a healthy, productive life.

References

Cohen, W.I., et al. "Down Syndrome Preventive Medical Checklist."
(National Down Syndrome Congress, 1605 Chantilly Drive, Suite
250, Atlanta, GA, 30324–3269; (800)232–6372. 1994).

Cooley, W.C. and Graham, J.M. "Down Syndrome—An Update and
Review for the Pediatrician." *Clinical Pediatrics,* Vol. 30, 1991,
233–53.

Crocker, A.C. and Rubin, I.L., eds. *Developmental Disabilities—Delivery of Medical Care for Children and Adults* (Philadelphia: Lea
and Febiger, 1989).

Pueschel, S.M. and Pueschel, J.K., eds. *Biomedical Concerns in the
Person with Down Syndrome* (Baltimore: Paul H. Brookes, 1992).

Wells, E., et al. *Paying the Bills: Tips for Families on Financing Health Care for Children with Special Needs* (Boston: New England SERVE, 101 Tremont Street, Suite 812, Boston, MA 02108. 1992).

3 | Heart Disease and Children with Down Syndrome

Anthony J. Cousineau, M.D.
Ronald M. Lauer, M.D.

While only about one percent of all people are born with heart disease, almost forty percent of babies with Down syndrome have it. In addition, the cardiac defects in children with Down syndrome tend to be more serious than the defects found in the general population. On the brighter side, studies also document progressive improvement during the past few decades in the treatment and survival rate of infants and children with Down syndrome who have heart disease. But early diagnosis and treatment of congenital heart disease in children with Down syndrome is crucial to their survival and well-being.

Improvements in the medical care of children with Down syndrome who have heart defects, and advances in surgery to repair these defects, have played a major role in adding to both the length and the quality of their life. Because early recognition and treatment of heart defects is very important, parents as well as medical professionals need to be well-informed about cardiac care for children with Down syndrome. This chapter discusses the types of heart disorders most often associated with Down syndrome and their treatment. It includes basic information about:

- how the heart works;
- the causes of heart defects in children with Down syndrome;
- the symptoms of heart disease;

- associated disorders of the heart and circulatory system;
- diseases of the circulatory system of the lungs; diagnosis;
- medical and surgical treatment; and
- the results of treatment.

To understand heart disease in children with Down syndrome, it helps to first understand how the heart and the circulatory system work.

How the Heart Works

The heart is a muscle designed to pump blood. There are four chambers in all, divided into the right and left side pumping systems. Each side has one collecting chamber, called an *atrium,* and one pumping chamber, called a *ventricle.* The chambers work in coordination during each heart beat. Figure 1A is an artist's rendition of the heart with its four chambers.

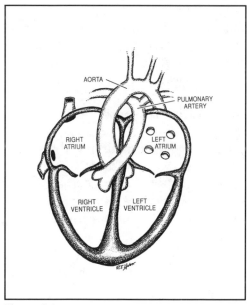

Figure 1A

Each heart beat, or cycle, has two parts. Oxygen-depleted blood is pumped to the heart from all over the body in the veins and collects in the right atria. In the first part of the cycle a valve opens to let this blood into the right ventricle, which then pumps the blood through another valve to the lungs. Figure 1B shows the right side of the heart. The second half of the cycle continues as oxygen-rich blood returning from the lungs first flows into the left atria and then is pumped through a third valve into the left ventricle. Figure 1C shows the left side of the heart. From there blood passes through the final valve, through

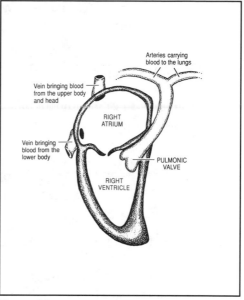

Figure 1B

the aorta (the body's largest blood vessel), and out to the body. As this oxygenated blood circulates through the body, it supplies oxygen to the body's tissues and organs. The blood already out in the arteries and veins is pushed along by the fresh blood on its way back to the heart.

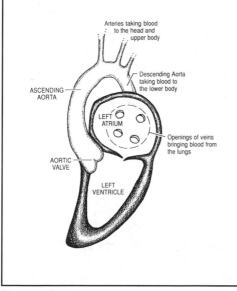

Figure 1C

Heart Disease in Children with Down Syndrome

Children with Down syndrome may have a variety of different kinds of heart disease. Most of these problems are referred to as *congenital heart disease*. *Congenital* means that the heart condition is present at birth. Usually, the seriousness of the heart disease depends upon how much the defect disrupts normal blood circulation. This section discusses the common types of heart disease in children with Down syndrome, and explains their effects on blood circulation and health.

AV Septal Defects

A group of congenital heart diseases known collectively as *atrioventricular (AV) septal defects* (also known as *endocardial cushion defects* and *atrioventricular canal defects*) account for the majority of heart problems in children with Down syndrome. AV septal defects occur in about one in five thousand people in the general population. In people with Down syndrome, however, the rate is nearly one in four. Males and females with Down syndrome are equally susceptible to this type of congenital heart disease.

To understand what AV septal defects are, it helps to know a little about the development of the human heart.

Heart Development. In the very early stages of life in the womb, the growing embryo has no circulation system. It absorbs the oxygen and nutrients it needs directly from its mother's placenta. While the embryo is very young and small, this system is adequate. With growth, however, the cells deep inside become too far away from the placenta for simple absorption to work very well. By that time the baby's circulatory system must begin to move blood to and from the placenta.

Around three weeks of growth, little groups of cells that will eventually become the heart, blood vessels, and blood begin to form. The heart itself begins as two tubes that grow to-

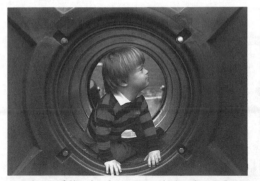

gether and develop pockets, flaps, and more tubes. Eventually these pockets and flaps develop to become the chambers and valves of the heart. As development continues and more blood is made, it fills the heart and the lengthening arteries and veins.

Early in development, when blood first begins to flow in the tubes, the heart is little more than a collecting sack. Blood moves from the placenta through the developing heart and out to the body. The first "beats" of the heart are not very co-ordinated. Blood moves more by the differences in pressure between the various parts of the system than by any pumping by the young heart muscle. As the heart becomes more completely formed, and the network of vessels more extensive, the heart pumping also becomes more effective.

By about 8 weeks of development, the four chambers of the heart are recognizable. Lumps of tissue on the sides of the fetal heart, called the *endocardial cushions,* grow toward each other at the middle of the heart and begin to separate the top from the bottom chambers (Figure 2). As this occurs, the walls between the atria and ventricles grow toward each other to separate right from left. The open space that remains is called the *atrioventricular canal.* Special tissue in this central region, called the *atrioventricular valve ring,* develop into atrioventricular (AV) valves. The valves separate the openings between the atria and ventricles (Figure 1A). The AV valves normally allow blood flow in one direction; they let blood pass through and then close to prevent any return.

Throughout the time in the womb, the baby continues to receive what it needs for growth, including oxygen, from the placenta. Blood flow is directed there through special vessels

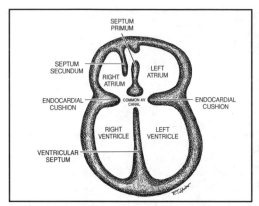

Figure 2. This diagram shows the developing heart and the location of the *atrioventricular canal* (AV canal). The *endocardial cushions* are growing into the AV canal in an effort to divide the heart into four separate chambers.

in the umbilical cord, which connects the heart and the placenta. There is very little flow of blood to the baby's lungs. At birth, however, as the baby starts to breathe, air fills the lungs and the pressures affecting the blood vessels in the lungs begin to fall. The volume of blood flowing into the vessels in the lungs increases. Oxygen taken in by the baby's lungs enters the bloodstream there. The special arteries and veins going to the placenta are clamped off as the umbilical cord is cut; they then tighten and close inside the baby as well. Thus, shortly after birth, your baby's breathing and circulation begins to provide her body with the oxygen it needs.

Eventually, the adult pattern of blood pressure in the lungs and the body is established. Normally, blood pressure in the lungs is lower than in the rest of body. This lower pressure makes it much easier for blood to flow to the lungs. The walls and valves of the heart become very important in keeping the flow of blood going in the right direction.

The heart's valves are each made up of 2 or 3 thin flaps of tough fibers that line the opening between the chambers. As the chamber fills and the muscles begin to squeeze, the valve opens to permit the blood to move into the next chamber or blood vessel. These flaps direct blood flow by "closing the door" on the pumping chamber so that blood can flow in only one direction. When the valves don't close well enough, blood can leak back. This condition is called *regurgitation*. In some cases of AV septal defects, one or more AV valves may leak. The leaking that results can add complications to any other defects, and may be difficult to repair.

Holes in the walls between the heart's chambers can let blood flow back toward the lungs instead of out to the body. As a result, the heart has to pump more times to get the same amount of blood circulated. These holes are named by their locations. A hole between the upper, collecting chambers of the heart is called an ASD, *or atrial septal defect.* A hole between the pumping chambers is called a VSD (*ventricular septal defect*). These are discussed in the next section.

Types of Septal Defects

As mentioned above, septal defects occur when the walls separating the heart's chambers do not develop normally, leaving gaps or holes. One of the more serious septal defects is the *partial atrioventricular septal defect.* This condition is also called a *primum atrial septal defect*, and is shown in Figure 3. In this defect, there is an opening in

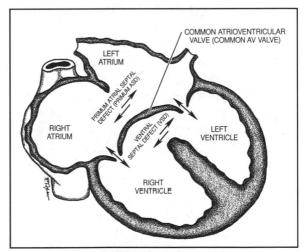

Figure 3. This diagram shows a complete *atrioventricular (AV) canal defect.* There is a large *primum atrial septal defect* (primum ASD), a large *ventricular septal defect* (VSD), and a common *atrioventricular valve* (AV valve). The arrows show the directions that the blood may flow through these defects.

the lower part of the wall between the right and left atria. Another type, a secundum ASD, is usually higher up on the atrial wall. The size of the holes varies, ranging from tiny and insignificant, to the point where the septum is completely absent.

In a complete atrioventricular septal defect, as shown in Figure 3, the atrioventricular valve ring fails to divide into separate right and left openings to keep the chambers separate. Instead, there is a single large opening bridged by a common AV valve, which allows mixing of blood from all four chambers.

Another variety of atrioventricular septal defect is called the *transitional* or *intermediate* defect. In this condition, the opening in the ventricular septum (the wall between the two lower heart chambers) is partially or totally blocked by AV valve tissue, so that the common valve appears to be attached to the top of the ventricular septum.

The Effects of AV Septal Defects. The primary physical consequence of any AV septal defect is that blood circulation is disrupted. With most AV septal defects, blood from the left side of the heart is forced, or shunted, into the right side (see Figure 3). This is called *intracardiac* (within the heart) *shunting.* As a result, too much blood is delivered to the lungs because they have lower pressure, and blood tends to flow toward areas of lower pressure. The increased flow to the lungs then returns to the left side of the heart. Ultimately the heart suffers from *volume overload,* a condition in which there is too much blood for the heart to pump effectively. How serious this is depends in part on the size of the defect. In general, the larger the opening in the AV septum, the greater the shunting. The greater the shunting, the greater the volume overload. The greater the volume overload, the greater the risk to the heart and lungs.

Other factors can affect the amount of shunting as well, such as the blood pressure of the pulmonary artery. As explained above, the pulmonary blood vessels (*pulmonary* means pertaining to the lungs) carry the oxygen-depleted blood from the heart's right ventricle to the lungs, and returns oxygen-filled blood from the lungs to the heart's left atrium. Heart defects cause the pressure inside the pulmonary artery to increase as a result of the increased blood volume being directed through it. This higher blood pressure in the pulmonary artery results in higher blood pressure throughout the lungs. If left untreated, the increased pressure can lead to fatal pulmonary disease (discussed below).

During gestation and early infancy, the pressure in the pulmonary artery is higher than it is later in life. Consequently, the amount of shunting in a newborn infant with an atrioventricular septal defect may be minimal—the higher lung pressure present at that time forces the blood to circulate more normally. As your infant develops, however, pulmonary pressure gradually decreases. By the time your child is two to three months old, the blood pressure in the lungs reaches normal, lower levels. As a result, shunting increases and produces the symptoms of heart disease.

Other Heart Conditions

Children with Down syndrome can have several other congenital heart defects, most of which are more common in children with Down syndrome than in the general population. These defects may be present in addition to an atrioventricular septal defect or they may be present alone.

Ventricular septal defect. The ventricular septal defect (VSD) is the second most common form of congenital heart disease in children with Down syndrome. A ventricular septal defect is an opening in the wall that separates the right and left ventricles. These holes can vary in size from a pinhole to an absence of the entire wall. Like an AV septal defect, a VSD allows left to right shunting of blood. And like an AV septal defect, the degree of shunting depends on the size of the hole in the septum as well as on the blood pressure in the pulmonary artery.

The particular types of VSDs children with Down syndrome have differ somewhat from those of the general population. In children with Down syndrome, these defects tend to be larger, and rarely close by themselves. They are usually

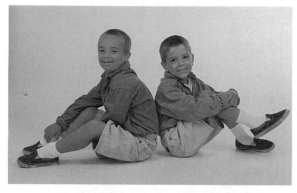

found in a part of the ventricular septum that is beneath the tricuspid valve, an area that is called the *inlet septum*. For this reason, they are often called an "inlet VSD or "VSD of the atrioventricular canal type."

Patent ductus arteriosus. Another relatively common cardiac defect children with Down syndrome have involves a structure that is present in the fetus, the *ductus arteriosus*. Before your child is born, the ductus arteriosus carries blood from the pulmonary artery to the aorta, bypassing the lungs, which are not used during gestation. After birth, when your child begins to breathe and to use her lungs, the ductus arteriosus closes. In about 10 percent of infants with Down syndrome, however, the ductus arteriosus remains open, a condition that is called *patent ductus arteriosus* (PDA). A PDA in an infant with Down syndrome is usually large and allows a significant amount of blood to shunt from left to right, from the aorta to the pulmonary blood vessels with the resulting volume overload and increase in pulmonary blood pressure. A PDA can often close by itself, but children with this condition require continued monitoring and possibly surgery.

Cyanotic Heart Diseases

Cardiologists divide the kinds of heart defects into two groups, based on whether or not they include *cyanosis*. Cyanosis is a condition in which a person has too much deoxygenated blood, or blood that is depleted of oxygen. This condition makes the lips and fingertips take on a bluish color. This is because deoxygenated blood is a bluish color. The lack of oxygen in the blood that cyanosis indicates can cause damage to the heart itself.

The conditions described above usually do not cause cyanosis (unless the heart is working very poorly) because blood flow into and out of the lungs is good enough to fully oxygenate the blood. In cyanotic heart diseases, flow into and out of the lungs is not as effective, so the oxygen level in the blood is too low.

A form of congenital heart disease called *tetralogy of Fallot* causes cyanosis in children with Down syndrome. *Tetralogy* means "having four parts"; the four components of this condition are:

1. a ventricular septal defect;
2. obstruction to pulmonary blood flow;
3. an aorta that overrides (lies over or sits on top of) the ventricular septum; and
4. enlargement of the right ventricle.

Tetralogy of Fallot results in cyanosis because blood that is on its way to the lungs to be reoxygenated cannot get there. Its flow is blocked by a narrowing of the outlet to the pulmonary artery. This obstruction, which is called *pulmonic* or *infundibular stenosis*, results in right to left shunting through the ventricular septal defect. As a result, deoxygenated blood is continually recirculated through the body, causing cyanosis.

Polycythemia. Polycythemia, often one of the complications of cyanotic heart disease, is a condition in which the blood contains too many red blood cells. These extra red blood cells thicken the blood, and make it more difficult for the heart to pump the blood through the body. In children with Down syndrome, polycythemia can appear in infancy, unrelated to heart disease, and can also appear with Eisenmenger's syndrome (discussed below).

Polycythemia is diagnosed if red blood cells make up more than 65 percent of your child's blood. This is determined by a blood test called a *hematocrit*. At birth the normal hematocrit count ranges from 40 to 60 percent, and over time lowers to 30 to 40 percent. Too many red blood cells may cause congestive heart failure (discussed below), poor flow of blood cells in the small blood vessels, and an increased heart rate. Because polycythemia can result in cardiac failure and other serious complications such as stroke, children who have symptoms typically require treatment. The usual treatment is to remove some of the blood, which may or may not be replaced by other fluids. Although there are some risks (such as blood clots in the artery into which the transfusion goes), the treatment is generally successful.

Pulmonary Artery Hypertension

Children with Down syndrome sometimes develop a type of high blood pressure called *pulmonary artery hypertension.* In this condition, blood pressure in the pulmonary artery is persistently higher than is normal. As explained above, pulmonary artery pressure is usually elevated before your child is born and during the first few weeks of life. Usually this increased pressure gradually decreases to normal levels by the time your child is two to three months old. However, when there is too much blood flow to the lungs, caused by left to right shunting inside the heart, the pulmonary blood vessels constrict in an effort to limit the extra blood flow. Over time the muscular tissues of the pulmonary vessels thicken because of this extra effort, creating a narrower passage for the blood to flow through. This leads in turn to increased pulmonary pressure, which can reverse the direction of shunting. Now the blood flows from right to left and bypasses the lungs, so that more deoxygenated blood is circulated. As with tetralogy of Fallot, cyanosis develops.

The most serious risk of pulmonary hypertension is that the process of thickening may be irreversible and can lead to a condition called *occlusive pulmonary vascular disease (OPVD)*. In this condition, the pulmonary blood vessels become so narrow from thickening that not enough blood can flow through to sustain life. When this disease becomes severe enough to cause reversal of left-to-right shunting, the condition is called *Eisenmenger's syndrome*. Pulmonary hypertension, OPVD, and Eisenmenger's syndrome are especially prevalent in children with Down syndrome.

Children with Down syndrome develop OPVD at an earlier age than other children. This condition has been found in infants with Down syndrome as young as six months old. We do not know why children with Down syndrome are more susceptible to this condition, or why they develop it at such an early age. We do know that it can be prevented if recognized and treated early in life.

Genetic Basis of Heart Defects

The genetic basis of heart defects in children with Down syndrome is unknown. It is generally believed that they are caused by a gene or genes on chromosome 21, the chromosome found in triplicate in Down syndrome. To date, no single gene or group of genes on chromosome 21, or on any other chromosome, have been conclusively linked to these heart defects. However, a number of possible genes for these defects have been identified on chromosome 21. These are located within a so-called "critical region for Down syndrome" on a particular part of chromosome 21.

Couples who have had a child with Down syndrome may be at increased risk to have another child with Down syndrome and heart defects. However, their other children who do not have Down syndrome are no more likely than the general population to have a congenital heart defect. In addition, no environmental agents (such as radiation or toxins) or drugs are known to cause Down syndrome or the heart defects associated with it.

Currently, no prenatal laboratory test is available to diagnose AV septal defects in utero. However, these defects are often detectable by a prenatal ultrasound technique called *fetal echocardiography*. This test can be used to evaluate any fetus at risk for congenital heart disease. If echocardiography indicates that the fetus has an AV septal defect, this does not necessarily indicate the fetus also has Down syndrome, because this heart defect is found with other congenital syndromes, as well as in the general population. Although AV septal defects cannot yet be repaired in utero, knowing before birth allows parents to prepare themselves and to choose the appropriate hospitals and doctors ahead of time.

Symptoms of Heart Disease

As explained above, most infants with Down syndrome who have congenital heart disease will not have symptoms at birth, due to the elevated pulmonary blood pressure present in early infancy. Often a child does not develop symptoms until a few months of age, when pulmonary pressure drops to normal levels. As pulmonary blood pressure drops, shunting of blood inside the heart increases.

In an adult, often the first sign of heart disease is easy tiring during work (because the heart cannot keep up with the increased need for oxygen). For an infant, work is eating and growing. The earliest symptoms of heart disease in a baby are usually difficulty in feeding and poor weight gain. Babies with heart disease have more trouble with the work of eating than do other babies. Your baby may perspire, have rapid or labored breathing, and become tired while eating. Some infants vomit after each meal. Some babies do not wake as often as usual for feedings. While resting or sleeping, your baby may have rapid, shallow breathing, and her ribs may retract noticeably with each breath. In addition, your baby's skin color may appear pale or somewhat bluish (cyanotic).

Children with heart defects often need to consume more calories than usual to make up for the extra strain placed on them by the defect. Often babies simply cannot consume enough, and the result is poor weight gain, or "failure to thrive." Heart disease often also leads to recurrent respiratory infections because the lungs tend to be somewhat "wetter" than normal due to the changes in blood flow. Fluid leaks into the lung's air pockets from the small blood vessels which are very full of slowly moving blood. These infections, such as respiratory syncytial virus (RSV) infection, are especially prevalent during the winter months.

Physical Examination for Heart Disease

Often a physical examination is the first step in the diagnosis of heart disease. During a physical examination of an infant with suspected heart disease, the doctor will begin by looking for poor weight gain. He or she will also look at your child's vital signs; a rapid heart rate and rapid or labored breathing are possible symptoms of heart disease. In children with heart disease, the chest wall over the heart is often *hyperdynamic*—it moves more than normal when the heart beats. When the doctor uses the stethoscope to listen to the heart, he or she may hear the characteristic sounds of intracardiac shunting, leaky valves, pulmonary congestion, and volume overload. These sounds are often referred to as *murmurs, crackles,* or *rales,* as well as *galloping rhythm.* Your child's pulse may be normal, weak, or irregular. Skin is often mottled (spotty coloration) or pale (although paleness is common in children with Down syndrome, it still should be considered as a possible symptom), and hands and feet may be cool due to poor circulation. The doctor will also feel the liver which is often enlarged in children with heart disease.

Congestive heart failure is the term used to describe these signs and symptoms. It means the heart is incapable of

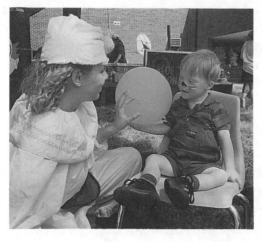

meeting the demands of the circulatory system; as a result, the lungs and liver become congested by excess fluids. When a child has congestive heart failure, fluid accumulates in the body because the kidneys are not able to dispose of it properly. Their function is impaired because they do not receive enough blood due to the heart defect. Fluid buildup is dangerous; it can cause *edema* (swelling) and high blood pressure, and can put even more strain on the heart. It is this congestion that poses the greatest health threat to children with heart disease.

While not all infants and children with congenital heart disease have the symptoms of congestive heart failure, many do. In older adults, congestive heart failure is often the result of an irreversibly exhausted heart for which there is no cure. In infants and children, on the other hand, congestive heart failure can usually be treated successfully with appropriate medicine and timely surgical repair.

Diagnosis and Evaluation of Heart Disease

A number of tests and procedures are available to evaluate a child with congenital heart disease and Down syndrome. A pediatrician who is caring for a baby with Down syndrome will often recommend these tests in early infancy, even if the baby appears to have none of the symptoms of heart disease. This is good preventive medicine.

Every infant with Down syndrome should be screened for congenital heart disease by a *pediatric cardiologist*, a physician with special training in the diagnosis and treatment of children with heart disease, or by a well-trained pediatrician. If there are no signs of heart disease in the hospital, you can wait until your child is settled at home. However, if there are any symptoms, consult a cardiologist immediately.

Screening for heart disease will usually include a chest x-ray and an electrocardiogram as well as the physical examination described above. The chest x-ray of an infant with significant left to right shunting usually reveals increased heart size and enlarged pulmonary blood vessels. An electrocardiogram, which graphs the electrical activity of the heart, can frequently identify an atrioventricular septal defect.

Echocardiograms and Catheterizations

If your child's diagnosis is unclear or if it becomes important to determine the degree of intracardiac shunting, pulmonary pressure, or AV valve regurgitation, an ultrasound study called an *echocardiogram* may be obtained. Because some defects can be quite small or silent, many physicians feel every baby with Down syndrome should have an echocardiogram. Ultrasounds are sound waves of a frequency higher than the human ear can hear; these sound waves are projected through the heart to provide a visual image of the inside of the heart and heart structure. They will not harm your child in any way. An echocardiogram should be done by a pediatric cardiologist or certified pediatric echocardiographer. An infant echocardiogram is a time-consuming process and requires your baby to be relatively motionless for a prolonged period of time. Sometimes the doctor will recommend that your child receive an oral sedative such as chloral hydrate. In most cases, a detailed echocardiogram will provide enough information to plan the best care for your child. However, in some cases a procedure called *cardiac catheterization* will be necessary to make absolutely clear what the defect looks like.

During cardiac catheterization, small flexible tubes are guided into the chambers of the heart. This is done by inserting the tubes into one of the major veins or arteries, usually in the area of the groin, through small skin incisions or needle punctures. Once the tubes are in position within the heart, measurements of oxygen levels and blood pressure are taken. Often during catheterization a fluid containing iodine (called a *contrast dye* because it appears on x-rays) is injected into the different chambers or vessels of the heart. This allows detailed x-ray films of the heart and of the blood flow in motion. These are called *cine-angiograms*.

Most pediatric cardiac catheterization procedures take several hours to complete. Although cardiac catheterization is considered safe, it is not completely without risks. In general, the smaller and more sick the infant, the greater the danger that she will have complications with the procedure. In most major hospitals that regularly perform pediatric cardiac catheterizations, the mortality rate is less than one percent.

Although complications may follow cardiac catheterization, they are rare. They may include stroke, infection, blood loss, and clots in the blood vessel used for the catheterization. Given these risks, the pediatric cardiologist is unlikely to recommend cardiac catheterization unless it is absolutely necessary.

Medical Treatment of Heart Disease

A pediatric cardiologist is usually in charge of the care of children with congenital heart disease. When a child is born with Down syndrome, a referral is usually made to a pediatric cardiologist to determine whether or not the infant has congenital heart disease. How soon after birth a referral is made depends on the symptoms present and on where you live. Even though your family's primary care physician may have already established a diagnosis, it is common to consult with a pediatric cardiologist in managing your child's health care.

If a diagnosis of congenital heart disease is confirmed, the pediatric cardiologist will provide detailed information about the specific nature of the defect. You will be educated about the signs and symptoms of congestive heart failure (discussed above). Children with heart disease need to be monitored closely; therefore, the pediatric cardiologist will recommend frequent follow-up visits.

If symptoms of congestive heart failure appear, the pediatric cardiologist may prescribe any one of a number of medications to help the heart do its job. Digoxin (Lanoxin)™, a medication often prescribed for congestive heart failure, increases the strength of the contractions of the heart muscle. Furosemide (Lasix)™, often used in combination with digoxin, helps the body dispose of excess fluid.

Because drugs like Lasix (called diuretics) sometimes cause the kidneys to waste potassium, a potassium supplement may be recommended. Maintaining normal potassium levels is especially important when using digoxin because low potassium levels can magnify the side effects of digoxin. If your child cannot tolerate potassium supplements (most are very strong tasting), a drug called spironolactone (Aldactone)™ may be prescribed instead of Lasix.

Captopril™ (Capoten) is another medication used in the treatment of congestive heart disease. This drug makes it easier for the heart to pump by lowering blood pressure throughout the body, which decreases the resistance against which the heart must pump. This medication is especially effective for children with significant AV valve regurgitation. One of the side effects of this medication is the retention of potassium. This means that children who are taking Digoxin, Lasix, and Capoten often do not require potassium supplements.

These medications, used alone or in combination, have been proven safe and effective for treating congestive heart failure in most children. However, some patients will not improve—in most cases, this is because their defects are too great. When this happens, surgery may be needed.

Treating Pulmonary Artery Hypertension. Identifying and treating pulmonary artery hypertension is one of the most important goals in managing the care of children with Down syndrome who have congenital heart disease. If an infant is at high risk for developing pulmonary artery hypertension, early surgery may be necessary. Before recommending it, however, most pediatric cardiologists will measure or estimate pulmonary artery pressure. They may do this by electrocardiogram, chest x-ray, echocardiogram, or cardiac catheterization. Abnormally high pulmonary artery pressure may make surgery too dangerous. In other cases, elevated pulmonary artery pressure may be treated with medicine, with surgery planned for a later date. Medical treatment for elevated pulmonary artery pressure includes the use of oxygen and certain nitrogen-based drugs. These agents relax the pulmonary blood vessels and increase pulmonary blood flow.

Surgery

Most children with Down syndrome who have congenital heart disease require surgery at some point in their lives. Most infants have surgery in early infancy because of the serious health risks posed by congestive heart failure or pulmonary artery hypertension. The dilemma in recommending early surgery is that the smaller the infant, the higher the risks are from surgery. But the longer surgery is postponed, the greater the risk of developing pulmonary hypertension and OPVD.

Many experienced pediatric heart surgeons estimate that among infants younger than three months, one child in ten will die during surgery to repair a complete AV septal defect. For this reason, the majority of surgeons prefer that surgery be delayed until the baby is six to nine months of age when the risks from surgery are lower.

Your child's weight and overall size are most often better predictors of survival than age. Ideally, most surgeons prefer to wait until your child weighs at least twenty pounds. However, most children with Down syndrome and congenital heart disease will not reach this weight until they are at least two years old. By this age, irreversible OPVD may already be present. Surgeons, therefore, will often choose to operate on children under two years of age who weigh less than twenty pounds.

For children with relatively well-controlled congestive heart failure, surgery is usually put off until they are of adequate size. In most cases, surgery will be recommended prior to one year of age. If there is no evidence of significant intracardiac shunting, congestive heart failure, or pulmonary artery hypertension, surgery can safely be delayed until about five years of age, as long as your child receives close monitoring and any needed medical treatment in the meantime.

In some children with complete atrioventricular canal defects, surgery may be difficult, or it may be delayed because the ventricles are not "balanced" (one is smaller than the other). In these cases, repair of the defect might leave the child with one side of the heart able to pump less blood than the other side. This is particularly a problem if the left side is smaller, causing volume overload as the extra flow from the right side backs up into the lungs. Sometimes surgery is delayed to allow the heart size to increase and hopefully balance. Surgeons may sometimes also be able to make the size of the two ventricles more equal during the operation. Unbalanced ventricles do not seem to be more common in children with Down syndrome than in children who have AV canals without Down syndrome.

For small infants with serious congestive heart failure who are not good candidates for complete surgical repair (because their weight and size are too small or because their heart defect is large or complicated), a procedure called *pulmonary artery banding* may be suggested. In this procedure a synthetic band is tied around the outside of the main pulmonary artery. The band is gradually tightened to increase the pressure or resistance in this artery until the pressure decreases left to right intracardiac shunting while allowing enough blood to flow to the lungs. The advantages of this technique are that it can buy time until your child is old enough for more complete surgical repair and it is safe for most small infants. However, this procedure has some drawbacks. Often it will not relieve the symptoms in children with significant AV valve regurgitation. In addition, as the pulmonary artery grows, the band becomes progressively tighter and may severely distort the pulmonary artery and cause severe cyanosis.

Surgical Procedures

There is no one surgical technique for repairing all types of heart defects. The exact nature of a child's heart defect determines the type of surgery. In general, the more extensive the defect, the more complicated, time-consuming, and risky the repair. For example, a partial atrioventricular septal defect consisting of a primum atrial septal defect and small cleft in the mitral valve usually requires a single patch to close the defect and only a few sutures to close the cleft in the valve. On the other hand, a complete AV septal defect, the most common heart defect associated with Down syndrome, may require a two-patch repair and perhaps extensive mitral valve repair. For ventricular septal defects, a single patch is usually used.

Complete surgical repair usually requires open-heart surgery using an incision down the middle of the chest. During surgery, the child's circulation will be maintained using cardiopulmonary bypass. To begin this bypass procedure, tubes are placed in the main arteries and veins leading to and from the heart. These tubes are then connected to a cardiopulmonary bypass machine which will do the work of the heart and lungs during the surgery. Then the heart is cooled (with ice and cold fluids) to stop the beating and protect it from injury (the heart's need for oxygen is less when it is very cold).

During the surgery, the bypass machine adds oxygen and removes carbon dioxide just as the lungs do. It also pumps the blood to the body and draws off the returning "used" blood. Medicines are added to the blood to keep it from clotting, and the chemicals in the blood are monitored very carefully. Adjustments to blood chemistry are made through IV tubes that are running into the veins.

As mentioned above, heart repairs vary from patient to patient. The size of the holes also vary widely, and may include valve defects as well. When patches are needed, they are often made of synthetic material (such as Dacron). Sometimes the lining of the sac around the heart (the *pericardium*) can be used for a patch; this can help avoid some of the clotting and infection complications synthetic materials can sometimes cause.

The patches are sewn in place using very small stitches of suture material. When a valve needs repair, again small stitches are used to change the shape of the valve leaflets. In each case, the surgeon needs to carefully place each stitch and to carefully cut the patch material in order to get the right shapes and dimensions of all the chambers and valves. Everything must fit together well, without extra tissue or tightness in the wrong places; otherwise the blood may not flow as effectively as it should or may flow in the wrong direction. Even the most experienced surgeons sometimes have to return the patient to the operating room for repeat surgery, to repair leaking valves or patches that do not fit properly.

Sometimes, repairing valve defects may require replacing the original tissue. This usually occurs later in life, as the child has grown, and new problems with the valve have developed. The new valve my be an artificial device or can be made from animal or human tissue. When a transplanted valve has been used, there is a higher risk of blood clotting problems. Anticoagulation medications will be needed permanently.

Once the surgical repairs have been completed, the heart is closed and rewarmed with warm fluids. As the heart temperature returns to normal, beating begins automatically. The bypass tubes are removed, and normal flow to and from the heart resumes.

The length of time for cardiac surgery varies tremendously depending upon the type of procedure done and any complications. Some simple operations may take an hour or less, and require more time getting ready and finishing up than the actual surgical repair. More commonly, the time needed ranges from 2 to 3 hours or more. Ask your child's surgical team for an estimate of the time expected to be necessary for your child's surgery. More important, ask that you be given regular progress reports as you wait. Sometimes, particularly before or after the actual repair, there are simple delays like placing IV lines or closing up incisions that take a lot of time. At those times, information can save a lot of anxiety See Chapter 16 for more information on preparing for and coping with surgery.

Many patients will require blood transfusion during or following open-heart surgery. Some centers allow directed donations from blood-type matched parents or relatives. This arrangement must be planned several weeks prior to the actual surgery; your pediatric cardiologist or surgeon can tell you how to arrange this.

Assessing Risk. Although there is always some degree of risk for complications or even death during heart surgery, fewer than ten percent of children with Down syndrome have serious complications. The degree of risk can be estimated by examining a number of risk factors, including pulmonary artery hypertension and the size of the ventricles of the heart. The surgeon will take these risk factors into consideration, and will talk with you about the risks involved. The major risks involved in heart surgery are that the repair will not work, that your child will go into shock, and that bleeding caused by the surgery will not stop (shock suppresses blood clotting). There is also a slight risk from anesthesia.

Other complications that can occur include rupture of the repaired tissues, failure or leakage of the valves, or disturbances to the electrical conduction of the heart. If conduction is damaged, the problem is usually treated with medications or by placing a pacemaker.

Post-operative care. Children recovering from open-heart surgery usually spend several days in a pediatric intensive care unit (PICU). When you see your child after surgery, you may be alarmed by the number of tubes, large and small, that surround your baby. These tubes are used to monitor her cardiac function, to help her breathe, and to drain excess fluids from her chest and body. Through these tubes, your child may be given analgesics to prevent pain, antibiotics to prevent infection, infusions to replace fluids, nutrition, and sedatives to promote rest. Nurses and physicians who are specialists in the management of children who have had heart surgery will closely monitor your child's care. They can answer your questions and calm your fears about your child and the technology which may seem intimidating.

When it is clear that recovery is going well, your child will be transferred to a pediatric cardiology unit. The average stay in the hospital for a child following open-heart surgery is about 7 to 10 days. Of course, the length of stay may vary, particularly if your child develops complications. Complications can include bleeding, infection, and leakage.

As you prepare to take your child home, you will want to arrange a follow-up appointment with your pediatric cardiologist and pediatric heart surgeon. This appointment should be scheduled for about four to six weeks after the date of the surgery. At the appointment the cardiologist may obtain an echocardiogram to view the results of the surgery. He or she will also obtain an electrocardiogram to measure the electrical forces in the heart and a chest x-ray to examine the heart's size and shape as well as the patterns of the blood vessels in the lungs. The doctor will also listen for heart murmurs and will measure your child's growth.

Preventing Subacute Bacterial Endocarditis (SBE)

Children who have congenital heart disease have an increased risk of acquiring bacterial infections of the heart, called *subacute bacterial endocarditis* (SBE), before and after surgery. These are infections that attack the heart, and are very serious medical conditions. They can occur when your child undergoes certain *invasive* procedures. An invasive procedure is a medical treatment that involves the puncture or cutting of the skin, or the insertion of an instrument such as a dental pick or other foreign material into the body. Certain types of dental care, such as cleaning the teeth, filling cavities, and tooth extraction, are invasive, as is any kind of surgery, however minor. These kinds of procedures can allow bacteria to enter the bloodstream. As the bacteria travels in the bloodstream, it can infect the heart, causing SBE.

Your child's cardiologist will determine whether your child is at risk for endocarditis because of the presence of a hole or leaky valve, or after certain types of repairs. If it is a concern, the standard treatment to prevent endocarditis is to give your child an antibiotic—usually amoxicillin (the currently preferred antibiotic for children)—one hour before a procedure, and again six hours later. This practice is called *SBE prophylaxis*. Special procedures are used with children who need more protection, who are allergic to penicillin, or who will be having invasive procedures affecting the gastrointestinal or genito-urinary tract.

You need to be sure that your dentist and any other physicians who care for your child are informed of your child needs for medication to ward off SBE prior to treatment. Even if your child is only suspected of having heart disease, talk with your physician about SBE. Some procedures that may require protection from SBE are:

adenoidectomy (removal of the adenoids);
bladder catheterization (during medical procedures);

rigid bronchoscopy (to view the airways);
dental procedures likely to cause even slight bleeding;
gall bladder surgery;
gastrointestinal tract surgery;
lung or other respiratory tract biopsy or surgery;
surgery on any infected tissue;
tonsillectomy; and
urinary tract surgery.

Long-Term Follow-Up

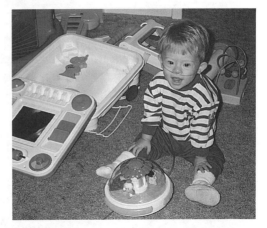

In most cases, heart surgery goes well, and the results are excellent. Normal heart function is restored and children attain good health. They are able to be normally active. When surgery is successful, follow-up is still necessary. Usually, your child will see the surgeon about six weeks after she leaves the hospital. She will also see the cardiologist for follow-up evaluations. The frequency of long-term follow-up evaluations with the cardiologist will depend on your child's progress.

In most cases, successful surgery will cause your child to go through a growth spurt. She will also likely have more energy. You may also, however, see some psychological trauma such as fear of doctors or hospitals or increased dependence or separation anxiety resulting from her memories of the surgery.

Even after heart surgery, some children will need ongoing, long-term medical treatment for congestive heart failure or irregular heartbeat. Sometimes surgery can only partially repair the heart defect or it can cause other problems. Some children can continue to have problems with valve regurgitation. And in some cases, a child who has had heart surgery will die long after returning home. When this happens, it is usually the result of continuing heart disease, typically involving severe AV valve regurgitation, persistent pulmonary artery hypertension, or abnormal cardiac rhythm.

Summary

Early diagnosis and treatment of congenital heart disease in children with Down syndrome is crucial to improving their quality and length of life. More than 40 percent of all people with Down syndrome have congenital heart disease. Because many infants with congenital heart disease will not have symptoms at birth, it is very important that all children with Down syndrome be carefully screened for heart disease early in infancy.

Pediatric cardiologists recommend the evaluation of every infant with Down syndrome for the presence of congenital heart disease. The outlook is very encouraging for children with Down syndrome with congenital heart disease who receive good medical care from early infancy. Without such care, most people with Down syndrome who have significant congenital heart defects will die of respiratory infections, congestive heart failure, or pulmonary artery hypertension before they reach the age of twenty. People with Down syndrome who receive appropriate and timely medical care can have a near normal lifespan and their quality of life is significantly better.

Resources

_____. *If Your Child Has a Congenital Heart Defect: A Guide for Parents* (Dallas: American Heart Association, pamphlet, 1991).

Gordon, L.S. "Cardiac Conditions", in Van Dyke, D.C., et al., eds, *Clinical Perspectives in the Management of Down Syndrome* (New York: Springer-Verlag, 1990).

Hallidie-Smith, K.A. "The Heart," in Lane, D. and Stratford, B., eds, *Current Approaches to Down's Syndrome* (New York: Holt, Rinehart and Winston, 1985).

Lott, I.T. and McCoy, E.E., eds. *Down Syndrome: Advances in Medical Care* (New York: Wiley-Liss, 1992).

Pueschel, S.M. and Pueschel, J.K., eds. *Biomedical Concerns in Persons with Down Syndrome* (Baltimore: Paul H. Brookes, 1992).

4 | Immune System Concerns for Children with Down Syndrome

Charles Steven Smith, M.D.

Overview

The human immune system is a remarkably complex and efficient blend of processes that function constantly to ensure our survival. This system protects our bodies from damage caused by invading microorganisms, including viruses, fungi, parasites, and bacteria. Although we are constantly exposed to these invaders, our immune system is usually capable of defending us. For example, it is our immune system that fights off the common cold, protects us from pneumonia, and prevents a cut on our finger from infecting our entire body.

This chapter explains what the immune system is, how it works, what science knows about how the system might work differently in people with Down syndrome, and what specific immune system problems they can have. Although the system is quite complex, science is beginning to understand more fully how it works.

What is the Immune System?

In order to understand the immune system, you first need to understand why it is needed. As mentioned above, the immune system fights against invaders like fungi, viruses, parasites, and bacteria. These organisms are always found in the environment, on our skin, in our hair, in our mouth, and in our digestive system.

The body is made up of many individual sterile compartments. Problems occur when one of the invaders, for example bacteria, go from a contaminated environment (such as the surface of the skin) into a sterile environment such as inside a joint or inside the abdomen. Commonly, this happens from a trauma, such as a puncture wound that causes an opening on the skin that allows bacteria to enter. Other causes can be diseases, such as inflammatory bowel disease where there may be damage to the mucous barrier in the gastrointestinal tract, allowing bacteria normally present in the bowel to make its way into the bloodstream or into the abdominal cavity. Other causes are malnutrition, a damaged or defective immune system, burns that cause skin breakdown, or allergic reactions. In fact, there are many ways for bacteria, fungi, parasites, and viruses to invade the sterile areas of the body.

If an organism gets in, it can proliferate rapidly. This type of invasion is called an infection. Infections can be local in a specific area (such as a joint) or generalized throughout the body.

The immune system exists to keep invaders at bay. To perform this function, the immune system has four major components, which are called *immune factors.* They are:

1. antibodies;
2. white blood cells;
3. special cells in the body (called *phagocytes*); and
4. special substances in the blood (called *complement*).

These different elements function in coordination to defend against invading organisms. They have one mission—to protect their world, the human body. Each of these different elements functions in a different way, but all have the same goal—to kill invaders and prevent their spread inside the body. The result of a properly functioning immune system is a state of immunity.

The immune system is constantly vigilant. Phagocytes and other cells travel in the blood stream and move in and out of the tissues of the body, ready to respond when invasions occur. Cells that make complement, antibodies, and other chemicals are always at work making small amounts of these substances; they are able to increase production quickly when necessary. Other elements of the immune system

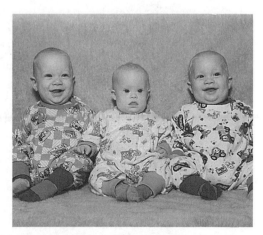

then react to this build-up, and in most cases, stop the invaders before any real infection can get started.

How the Immune System Works

The immune system works in three remarkable ways. First, it is able to recognize invaders, some of which are no bigger than a single cell. The system is usually able to identify foreign organisms, and can even find them when they hide inside cells. Second, the immune system kills invaders. It is capable of killing in many different ways depending on the particular type of invader it confronts. Third, and most amazing, the system remembers. Usually, if an invader is killed once, the immune system is armed and ready if a similar organism ever appears again. Each of these critical functions is explained below.

Recognition

The first step the body takes to fight an infection is to recognize when an invader is present and, most importantly, recognize when one is *not* present. Each cell in the body has its own individual molecular structure; it carries within it or on its surface substances which label it with a unique identity or "fingerprint." The immune system "knows" the identity of all of the cells in its world, the body. It recognizes these cells as "self." Any cell not matching its records is considered "non-self." The system responds to non-self cells by dispatching agents to kill them, but leaves "self" cells unharmed. An example of self cells are your skin cells. Examples of non-self cells are bacteria that have made their way from your skin into a joint space, or a graft of someone else's skin on to your skin. Cells identified as non-self are called *antigens*, which stands for "antibody generating substance." Thus non-self cells, or antigens, are recognized, and the immune system gears up to attack them.

In most cases the immune system accurately identifies both self and non-self cells, and attacks only non-self cells. Many cases, however, are close calls because some self and non-self cells have very similar fingerprints. This is the case with some viruses which can mimic the molecular structure of self cells. In this case, the body erroneously manufactures antibodies to attack some of its own cells. This is called *viral induced autoimmunity*. In addition, the immune system can sometimes have a defect that causes it to mistake self cells for non-self cells and to attack them. There are a number of *autoimmune disorders*. Scientists are just beginning to learn about some of them. Most of them are not common, but can be chronic and debilitating. An example of an autoimmune disorder is *systemic lupus erythematosus* (SLE). In this disorder the body develops antibodies against the DNA of its own cells. Another disorder thought to have an autoimmune component is multiple sclerosis in whichcells attack and destroy the insulation (called *myelin*) that covers and protects nerve cells.

Killing

Once the immune system identifies a cell as non-self, it mobilizes to kill the invader. The system is capable of picking different methods to kill invaders based on the nature of the invader. That is, the immune system can tailor its killing method to be effective against almost any kind of defense that the invading organism might have.

There are four ways the immune system kills invaders:

Antibodies. An antibody is a substance produced in the body and known as *immunoglobulin* (Ig). Each antibody responds to and interacts with a specific antigen. There are five primary types of antibodies, named immunoglobulin A, D, E, G, and M, along with some subtypes. Each fights antigens differently. Antibodies are produced by special cells called *B cells,* located in the bone marrow. The human body is capable of producing about 100 million different kinds of antibodies, each with its own unique structure and purpose. There are a number of categories of antibodies, and a number of types of antibodies.

When the immune system detects an invader that can be killed by antibodies it dispatches them into the bloodstream. These antibodies travel to the invader, attach themselves to it, and then kill it, in one of several ways. First, some antigens may be killed directly by the antibody. It may combine with the invader in a manner that prevents or interferes with a critical biological function of the cell, such as the manufacturing of the cell wall. Second, antibodies can coat invading cells and cause them to clump together. When this happens, other cells in the immune system can more easily destroy them. Clumps of cells are easier to grab onto than individual cells. Third, antibodies, in combination with another part of the immune system called *complement,* can actually disintegrate an invader very quickly. Some antibodies label invaders by damaging their cell membranes. By marking them, these cells can be more easily identified and killed by *phagocytic cells* (discussed below).

T-cells. *T-cells* are important killing agents of the immune system. Like antibodies, T-cells are produced in the bone marrow, but are then sent to the *thymus* (a small organ high in the chest) to complete their development. Unlike antibodies, T-cells do not kill invaders directly. Their specialty is finding invaders, usually viruses, when they are hidden inside a cell. For example, many viruses multiply inside normal cells. When this occurs, the normal cell reveals the presence of the virus. T-cells pierce the cell, exposing the viruses inside to antibodies. This type of immune response is called *cell-mediated response.*

Phagocytes. Another weapon to combat invading cells is phagocytes, special white blood cells that flow in the bloodstream. When certain bacteria invade, the immune system responds by dispatching specific antibodies. These antibodies mark the bacteria, and then phagocytes engulf and literally digest them.

Complement. The complement system is the fast emergency response system of the immune system. The complement system consists of small proteins in the bloodstream that act as a quick-response system. Combined with antibodies, it directly destroys foreign cells. In some cases complement combines with antigens that have been clumped together by antibodies to enhance their destruction by phagocytic cells. Thus, the complement system kills directly and also enables other weapons to kill invaders. In addition, complement can label foreign cells so that when they pass through certain organs, such as the spleen, they are identified, killed, and removed.

The result of these four methods of fighting foreign cells is a comprehensive immune system involving billions of cells that can confront and destroy harmful invading organisms. These four methods are highly coordinated and extremely effective in protecting the body from harm.

Memory

Once the immune system has identified and killed a foreign cell, it is capable of "remembering" that cell's identity so similar cells can be killed more rapidly if they appear in the future. The immune system produces cells called *T-lympho-*

cytes that specialize in killing the specific invaders confronted before. Through this process, the human body 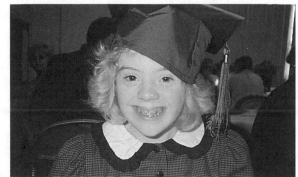 is prepared to quickly fend off invasion of cells or microorganisms similar to those it has encountered in the past. Speed in killing invaders is important because it prevents an organism from rapidly reproducing in the body.

After exposure to an organism or following immunization with a vaccine, our immune system develops defenses that it will use in any future encounters with these organisms. For example, if we have German measles, we develop antibodies to German measles. These antibodies remain even after we recover from the measles. If we are again exposed to the German measles virus, antibodies are already present. In addition, the immune system's memory triggers immediate additional production of antibodies. Thus, we never get German measles again.

Vaccinations stimulate the immune system's memory and antibody production so that in the future when we are exposed to the offending invader, we rapidly mount a defense and do not develop an infection. The development of vaccines has become very important in preventing disease. It has led to the rapid decrease in many serious childhood and adult illness that previously resulted in death. There are vaccines against both bacteria and viruses. The most commonly used are those against viruses such as mumps, measles, German measles, and polio. There are also vaccines against bacteria such as hemophilus influenza, diphtheria, tetanus, and pertussis (whooping cough).

Immunizations can be given by injection, nasally, or by swallowing. The optimal way to administer a vaccine depends on the particular vaccine. Vaccine production in this age of molecular genetics has become very sophisticated. Vaccines were made originally of killed organisms. For example, a virus was killed either by heating it or treating it with chemicals, and then it was administered in the killed state. Later, researchers learned how to make vaccines without killing the virus, by decreasing its *virulence*. Lack of virulence means that the virus, while still present, no longer is capable of causing disease. These non-virulent or *attenuated viruses* (live viruses) are given to stimulate the immune system in the same ways an active (virulent) virus would. In addition, through molecular genetics, we have learned how to make vaccines with certain portions of the virus structure that stimulate immunity without causing disease.

Immune System Problems in Children with Down Syndrome and Their Treatment

When a defect occurs in our immune system, it can change the way our bodies respond to invading organisms. If there are defects, the immune system may attack our body's own cells, called autoimmunity, or may create unneeded antibodies that may damage some of our cells rather than protect them. For example, defects in the immune system can cause the destruction of bone marrow cells in SLE (described above). Defects can also result in allergies, the result of an over-reactive immune system that leads to the release of substances that cause itching, tearing, or swelling. Defects in the cell-mediated immune system can result in recurrent infections, malignancies, and autoimmune disease. When the phagocytic cell system functions abnormally and these special cells do not destroy invaders, abscesses and recurrent infections occur. When the complement system is defective, *angioedema* (swelling of tissue), recurrent infections, and autoimmune problems appear.

Some children, including children with Down syndrome, may have immune system disorders. However, without doing specific individual evaluations, it is not possible to determine which child with or without Down syndrome has a specific immune problem. The following sections discuss the immune system problems that can affect children with Down syndrome.

Antibody Disorders

As discussed above, antibodies are made from five types of immunoglobulin. Each type is specialized by the timing of its actions, the part of the body where it is most effective, or the type of allergen it responds to. Having too much or too little of any type of immunoglobulin can cause problems with the immune system.

One type of immunoglobulin that can cause immune system problems is lack of or low levels of immunoglobulin A (IgA). IgA is called the *secretory antibody* because it is found in many of the secretions of our body's mucous membranes, such as tears and respiratory tract secretions. It serves as our body's first line of defense against invading organisms. Disorders that affect the production of this antibody usually do not present a threat to life, but can make your child's life more unpleasant because it makes him more susceptible to infections. Many children with secretory or IgA deficiency have frequent respiratory infections. The respiratory system is one of the areas in which antibodies are extremely active.

Immunoglobulin A deficiency is found in approximately one in every 200 to 500 people. It may be increased in children with Down syndrome but we do not know its exact incidence. It can be congenital (present from birth), or can be acquired later in life.

Immunoglobulin G (IgG) is the primary type of antibody that responds to problems. When the body's immune responses are in full swing, most of the antibodies present are IgG. Defects in the production of IgG can be life-threatening, especially if there is a complete absence of IgG. Doctors think IgG deficiency is more common among people with Down syndrome but its exact incidence is not known. As mentioned above, IgG has different varieties, called *subclasses*. If one of the less important subclasses of IgG is absent, it may cause only minor problems. Some people with Down syndrome may be deficient in IgG subclasses 2 and 4. Because the overall IgG level may be normal, this deficiency can only be detected by analysis of the specific subclass.

Children with a deficiency of immunoglobulin G or one of its subclasses can receive replacement therapy with intravenous (into the vein) or intramuscular (into the muscle) injections of *human immune globulin*. Human immune globulin is derived from human plasma, the liquid part of blood, by a special separation process. It consists primarily of at least 95 percent IgG and trace amounts of IgA and IgM. It is a sterile preparation and does not transmit hepatitis, HIV, or other infectious diseases. In addition, children with IgG deficiency may need aggressive antibiotic therapy. While this treatment is typically successful, it usually requires life long administration. Treatment of children with IgG or a subclass deficiency should be monitored by a physician who specializes in immunology and is familiar with the highly technical, newer, and more sensitive methods used to detect subclass antibody levels in infants and children.

Much less is known about IgM and IgD. The exact function of IgD is not known. IgM antibodies are very large, and are able to attach to many antigens at once. Early in a response to an infection, most of the antibodies made are likely to be IgM, with IgG levels increasing later. A deficiency in IgM is rare; children with this deficiency will have recurrent bacterial infections.

Cell-Mediated Disorders

Problems with cell-mediated immunity are more difficult to diagnose in the laboratory than antibody disorders. Diagnosis usually requires sophisticated laboratory tests by special laboratories. Because T-cells are critical in the defense against viruses and fungi, this type of immune system disorder often results in recurrent fungal infections; one of the most common of these is the yeast infection, *candida. Candidiasis* affects the skin and mucous membranes primarily of the gastrointestinal system. Viral infections are also more frequent and may be very severe and sometimes life-threatening. Doctors believe that the incidence of cell-mediated dysfunction in Down syndrome is increased but the exact incidence is not known.

Treatment for cell-mediated immune dysfunction is in its infancy. Techniques such as bone marrow transplants and thymus gland supplements have been successful with some children. Treatment with antibiotics may also prevent recurrent infections.

Special techniques must be used to prepare blood for transfusion to children with cell-mediated deficiencies. Blood must be treated so that there is only a very remote possibility that viruses, even in small amounts, could be transmitted. In addition, the blood must be treated so that it will not cause a severe immune reaction due to the presence of antibodies.

A child with cell-mediated immune dysfunction must also avoid immunization with live viral vaccines, such as oral polio vaccines and the live vaccines for measles, mumps, and rubella (MMR). In these children, use of a live attenuated viral vaccination could result in an overwhelming viral infection that might cause death. While attenuated viruses do not cause disease in children with normal immune systems, there is a significant risk that they could cause significant infection in people with compromised immune systems.

Another function of normal white blood cells is to travel to infection sites to destroy disease organisms. In children with Down syndrome, the white blood cells may not travel as quickly as they should. This results in an increase in infections, especially in the respiratory tract. In combination with cardiac defects, this may have life-threatening consequences. For this reason, prompt antibiotic therapy is very important in people with Down syndrome. Daily antibiotic therapies may be warranted for some children who have significant recurrent infections or have been diagnosed with immune problems by laboratory testing. It is also particularly important for children with underlying problems, such as heart defects that could result in a bacterial infection of the heart, to receive antibiotics prior to procedures such as dental exams or other invasive studies. This is because these procedures may result in small amounts of bacteria being released into the blood. While these small amounts of bacteria may not cause infection in people with normal immunity, in some children with Down syndrome they could rapidly result in an overwhelming bacterial infection of the heart called *bacterial endocarditis*.

In order to prevent infections in the past, oral zinc supplements were given to treat immune dysfunction in some children. However, the results of this procedure have been shown to be disappointing and it is not presently recommended. At the present time, disorders of the phagocytic system can only be treated with antibiotic therapy to prevent infection. Treatment with phagocytic cell transfusions such as white blood cell transfusion has had only limited success.

Autoimmunity Problems

Children with Down syndrome seem to have a greater tendency to develop auto-antibodies. That is, they develop antibodies that attack their own cells, including the cells of the pancreas, thyroid, and parathyroid. This can cause serious pancreatic dysfunction, resulting in malabsorption of food; or thyroid dysfunction, with the most common result being hypothyroidism, underactive functioning of the thyroid gland (hypothyroidism is discussed in detail in Chapter 5). Some investigators believe that the development of auto-antibodies results from premature aging of the immune system. However, much more research needs to be done in this area. Treatment involves replacing the deficient hormones (such as thyroid

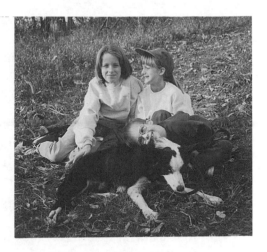

hormone) in people who have hypothyroidism or the treatment of malabsorption that results from pancreatic dysfunction. The exact incidence of these symptoms is not known. Specifically, the incidence of hypothyroidism which may be due to auto antibodies in people with Down syndrome may be as high as 15 to 20 percent. Autoimmune problems may also affect the skin and joints.

Allergies

In approximately 20 percent of all people, the body makes unnecessary IgE antibodies in response to normally harmless substances. These normal, harmless substances are called *allergens;* they may be foods, pollens, mold spores, animal dander, insect body parts or venom, or medications. Once exposed, an allergic person creates so much IgE antibody that on later exposure the IgE and the allergen bond together. They then attach to certain cells that cause the release of specific chemical compounds called *histamines.* It is histamines that result in the miserable symptoms of allergy such as coughing, drippy nose, red eyes, sinus and middle ear infections, asthma, hives, eczema, and problems with the digestive system. In many cases allergies can lead to an increase in respiratory infections. The exact incidence of allergies in children with Down syndrome is not known.

An allergy may be evaluated with skin tests or, if skin tests are impossible for one reason or another, with specific IgE allergy blood tests. IgE dysfunction, called allergic illness, can be treated in three ways. First, your child's environment can be controlled to avoid contact with the offending allergen. Of course, this may not always be possible if the allergen is very common. Second, allergies can be treated with medications to control symptoms. These medications include:

- **antihistamines**—drugs that counteract the effects of histamines;
- **bronchodilators**—drugs that counteract the effects of *vasoactive substances,* chemicals that occur with allergies that can cause airways to constrict; and
- **steroids**—chemical compounds that decrease the swelling and inflammation of the lining of the respiratory tract that allergens can cause.

The third treatment for allergies is *immunotherapy* (often called "allergy shots"). Immunotherapy involves injecting a person with increasing amounts of the allergens that make their bodies produce IgE antibodies. Gradually increasing the strength of these shots encourages the body to decrease its production of IgE and to increase the production of a blocking or protective antibody in the immunoglobulin G group. In 75 to 80 percent of people, this procedure decreases their allergies to a tolerable level. This therapy can be used for airborne allergens and in some cases for allergies to medications, but it is not effective for food allergy. To be effective, the injections have to be repeated regularly. When doses are missed, protection is rapidly lost.

Children with Down syndrome with allergies or unexplained recurrent infections should be evaluated by an allergist or an immunologist. Allergic conditions may be permanent; long-term follow-up care is important.

Problems with the Complement System

As discussed above, the complement system consists of small proteins in the bloodstream that act as a quick response force for the immune system. Complement works by combining with antibodies to directly destroy foreign cells and by combining with antibody-antigen clumps to enhance destruction by phagocytic cells. Defects in these small proteins lead to problems in the operation of the complement system. At the present time, defects of the blood cell complement system cannot be treated using replacement therapy; however, treating children with medications to slow down the body's use of complement has been successful in some cases. The use of fresh frozen plasma that contains complement to treat episodes of severe infections has also been somewhat successful. Children can also sometimes be helped by preventive treatment with oral antibiotics.

Childhood Immunizations

Your child with Down syndrome should receive all the routine childhood immunizations unless he has a cell-mediated immune deficiency. Tables 1 and 2 show immunization schedules. As discussed above, some vaccinations pose a danger to children with cell-mediated immune deficiency.

If your child has recurrent infections (most of which are respiratory), he should receive three additional immunizations: the pneumococcal vaccine, the hepatitis type B vaccine, and yearly immunization for influenza. These immunizations can protect your child against an important group of bacterial and viral infections. All children with Down syndrome should get these vaccines on a regular schedule, even though some decrease in immune response may occur—especially to influenza A.

The pneumococcal immunization protects against 23 different types of pneumococcal bacteria, organisms that cause 88 percent of all pneumococcal blood infections. However,

Table 1: Recommended Schedule for Immunization of Healthy Infants and Children.		
Recommended Age	**Immunizations**	**Comments**
2 months	DTP, HbCV, OPV	Diphtheria-tetanus-pertussis (DTP) and oral polio vaccine (OPV) can be initiated as early as 4 weeks after birth in areas where they are widespread or during epidemics; as of 1990, only one Haemophilus B conjugate vaccine (HbCV) is approved for children younger than 15 months
4 months	DTP, HbCV, OPV	A 2-month interval (minimum of 6 weeks) desired for OPV to avoid interference from previous dose
6 months	DTP, HbCV	Third dose of OPV is not indicated in the U.S., but is desirable in other geographic areas where polio is widespread
15 months	MMR, HbCV	Tuberculin testing may be done at the same visit
15-18 months	DTP, OPV	DTP should be given 6-12 months after the third dose; may be given simultaneously with live measles-mumps-rubella (MMR) and HbCV at 15 months or at any time between 12 and 24 months; priority should be given to administering MMR at the recommended age
4-6 years	DTP, OPV	At or before school entry; DTP can be given up to 7th birthday
11-12 years	MMR	At entry to middle school or junior high school unless second dose previously given
14-16 years	Td	Adult tetanus toxoid and diphtheria toxoid (Td), repeat every 10 years throughout life

Adapted from the 1991 Report of the Committee on Infectious Disease, American Academy of Pediatrics

children under two years of age, as well as some people who are older or who have chronic illnesses, may not respond as well or at all. The vaccine probably provides long-term protection for most people; however, it is recommended that some people be revaccinated every six years. Children who will benefit most from a pneumococcal vaccine are those with heart disease, lung disease, kidney disease, diabetes, or cancer; and those whose spleens have been removed. Children with Down syndrome often meet one or more of these criteria, and should be vaccinated after two years of age.

Influenza A, a virus, is a threat to both healthy children and children with chronic, underlying health conditions. It has been estimated that about 10 to 40 percent of all healthy children develop influenza each year. About 1 percent of these infections result in hospitalization. A wide variety of complications, including Reye's syndrome, myelitis (severe muscle inflammation), and central nervous system disorders can occur. Of the children who get these serious complications, between 1 to 5 percent die.

Because

Table 2: Recommended Immunization Schedules for Children Not Immunized in the First Year of Life.		
Recommended Time/Age	Immunizations	Comments
Younger Than 7 Years		
First visit	DTP, OPV, MMR	Diphtheria-tetanus-pertussis (DTP) and oral polio vaccine (OPV). Measles-mumps-rubella (MMR) if child is more than 15 months old; tuberculin testing may be done at same visit; minimum interval between doses of MMR is one month
	HbCV	For children aged 15-59 months, Haemophilus B conjugate virus vaccine (HbCV) can be given simultaneously with DTP and other vaccines *(at separate sites)*
Interval after first visit		
2 months	DTP, OPV (HbCV)	Second dose of HbVC is indicated only in children whose first dose was received when younger than 15 months
4 months	DTP	Third dose of OPV is not indicated in the U.S. but is desirable in other geographic areas where polio is common; not generally given if person is older than 18 and living in U.S.
10-16 months	DTP, OPV	OPV is not given if third dose was given earlier
4-6 years *(at or before school entry)*	DTP, OPV	DTP is not necessary if the fourth dose was given after the fourth birthday; OPV is not necessary if third dose was given after the fourth birthday
11-12 years	MMR	At entry to middle school or junior high
10 years later	Td	Repeat tetanus toxoid (Td) every 10 years throughout life
7 Years and Older		
First visit	Td, OPV, MMR	
Interval after first visit		
2 months	Td, OPV	
8-14 months	Td, OPV	
11-12 years	MMR	At entry to middle school or junior high
10 years later	Td	Repeat tetanus toxoid (Td) every 10 years throughout life

Adapted from the 1991 Report of the Committee on Infectious Disease, American Academy of Pediatrics

of some of the immune problems described above, children with Down syndrome are at a much higher risk for chronic respiratory infections such as influenza. For this reason, you should to make yearly influenza A vaccinations part of your child's health care plan. Alternative methods of protecting against influenza may also be considered, such as the use of an antiviral medication. Amantadine is an antiviral medication which seems to work well to protect against influenza A infection.

Children who have Down syndrome have also been found to be at a higher risk for developing chronic active hepatitis B, a serious infection of the liver. It is difficult to determine the exact incidence of chronic active hepatitis B in people with Down syndrome because the incidence at the present time seems to be changing. This may be a result of the fact that many people with Down syndrome are no longer institutionalized, a source of hepatitis B exposure. This illness is usually caused by the hepatitis B virus, though in a few children its results from an autoimmune disorder that destroys their livers. Hepatitis B can cause serious liver disease, liver cancer, and death. About two of every twenty individuals in the United States have been infected with hepatitis B. A certain percentage become chronic carriers, usually with no symptoms until later. These individuals can spread the infection to others throughout their lifetime. They can also develop long term liver disease such as *cirrhosis* (scarring of the liver) and liver cancer.

Because they are at higher risk for chronic, active hepatitis, children with Down syndrome are candidates for the hepatitis B vaccine. In fact, the American Academy of Pediatrics has recommended that all children receive hepatitis B immunization. The hepatitis B vaccine is given in three doses on three different dates (see Table 3). Infants can get the vaccine at the same time as their other baby shots. The hepatitis B vaccine prevents infection in 85 to 95 percent of people who get all three shots. Studies have shown that protection lasts at least ten years; booster doses are not currently recommended.

Table 3: Recommended Doses (Given Intramuscularly) and Schedules of Currently Licensed Hepatitis B Vaccines.

Vaccine
Usual schedule for each vaccine is three doses, given at 0,1, and 6 months

Group	Heptavax B (Merck) Dose (ug)(mL)	Recombivax HB (Merck) Dose (ug)(mL)	Engerix-B (SmithKline) Dose (ug)(mL)
Infants of mothers who are viral hepatitis (HBV) carriers	10 (0.5)	5(0.5)	10 (0.5)
Other infants and children younger than 11 years	10 (0.5)	2.5 (0.25)	10 (0.5)
Children and adolescents 11-19 years	20 (1.0)	5 (0.5)	20 (1.0)
Adults older than 19 years	20 (1.0)	10 (1.0)	20 (1.0)
Dialysis patients and other immunocompromised persons	40 (2.0) (Given as two 1.0 mL doses at different sites)	40 (1.0) (Special formula for dialysis patients)	40 (2.0) (Given as two 1.0 mL doses at different sites; on a five dose schedule, given at 0, 1, 2, and 12 months)

Adapted from the 1991 Report of the Committee on Infectious Disease, American Academy of Pediatrics

Most of the side effects are minimal and include redness and soreness at the site of injection.

Summary

Some children with Down syndrome have immune system disorders which, if not treated, can lead to serious chronic illness and poor health. Not all of these immune system disorders can be treated, but identifying them may lead to better control of the symptoms. Health care for your child, especially if your child has recurrent infections, may need to include: screening by an allergist, or an immunologist, for allergies or immune system disorders; allergy testing; pneumococcal, hepatitis B, and influenza A immunizations, in addition to normal childhood immunizations. Your child's pediatrician can be your first source for information about your child's immune system and can refer you to a specialist if that is necessary.

Resources

The Centers for Disease Control (CDC), United States Public Health Service, Department of Health and Human Services, Atlanta,

Georgia 30333. Provides publications for parents and children about all types of immunizations, prevention and control of infectious disease, injury, chronic diseases, and environment-related injury and illness.

American Academy of Allergy and Immunology, 611 East Wells Street, Milwaukee, Wisconsin 53202; 410/227–6071 or 800/822–2762. Provides general allergy and immunology information and referrals if necessary.

National Institutes of Health, Division of Allergy and Immunology, NAIAD Solar Building, Room 4A-18, Bethesda, Maryland 20892; 301/496–5717.

References

_____. *Report of the Committee on Infectious Diseases.* American Academy of Pediatrics, 1991, 275–281.

_____. *Report on Pneumococcal Vaccine.* (Atlanta, GA: The Centers for Disease Control, U.S. Public Health Service, Department of Health and Human Services, 1989).

_____. *Report on Hepatitis B.* (Atlanta, GA: The Centers for Disease Control, U.S. Public Health Service, Department of Health and Human Services, 1992).

Kass, E.H. and Platt, R. *Current Therapy in Infectious Diseases.* (Mosby Year Book, 1990), 57.

Loh, R. K., et al. "Immunoglobulin G Subclass Deficiency and Predisposition to Infection in Down Syndrome." *Pediatric Infectious Disease Journal,* Vol. 9, No. 8, 1990, 547–551.

O'Mahony, D., et. al. "Down Syndrome and Autoimmune Chronic Active Hepatitis." *The Irish Journal of Medical Science,* Vol. 159, No. 1, 1990, 21–21.

Rabinowe, S.L., et. al. "Trisomy 21 (Down Syndrome): Autoimmunity, Aging and Monoclonal Antibody-defined T-Cell Abnormalities." *Journal of Autoimmunity,* Vol. 2, No. 1, 1989, 25–30.

Stiehm and Fulginiti. *Immunologic Disorders of Infants and Children* (Philadelphia: W.B. Saunders, 1980), 266–267.

5 | Thyroid Conditions and Other Endocrine Concerns in Children with Down Syndrome

Thomas P. Foley, Jr., M.D.

Introduction

The *endocrine system* is one of the human body's most important regulatory systems. It is made up of a number of glands found throughout the body, including the adrenal glands, ovaries (in females), pancreas, parathyroid glands, pituitary gland, testes (in males), and thyroid gland. These glands produce and secrete *hormones*, chemical messengers that control and regulate the activities of the cells of certain organs or other body parts. For example, hormones control sexual maturation, growth, and the body's use of nutrients (metabolism).

Hormones work to trigger responses in cells in the body. When the body senses a need for something to occur (for example, to control the level of sugar in the blood), it secretes hormones. These hormones travel in the bloodstream to target cells that have receptors that then respond to the hormone. The hormones do not perform the needed action; they just they trigger it. They are the body's messengers to cells to perform needed work. When the body senses the work has been completed (for example, when the blood sugar level reaches the proper level), it shuts off the hormone. This process of the body first sensing a need; second, secreting hormones to trigger the required work; and third, sensing when the work is finished and shutting off the hormone, is called a *feedback loop.* Thus, the body is continually sensing its needs, and secreting hormones to trigger cells to meet them. Hormones can also have multiple effects on different cells in the body. For example, insulin, which controls blood sugar, affects the liver and the muscles in different ways.

Usually, the endocrine system operates in balance with the body's needs, producing all the hormones needed in just the right amounts. When hormones are produced in abnormal amounts, however— whether too much or too little—a variety of mild to quite serious disorders can result. Some of these disorders are hard to detect, and may exist for many years before they are recognized. Consequently, close monitoring is important for children with Down syndrome.

The endocrine problems that affect children with Down syndrome more than other children are thyroid disorders, discussed below. Aside from thyroid problems, however, other endocrine disorders are no more common in children with Down syndrome than in other children. There are, however, some other concerns related to the endocrine system of children with Down syndrome that are discussed briefly in this chapter.

Thyroid Disease

The most common endocrine disorder in people with Down syndrome occurs when the thyroid gland produces too little (*hypo*) or too much (*hyper*) thyroid hormone. We do not know what causes this, but we do know that people with Down syndrome are much more likely to have thyroid problems than are other people. By adulthood, as many as 20 percent of all people with Down syndrome, or 1 in 5, will have abnormal thyroid function. This section discusses the thyroid problems children with Down syndrome have.

To understand thyroid disease, however, you need to first understand what the thyroid gland does and how it works. The thyroid gland is the largest endocrine gland in the human body. It is located in the throat just below the voice box. The hormones it secretes have very wide ranging affects throughout the body. They regulate metabolism, and affect heart rate and growth.

The thyroid gland secretes a hormone called *thyroxine* (also called *T4*). Thyroxine is one of the most important hormones used throughout the body, and keeping the body supplied (but not over-supplied) is the thyroid gland's job. The thyroid gland secretes thyroxine when it receives a signal—in the form of another hormone called *thyrotropin*, which is also called *thyroid stimulating hormone (TSH)*—secreted by the *pituitary gland*. The pituitary gland, a small gland located at the base of the brain, secretes TSH when the brain detects low levels of T4 in the blood. The brain releases a hormone, called *thyrotropin releasing hormone (TRH),* to stimulate the pituitary gland to secrete TSH. In short, the thyroid gland's release of T4 is controlled by the brain and the pituitary gland, which sense the level of T4 in the blood, and send instructions.

Although this chapter refers to thyroxine (T4), it is actually another form of thyroid hormone, called *T3,* which the thyroid releases. T4, which is not active, is converted after release into T3 which is the active thyroid hormone. TSH is the switch that turns on the thyroid gland to release T4 (which turns into T3). When the brain senses adequate levels of T4 in the blood, it turns off the TSH switch. The result of this system is that the levels of T4 are regulated. However, because the body's mechanism for controlling T4 requires first releasing two other hormones, the regulation of T4 is consequently slower and less precise than the control of other hormones.

Hypothyroidism

The most common form of thyroid disease—both in children with Down syndrome and in the general population—is *hypothyroidism.* This is a condition in which the thyroid does not produce enough thyroid hormone (T4) to meet the body's needs. This disease can be treated easily in a number of ways,

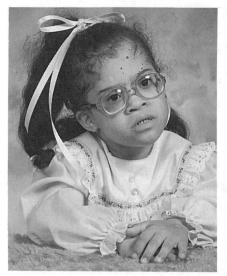

but it is important to monitor your child because children with Down syndrome are prone to this problem. Untreated thyroid disease can lead to serious health problems—slow growth, skin disorders, blood disorders like anemia, learning disorders, constipation, sleep disorders, and feeding disorders. In some circumstances, such as during anesthesia or surgery, untreated hypothyroidism can be life-threatening.

Hypothyroidism may be discovered during routine newborn blood testing. It may be found later, during a physical examination of a child's thyroid gland. Or it may be discovered by blood tests given to find the cause of symptoms of thyroid disease, such as fatigue, poor growth (see Figure 1), sleep disturbances, or changes in appetite. Sometimes, thyroid disease is discovered through blood tests done in the first week of a child's life. These tests are part of the routine testing required by law to be done on all newborns in the United States.

Congenital thyroid disorders. When a child is born with a thyroid that does not secrete enough thyroid hormone, this condition is called *congenital hypothyroidism* (congenital means that the condition exists at birth). Congenital hypothyroidism seems to occur more often in newborns who have Down syndrome than it does in other infants. Routine screening tests that are performed on every newborn can detect this disorder when thyroid screening is part of the test. Although every state and province in the U.S.A. and Canada screen newborns for hypothyroidism, not all countries in the world in-

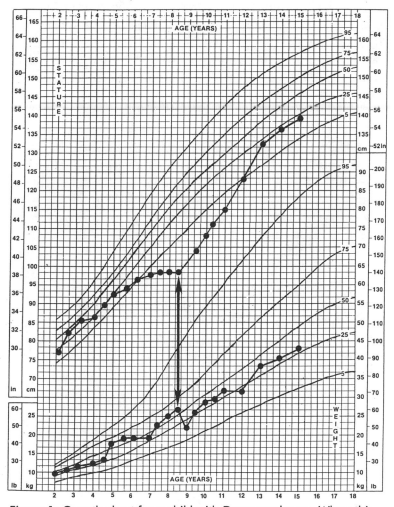

Figure 1: Growth chart for a child with Down syndrome. When this child was five years old, growth began to be delayed due to hypothyroidism. A diagnosis of hypothyroidism was confirmed when the child was 8½ years old (shown by arrows on the chart). With the start of thyroxine treatment, growth increased steadily until the child's height again reached the twenty-fifth percentile—the growth percentile achieved prior to the development of thyroid disease. The child's weight dropped slightly at the beginning of treatment due to loss of fluid (which had been retained as a result of thyroid disease).

clude thyroid screening as part of their newborn screening tests. Babies with hypothyroid disease who have high levels of thyroid stimulating hormone (TSH) and low levels of thyroxine (T4) need to begin treatment with thyroxine immediately. High TSH levels paired with low T4 levels usually mean that the brain is detecting the need for more T4 and trying to instruct the thyroid gland to produce it, but that the thyroid gland is not responding properly to the body's signals.

Acquired Hypothyroidism. Thyroid disease, including hypothyroidism, can be absent at birth, but appear later at any time. In people who develop thyroid disease later in life, the condition is often linked to a problem with the immune system known as *autoimmunity*. This process occurs when the body does not recognize its own tissue and generates an immune response to attack it.

Children with Down syndrome are more likely than other children to have acquired thyroid disease. After three years of age, your child may acquire thyroid disease as a result of an autoimmune disorder. Other autoimmune diseases may occur with thyroid disease, including *diabetes mellitus* (abnormal glucose metabolism, discussed below), *pernicious anemia* (low red blood cell count), and *alopecia* (loss of hair, discussed in Chapter 7). Autoimmune disorders are discussed in more detail in Chapter 4.

Thyroiditis is another form of acquired thyroid disease. It is an inflammation of the thyroid gland, and it may cause either too much or too little thyroid hormone to be produced. This condition can be puzzling because most children with thyroiditis have normal thyroid hormone levels. The most common form of thyroiditis with hypothyroidism is *chronic lymphocytic thyroiditis*. This condition is also known as *Hashimoto's disease*, named for Dr. Hakura Hashimoto, the physician who first reported the disease. There are two common signs of thyroiditis with hypothyroidism: 1) enlargement of the thyroid gland and 2) a slowing of linear growth (growth in height). The effects of Hashimoto's disease are treated like hypothyroidism—with monitoring of thyroid levels and with thyroid hormone supplements when levels are too low.

Symptoms of Hypothyroidism. There are many symptoms children with hypothyroidism may have. They include:

- dry skin;
- decreased muscle tone;
- fluid retention in the tissues (edema);
- anemia;
- reduced appetite;
- increased sleep;
- constipation;
- intolerance to cold;
- hair loss;
- slowed speech;
- cool skin; and
- decreased activity level.

These symptoms may appear at any age. Children with hypothyroidism may maintain the same weight, or may show a slight gain. Contrary to belief, serious obesity is *not* an early sign of hypothyroidism. Obesity is usually found in children with severe, long-term hypothyroid disease whose linear growth has very nearly stopped.

Acquired hypothyroidism may develop slowly over a long period of time. Symptoms can appear so gradually that they are very difficult to detect. This is especially true for children with Down syndrome, because the symptoms of Down syndrome are often similar to those of thyroid disease listed above. For this reason, parents are usually advised to have their child with Down syndrome tested for TSH and T4 levels every one to three years. These tests are highly sensitive ways to screen for hypothyroidism, and can often detect the disease even before the symptoms appear.

Diagnosing hypothyroidism can be tricky. The levels of TSH and T4 both need to be measured carefully. Sometimes T4 levels measure normal, but TSH levels are high. This can mean that the thyroid is producing sufficient T4, but that the brain is not sensing its presence. It can also mean that the thyroid is not responding to the TSH normally and that the pituitary gland must secrete extra TSH to get the thyroid gland to secrete enough T4. This condition requires careful monitoring.

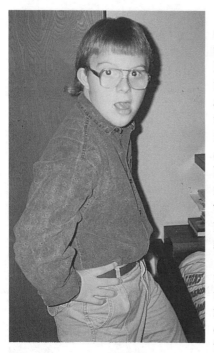

Your child's pediatrician can perform the routine screening blood test for hypothyroidism. Your doctor can also tell you when an endocrinologist—a doctor who specializes in treating problems of the endocrine system—should be consulted. The endocrinologist can thoroughly investigate any thyroid problems, diagnose, and begin treatment.

Treatment. Once diagnosed, hypothyroidism can usually be treated successfully. The treatment of choice is the oral medication, L-thyroxine, which is T4. L-thyroxine is an inexpensive medicine, given once daily by mouth, at least 30 minutes before a meal. The tablets can be crushed and mixed with milk. It is important that your child not eat for at least 30 minutes after taking this medication. With proper dosage, there are few if any side effects or allergic reactions. Your child will need a few blood tests during the first two years of thyroxine therapy. These tests will enable your doctor to check the levels of TSH and T4 in your child's system. L-thyroxine increases the level of T4; in most cases the levels of TSH will drop as the body senses sufficient T4. Before thyroxine therapy is started, your doctor should brief you on what to watch for during the first year or two of treatment, especially the symptoms that the dose is too large or small.

Idiopathic Hyperthyrotropinemia. During or shortly after newborn screening, some infants with Down syndrome are found to have high TSH levels, but normal levels of T4 and T3. When tests are repeated later, the levels of TSH remain the same or are closer to normal. This disorder is called *idiopathic* (no known cause) *hyperthyrotropinemia* (high serum TSH levels). In this condition, doctors may often find that TSH levels may be high on one occasion and normal when tested again. This suggests that the cause is a problem in the *regulation* of TSH secretion, and not a disease of the thyroid gland.

Idiopathic hyperthyrotropinemia usually disappears by the time a child is three to four years old. Treatment does not seem to be useful and is not recommended unless TSH levels increase and T4 levels steadily decrease. If treatment appears to be necessary, thyroxine medication is the treatment of choice. You should ask how long thyroxine therapy should continue and what symptoms may appear if too little or too much thyroxine is given.

Some doctors call idiopathic hyperthyrotropinemia *compensated hypothyroidism* when it develops during childhood, and think that at least some of the children with it may go on to develop thyroid failure. Your doctor may recommend further studies, and may begin treatment. Because not enough is known about what happens in the long run, it is impossible to say which approach is correct. If there are any symptoms of thyroid failure in a child who has high TSH and normal T4 levels, treatment with thyroxine can be considered. This is an area needing further research.

Hyperthyroidism

There are several thyroid disorders that result in too much thyroid hormone being produced.

Graves Disease. One form of hyperthyroidism is called Graves disease, named for Dr. Robert Graves, who described this disorder in 1835. It occurs most often in women, and is believed to be the result of an autoimmune disorder (discussed above). In Graves disease, the immune system stimulates rather than attacks the thyroid gland. It is slightly more common in children with Down syndrome than in the general population. Graves disease causes the thyroid to produce too much thyroid hormone. Some of its unique symptoms are bulging eyes (*exophthalmos*), goiter (or enlarged thyroid gland), weight loss, and mood swings.

Symptoms of Hyperthyroidism. Hyperthyroidism is found more often in children with Down syndrome than in other children. It is not as common as other forms of thyroid dysfunction. In addition, sometimes a child may have hyperthyroidism initially and years later may have hypothyroidism. The signs and symptoms of hyperthyroidism include:

- increased appetite, with weight remaining the same or dropping;
- shortened attention span;
- bulging eyes (but *exophthalmos* is less common and less severe in children than in adults);
- thinning hair;
- heat intolerance (removing clothing to be cooler when others are comfortable);
- irritability;
- nervousness;
- increased perspiration;
- flushed skin, with warm, smooth texture;
- disturbed sleep;
- infrequent stools;
- enlarged thyroid gland; and
- increased urination (and bed wetting).

Diagnosing Hyperthyroidism. Hyperthyroidism is more complicated to diagnose and treat than is hypothyroidism. In more obvious cases of Graves disease, only blood tests will be needed to confirm a diagnosis. These tests will measure the levels of T3, T4, and TSH. Test results showing elevated T3 and T4 levels and an absence of TSH indicate hyperthyroidism that is caused by a problem with the thyroid gland. High levels of T3, T4, *and* TSH may indicate hyperthyroidism that is caused by a problem with how the brain is sensing hormone levels. A TSH receptor antibody test, or TRAb, may also be used to confirm a diagnosis of Graves disease.

An enlarged thyroid is the most common clue to hyperthyroidism. Children with hyperthyroidism who do not have clear symptoms may need additional tests to measure how the body is making and using thyroid hormone. As with hypothyroidism, your pediatrician, in consultation with an endocrinologist, can diagnose hyperthyroidism. An endocrinologist can begin and monitor treatment.

Treating Hyperthyroidism. Children with hyperthyroid disease are usually treated with drugs that block the thyroid's production of the hormones T3 and T4. One of these drugs is methimazole, or MTZ. In the United States, its trade name is Tapazole™. The other drug used to treat hyperthyroidism is propylthiouracil, or PTU. About five percent of children who take these drugs have side effects. One possible side effect is a decrease in the number of white blood cells (WBC), specifically the neutrophils, white blood cells that help fight bacterial infections in the body. Before your child begins treatment, a blood test should be done to be sure that she does not already have a low WBC count due to *neutropenia* (low neutrophil count) or *anemia* (low red blood cell count).

If a child taking MTZ or PTU develops a bacterial (not viral) infection, WBC and neutrophil counts should be checked. It is important that the medication not increase the risk for very serious bacterial infections. Switching to different medications and using antibiotics can help avoid this problem. Signs of a low neutrophil count include recurrent sores in the mouth, on the tongue, or on the gums. Other side effects of MTZ or PTU may include persistent rashes, joint pain or swelling, and muscle aches. A loss of appetite, reduced energy, and the development of yellow, itchy skin may signal liver inflammation, a rare side effect. Some children may also have an allergic reaction to MTZ or PTU; it is important that any changes in your child's health be reported promptly to your doctor.

If your child has mild side effects with one of these drugs, the doctor may recommend treatment with the other. Your child will be then carefully monitored to be certain that the side effects do not reappear. If treatment with MTZ or PTU is not an option (because of infection or immune system problems), or serious side effects occur, two alternative treatments may be suggested: destruction of the thyroid with radioactive iodine or surgical removal of the thyroid.

For children with Down syndrome who are very young surgical removal of the thyroid is usually the preferred treatment if treatment with medication is not possible or successful. This procedure is called *subtotal thyroidectomy*. It is called *subtotal* because the surgery leaves some thyroid tissue and smaller glands surrounding of the thyroid—called the *parathyroid*—in place. During this surgery, which should be performed by an experienced pediatric surgeon, the thyroid itself is removed. This surgery has generally good results. Healing of the incisions is usually problem-free, and thyroid replacement therapy is started. One variation of this surgery is to leave some of the thyroid gland in the hope that it will produce normal amounts of thyroid hormone, thereby eliminating the need for thyroid replacement therapy.

For young children with Down syndrome, surgery is preferred over treating the problem with radioactive iodine (I-131). This is because little is known about the long-term effects of radioactive iodine treatment in young children. With children who have Down syndrome, this is a special concern because they have a higher risk of developing leukemia than do other children (see Chapter 11). More research is needed to determine the safety of radioactive iodine treatment in young children with Down syndrome. For older children, adolescents, and adults, treatment with radioactive iodine is preferred. It is less expensive than surgery, less painful, has fewer side effects, and is highly effective.

Radioactive iodine treatment works as follows: Normally, the thyroid gland absorbs iodine from the blood in order to make T4. When radioactive iodine is given, the thyroid absorbs it, too, and this iodine kills the cells of the thyroid. This treatment usually makes lifelong thyroid replacements necessary whenever it completely eliminates thyroid function.

The hormones produced by the thyroid are essential to the body. Removing the thyroid gland permanently ends the production of these hormones. In order to prevent your child from developing hypothyroid disease, lifelong hormone replacement therapy with L-thyroxine will be needed. Lifelong thyroid replacement is safe and effective for children with Down syndrome. L-thyroxine is very effective in replacing the body's natural thyroid hormone.

Other Endocrine-Related Problems

Children with Down syndrome can have problems with other endocrine glands in their body, but are no more likely than other children to have them. This section reviews two endocrine-related areas of concern to parents: stature and the reproductive system.

Stature

Many children with chromosomal disorders, including Down syndrome, have small stature, regardless of how tall their parents are. Because this is so common, special growth charts have been developed for children with Down syndrome (see Figures 2 and 3). These growth charts provide information on typical growth for babies with Down syndrome who are between the ages of one month to 36 months, and also for children with Down syndrome who are between the ages of 2 years and 18 years. If you compare these charts to the charts used for children who do not have Down syndrome, you will notice the differences between the growth patterns. In general, the growth rates are similar, although the actual height

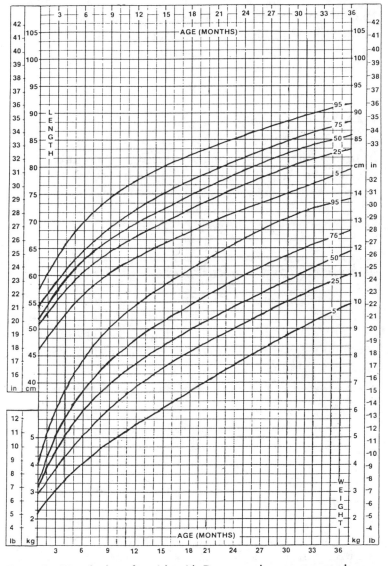

Figure 2: Growth chart for girls with Down syndrome, age newborn to 36 months. Reprinted by permission of *Pediatrics,* Vol. 81, 1988, 102–110.

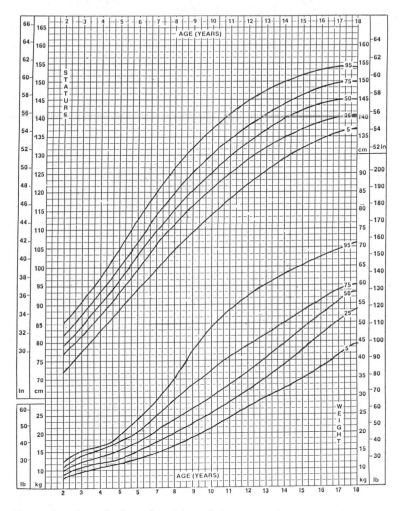

Figure 2a: Growth chart for girls with Down syndrome, age 2 years to 18 years. Reprinted by permission of *Pediatrics,* Vol 81, 1988, 102–110.

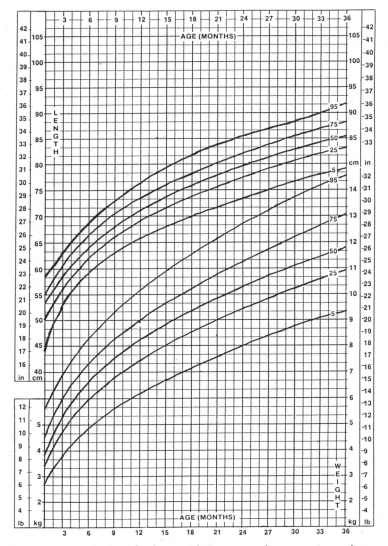

Figure 3: Growth chart for boys with Down syndrome, age newborn to 36 months. Reprinted by permission of *Pediatrics*, Vol 81, 1988, 102–110.

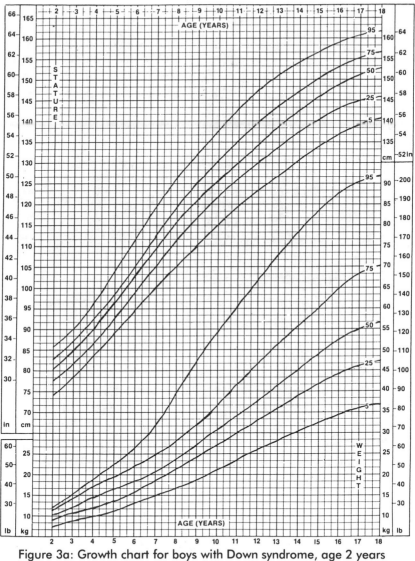

Figure 3a: Growth chart for boys with Down syndrome, age 2 years to 18 years. Reprinted by permission of *Pediatrics*, Vol 81, 1988, 102–110.

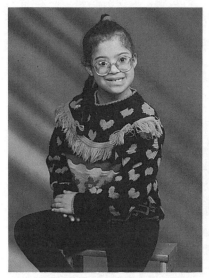

and weight at particular ages is less for the child with Down syndrome.

After your child celebrates her second birthday, her height and weight should be measured at least annually, and plotted on the appropriate growth chart. By the age of 2 to 3 years, children typically maintain a fixed rate of growth. If the rate of growth declines, it could be a symptom of a serious disorder, such as thyroid disease, a malabsorption syndrome (see Chapter 9), or a chronic disease (such as heart, kidney, lung, or liver disease). It is rare, but sometimes a shortage of *growth hormone (hGH)* secreted by the pituitary gland can be the cause of decreased growth.

The pituitary gland is located at the base of the brain, just behind the bridge of the nose. In addition to the pituitary gland's role in thyroid function, it controls growth by distributing growth hormone. The brain manufactures growth hormone and sends it to the pituitary gland, which then releases it into the bloodstream.

Current research has not shown that children with Down syndrome are more likely than other children to have *hypopituitarism*— a shortage of growth hormone (hGH). However, when growth slows and tests do not identify any of the more common causes, it makes sense to test for hGH levels.

Treating children with Down syndrome with human growth hormone (hGH) is controversial. Because slow growth in children with Down syndrome is *not* usually caused by a shortage of hGH, most physicians are reluctant to use this hormone to increase rates of growth. They prefer to use human growth hormone only when a child does not produce enough of it himself. There is some evidence from research that giving growth hormone to children who are not deficient in growth hormone does make them grow faster for a while, but their final adult height is not changed. These studies are limited, and too recent, to draw many conclusions about the long-term effects of hGH.

Treatment with hGH has not been shown to cause children with Down syndrome to become taller adults. Neither does hGH replacement therapy lead to increased brain growth or improved cognitive function, despite some claims. There are parents who report that their children with Down syndrome improved in speech and other areas of development after receiving hGH, but no carefully controlled studies have yet been done. As with all new treatments in Down syndrome, the reasons for change in a child have to be carefully evaluated. This issue is discussed in detail in Chapter 15.

A child with Down syndrome and a slow rate of growth should be considered for hGH replacement therapy when tests clearly indicate that she has hGH deficiency. Treatment with hGH is by daily injection of hGH beneath the skin at a dose of no higher than 0.2–0.3 mg/kg/week. If the slow rate of growth is indeed due to hGH deficiency, the child's rate of growth should double or triple in the first year. If the rate of growth does not at least double, the slow growth rate most likely was not caused by hGH deficiency, and hGH replacement therapy should be stopped. This is an area of medical research that bears close watching.

The risks accompanying hGH therapy may be higher for a child with Down syndrome than for other children. Pediatric endocrinologists are concerned that hGH treatment, which may increase the risk of leukemia in certain children, may be particularly risky for children with Down syndrome, who already have a higher incidence of this disease. Until the questions surrounding the use of hGH treatment in children at risk for leukemia have been answered, caution is needed.

When considering therapy to treat short stature, you and your child's doctor need to ask whether your child's height is due to hypothyroidism, shortage of growth hormone (hypopituitarism), malabsorption, chronic illness, or simply because of Down syndrome. An appropriate therapy cannot be decided on until the cause is identified. If the cause is a shortage of growth hormone, you need to carefully evaluate the risks and benefits of each therapy. What are the side effects? How long should treatment be continued? What constitutes a successful outcome? Hopefully, research will soon be able to provide answers to the many perplexing questions that surround growth hormone therapy. Until then, caution is necessary.

Endocrine-Related Reproductive Problems

Male adolescents and adults with Down syndrome are usually not fertile. No one knows exactly what causes this. One endocrine-related problem that may contribute to their infertility is low *testosterone* levels. Testosterone is a hormone produced by the testes. It stimulates young males to mature with the characteristics of males, including facial and body hair, sweat, and genitalia. Testosterone also influences reproductive function and fertility.

Low testosterone levels can be treated with regular injections of a long-acting synthetic testosterone. This treatment is used because low testosterone levels impede sexual development—it is not used to cure infertility. However, this treatment also increases aggressive behavior, strength, and sex drive. When considering the use of testosterone replacement therapy, you should consider the risks and benefits. Ask how long treatment will need to be continued, and what the side effects will be over the course of many years. Testosterone is an anabolic steroid; long-term side effects from high doses can include heart and central nervous system problems in addition to aggression.

Young women with Down syndrome are usually fertile, although they often have reduced levels of fertility. Both young men and young women with Down syndrome should be taught about reproduction, sexuality, and safe sex. They should be provided with appropriate contraceptives. More information about these issues appears in Chapter 13.

Diabetes Mellitus

Children with Down syndrome are more likely than other children to develop diabetes. It is thought that an autoimmune problem causes this to occur, and children with Down syndrome are more susceptible to autoimmune problems. How the disease affects children with Down syndrome and how it progresses is the same as for other children.

Insulin is a hormone that is produced by the pancreas to help the body store the sugars digested from food. In *diabetes mellitus,* the effects of insulin are reduced. In the childhood type of the disease, (Type 1 or *insulin-dependent diabetes mellitus*), not enough insulin is made, and the amount of sugar in the blood becomes much too high. Consequently, the body tries to get rid of the extra sugar by increasing the amount of urine. A child with this condition will often begin drinking more and more fluid and have increased urine output. There will also be poor weight gain or even weight loss as most of the calories from food are wasted in the urine sugars.

Diabetes mellitus is easy to diagnose but often difficult to treat. The symptoms, which appear over a period of a few weeks, include:

- increased appetite without weight gain (and often with weight loss);
- increased thirst;
- increased urination (often with bed wetting); and
- general weakness and fatigue.

Sometimes diabetes is brought on by an infection; this can cause the disease to progress very rapidly. Treatment includes a special diet and insulin injections, which ease the symptoms but do not cure the disease. Insulin is usually injected two or three times a day, just beneath the skin. It directly affects the amount of sugar in the blood. People with diabetes who have blood sugars that remain close to normal have the least complications from the disease. The level of blood sugar is monitored by drawing blood from the tip of the finger several times each day, and testing it. This monitoring allows the medical team to adjust the doses of insulin to adapt to your child's diet and level of activity. The medical team should include an endocrinologist with experience in treating childhood diabetes and a specialized nurse educator and dietician. These specialists are often needed to get the diabetes under control, especially when it is first diagnosed.

Juvenile diabetes is a serious health concern, and should be monitored carefully and treated aggressively. Many health problems can appear and worsen rapidly if the condition is not well-controlled. These problems can affect the eyes, kidneys, heart, and other organs. Sometimes even careful control is not enough to prevent some of these problems. With effort and support, however, children with diabetes can lead full lives. There are national and local organizations to help you with information and support.

Summary

Children with Down syndrome are more likely than other children to have certain endocrine diseases, particularly those caused by autoimmunity. Newborn screening tests may reveal hypothyroidism, a missing or abnormal thyroid gland, or an unexplained mild elevation of thyroid stimulating hormone (TSH). A TSH measurement every one to three years will allow the early detection of hypothyroidism.

All children with Down syndrome need to be measured each year, and their height and weight plotted on an appropriate growth charts. When growth failure is found, further tests need to be made. Growth failure and the use of human growth hormone (hGH) are areas of ongoing research.

Endocrine problems can pose serious health risks. Fortunately, however, most endocrine system disorders in children with Down syndrome are mild and easy to treat. If you work closely with your doctor, endocrine problems can be diagnosed and treated effectively.*

Resources

The following are some medical organizations that may be able to help with specific questions you might have about thyroid problems, growth, and the use of growth hormone.

American Thyroid Foundation, Martin Surks, M.D., Secretary, Department of Medicine, Montefiore Medical Center, 111 East 210th Street, Bronx, New York, 10467; 212/920–4331.

Human Growth Foundation, 7777 Leesburg Pike, P.O. Box 3090, Falls Church, VA, 22043; 800/451–6434.

Lawson Wilkins Pediatric Endocrine Society, Barbara Lippe, M.D., Secretary, Department of Pediatrics, UCLA Center for Health Science, 10833 LeConte Avenue, Los Angeles, CA, 90024; 310/825–6244.

References

Allen, D.B. "Growth Hormone Therapy for Children with Down Syndrome" (editorial correspondence). *Journal of Pediatrics,* Vol. 120, 1992, 332–333.

Cronk, C.E. "Growth in Children with Down Syndrome: Birth to Age Three Years." *Pediatrics,* Vol. 61, (1978), 564.

---

* *The research on which some of this chapter is based was supported in part by grants from the Swiss National Science Foundation (number 32–9506–88), the Roche Research Foundation, the Renziehausen Trust, the Pediatric Endocrine Research Fund, and USPHS (grant number RR-84) for the General Clinical Research Center at Children's Hospital of Pittsburgh.*

Ershow, A.G. "Growth in Black and White Children with Down Syndrome." *American Journal of Mental Deficiency*, Vol. 90, 1986, 507–512.

Torrado, C., Bastian, W., et al. "Treatment of Children with Down Syndrome and Growth Retardation with Recombinant Human Growth Hormone." *Journal of Pediatrics*, Vol. 119, 1991, 478–83.

6 | Common Eye Conditions of Children with Down Syndrome

Robert A. Sargent, M.D.

Introduction

Clear vision is vital for good development and learning. We all depend on our eyes enormously because so much of our world is visual. For children with Down syndrome, this is equally true. Because of Down syndrome, however, they are more likely than other children to encounter some problem with their eyes that could threaten the clear vision they need.

All of the eye conditions that affect children with Down syndrome are seen in other children as well. However, they affect children with Down syndrome more frequently than other children. Fortunately, because eye conditions are so common among everyone, a lot of information and good treatment options are available. Understanding how the eye works and the effect and treatment of different eye conditions is a useful first step.

The Appearance of Eyes in Children with Down Syndrome

The eyes of children with Down syndrome tend to have a unique appearance. In the past, these eye characteristics were used to identify and even diagnose Down syndrome. Dr. Langdon Down used them to first identify the syndrome that bears his name, although he used the term "mongoloid" to describe the appearance. After more than a century of work to overcome the negative stereotypes of the label "mongoloid," caution is still important. Every child with Down syndrome is individual; some may not have all or even any of the eye characteristics discussed in this section. However, it is important to understand how these characteristics affect eye function.

Shape, Size, and Position

One of the obvious signs of Down syndrome is the shape, size, and position of the eyelids. The outer corners of the eyes are typically higher on the face than the inner corners, giving the eyes an upward slant. The highest elevation of the upper lid is midway between the inner and outer corners of the eye, so that the upper lid is symmetrical. Medical textbooks often call the eyes "almond shaped" because the maximum width is greatest in the middle of the eye, rather than toward the nose. None of these characteristics, however, has any effect on the function of the eye.

Epicanthal Folds

Many children with Down syndrome have noticeable skin folds at the inner corner of each eye, called *epicanthal folds.* The corner of the eye is called the *canthus,* and the skin covering the inside corner is the *epicanthus.* In children with Down syndrome epicanthal folds sometimes cover the white outer lining of the eye, called the *sclera.* This is commonly seen in newborn babies because the bridge of their nose has not yet grown forward. Children with Down syndrome have prominent epicanthal folds well into childhood when nasal bridges finally develop.

When epicanthal folds cover the white sclera, it creates the appearance of crossed eyes. It appears as if the colored iris of each eye is closer to the nose than it actually is. Sometimes there is a difference between each eye in the amount of whiteness showing on the inner part of the eyes, suggesting crossed eyes. This appearance is entirely cosmetic, and does not affect vision.

Brushfield Spots

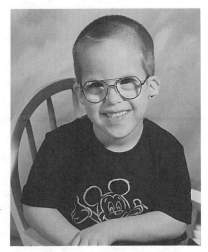

In 1924 a physician named Brushfield first described yellow or white spots on the colored portion of the eye (iris) which he thought could be used to confirm a diagnosis of Down syndrome. These spots, speckles, or dots occur in other children, particularly in those with blue eyes. Children with Down syndrome usually have blue irises. Brushfield spots are strands of connective tissue that are clustered together. They are less likely to be seen in brown-eyed children. Brushfield spots are common to children with Down syndrome, but may not always be present. Children with Down syndrome often have, in addition to Brushfield spots, a thin, wavy texture to the peripheral iris tissue. None of these characteristics have any effect on vision.

Vision Development and Amblyopia

Children are not born with fully functioning vision. Vision actually develops over time, and this occurs during the first 8 to 9 years of life. *Vision* is the combination of the eye (the camera) and interpretation by the brain (the computer). Although the eye's camera is almost mature at birth and delivers images to the brain, the brain must learn to interpret and understand them. This learning is the result of an intricate process of maturation of the cells in the brain where vision is perceived, called the *occipital cortex*. These cells are in the posterior (back) part of the brain, and they mature in the first 8 to 9 years of life.

Input from the eyes guides the development of the occipital cortex, and determines whether vision will develop normally. Each eye must send a clear, crisp image to the brain in order for that eye to be able "see" clearly later in life. If the brain cells are not stimulated by clear visual input from the eyes, they do not develop normally, and visual perception is stunted. This leads to lazy or weak vision, called *amblyopia*. In amblyopia, the brain ignores the images from one of the eyes. Although often called *lazy eye*, the problem actually lies in the understimulated brain cells.

There are three main components that allow each eye to stimulate the brain, and thereby foster normal vision. First, the eyes must be straight so that each eye is on the same target, or *object of visual regard*. If, in early childhood, one eye is deviated or crooked (as in *strabismus,* discussed below), it does not stimulate the brain cells properly. Thus, the eye can become weak or lazy in its vision (amblyopia). Crooked eyes are of concern to children with Down syndrome because they are more common than with other children.

Second, each eye must be in approximately equal focus in order to send crisp, sharp images to the brain. Rays of light enter the eye and focus on the back surface called the *retina*; here they are converted into nerve impulses, and then transmitted through the optic nerve to the occipital cortex in the brain. When one eye is excessively nearsighted, farsighted, or astigmatic (discussed below), the retinal image is blurry, similar to a fuzzy photographic film. This does not allow for a clear image to be sent to the brain, which leads to amblyopia. The technical medical term for being out of focus is *anisometropia* which means "not the same focus." Children with Down syndrome are more likely to have anisometropia than are other children.

Third, from birth through age 9, any defect in eye anatomy or any disease that prevents stimulation of the retina or interrupts transmission of nerve impulses to the brain can lead to amblyopia. For example, cataracts (discussed below) that do not allow clear visual images to reach the retina can cause amblyopia. This type of amblyopia may require removal of the cataract (or appropriate treatment for other conditions) in order to allow for normal visual input to the brain. Children with Down syndrome are more likely to have cataracts, most of which form over a period of years, rather than a congenital cataract from birth. Cataracts are discussed later in this chapter.

How do you correct amblyopia? First, you must correct the underlying cause of the amblyopia, such as strabismus, farsightedness, or cataracts. That is not enough, however. It is still necessary to undo the abnormal development the problems have caused, and to enable the brain cells to mature normally.

Treatment of amblyopia involves patching the better eye in order to "strengthen" the amblyopic eye. By cutting off the images from the "good eye," the brain is forced to use the images from the unpatched eye. This helps to complete development of the brain cells. The duration of patching depends upon both the severity of amblyopia, and the age of your child. Younger children in the first few years of life can loose vision easily, but regain the vision readily with patching. Patching usually lasts a few weeks. In contrast, a child of 6–9 years of age does not gain or loose vision readily. Thus, regaining good vision at this late stage requires patching for months. There are many variations in the duration or frequency of patching; for example, sometimes patching is only used for several hours a day, or for several days a week. Part-time patching is usually used to prevent recurrence of amblyopia after daily full-time therapy has already achieved equal vision.

Sometimes children refuse to wear patches, simply because of personality differences, stubbornness, or lack of understanding. Children with Down syndrome are more likely to resist patching, and require understanding, encouragement, and patience from you and your child's doctor. One other

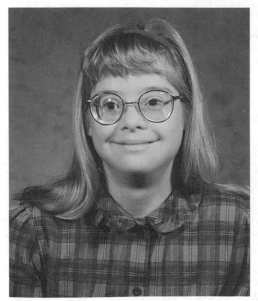

therapy is to put atropine eye drops in the better eye. These drops temporarily paralyze focusing so that your child cannot see clearly up close. Consequently, he may use the weaker eye in order to read or focus up close. A side effect of this atropine is pupil dilatation; this does not harm the eye even in bright sunlight, although your child may sense greater light.

After age nine patching the better eye does not correct amblyopia; improvement in visual acuity does not occur. The cells in the occipital cortex are no longer able to adapt to new input. Thus, it is important to diagnose amblyopia in children as early as possible in order to start patching therapy.

Early diagnosis means early eye and vision examinations. Guidelines set by the American Academies of Ophthalmology and Pediatrics recommend an eye check of most children by approximately three years of age. This age is chosen because children at this age will have verbal responses. However, some children with Down syndrome may not be reliable on verbal feedback, even at an older age. Thus, I recommend that children with Down syndrome be checked in the first year or two of life. This involves an examination with eye drops by an ophthalmologist who is comfortable in examining young infants.

Binocular Fusion and Depth Perception

People see in three dimensions. We are able to perceive how close or far away objects are from us. For example, we can perceive that a creek is too wide to jump across or that a car is far enough away to cross in front of safely. Usually, both eyes send messages to the brain and the brain integrates, or fuses, them into one three-dimensional picture. This is what is meant by *binocular fusion.*

Binocular fusion and depth perception require properly aligned eyes. It requires approximately straight eyes (but not necessarily exactly straight) in order for the brain to fuse the images from each eye into one picture. In strabismus, however, one eye is crooked, and consequently the brain cannot integrate the two images. Both eyes are not able to view the same object simultaneously. When this occurs, two things can happen: 1) the brain can see double, or 2) the brain can suppress the image from the deviated eye. Most all children, including children with Down syndrome, learn to suppress the deviated eye, resulting in loss of depth perception.

There are three types of strabismus, *esotropia* (when one or both eyes crosses inward), *exotropia* (when one or both eyes looks to the outside), and *hyper- or hypotropia* (when one eye looks up or down).

Besides the benefit of depth perception, straight eyes are also desirable for emotional and psychological reasons. Crooked eyes, especially in children with Down syndrome, convey a stereotypical image of mental retardation, and hinder other areas of development. For example, lack of depth perception would make learning games and sports much more difficult, and consequently would limit opportunities for these activities in the community. It is well worth the extra effort required in children with Down syndrome to enable them to function and be perceived as equals of other children. Absent crooked eyes, children with Down syndrome have the same ability for binocular fusion and depth perception as other children. Thus, I highly recommend aggressive treatment to obtain straight eye alignment.

Some children, who have good motor control, have strabismus only intermittently. However with fatigue, illness, anxiety, or stress, they cannot employ the necessary neuromuscular control that maintains straight eye alignment. Thus, you may see your child's eyes cross at bedtime, or when he is upset. How and when to treat children with this intermittent strabismus is controversial among specialists in this field. In general, if your child's eyes are usually straight, you can defer treatment; if your child is usually strabismic, something should be done to correct the eye alignment. If you don't, it could lead to lack of depth perception.

The usual treatments for strabismus are glasses or eye muscle surgery. Eye muscle surgery involves changing the muscles that control eye movement, either by lengthening or shortening them, or by altering how they attach to the eye or eye socket. The choice between glasses and surgery depends upon what your child's ophthalmologist finds during the eye exam. Eye exercises are not usually necessary or beneficial.

Refraction

The human eye works like a camera. Light enters through the cornea and is projected by the lens to the retina at the back of the eye. The retina acts like the film in a camera; it converts the visual picture to nerve impulses and sends them to the brain. Just as a camera must be properly focused for clear pictures, the eye must be able to focus images clearly on the retina.

Refraction is the term used to describe how the lens projects and bends light rays that enter the eye. Ideally, the lens bends light rays so that their clearest point of focus is on the retina. When this happens, vision is crisp and clear. However, not all eyes have the correct shape to permit proper focus.

When light rays are focused either in front of or behind the retina, vision is blurry. These are called *refractive errors.*

There are three types of refractive errors. First, some eyes are too elongated; they focus images in front of the retina. This causes *myopia,* which means nearsightedness. Nearsighted people see well up close but objects in the distance appear blurry. Glasses which are thick on the edge and thin in the middle (concave) are used to correct this problem.

Second, some eyes may be too short from front to back; they focus images behind the retina. This causes *hyperopia,* which means farsightedness. Usually farsighted people see well in the distance, but need extra straining for vision up close. Many people with hyperopia have difficulty reading, and need glasses for close work. Glasses which are thick in the middle and thin on the edge (convex) are used to correct this problem.

The third cause of refractive errors is misshapen or uneven corneas. Misshapen corneas cause individual light rays to have different focal points. That is, when rays of light strike a cornea at 12 and 6 o'clock they usually bend to a focal point at the same spot as those rays which pass through the cornea at 3 and 9 o'clock. The vertical and horizontal planes all focus at one point. In *astigmatism* the cornea has a shape like a football lying on the ground. The rays of light that strike at 12 and 6 o'clock have a shorter focal point than the rays that strike at 3 and 9 o'clock. Thus, there are no two planes that focus at exactly the same point. As a result, vision is blurred both close up and far away. Astigmatism can be minimal and not require glasses or it can be significant and require glasses for both reading and distance vision.

Young people have the ability to change the thickness of their own lens within the eye. This changes the point of focus in the eye, and enables them to compensate for refractive errors. This unique ability allows babies to focus on fingers thrust right up to their nose and eyes. As they age, their lenses become less flexible, and their ability to compensate decreases.

It is actually desirable for children to be somewhat far-

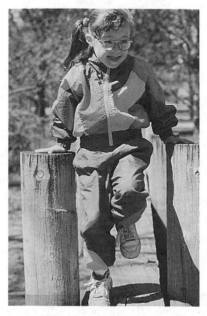

sighted because the eye grows for all people during the first few decades of life. Typically eyes reach their ultimate shape by late adolescence. As the eye grows, it elongates, and its focus mechanism becomes less farsighted and more nearsighted. By starting with a "farsighted reserve" as a young person, an adult is more likely to have clear focus. On the other hand a child whose vision is perfectly focused without any farsighted reserve will eventually become nearsighted. This is why nearsighted people start out without glasses but need progressively thicker lenses as they get older. The farsighted child usually does not need glasses for farsightedness, unless it is moderate to significant.

Refractive errors are measured by having an individual read an eye chart. "20/20" or "normal" vision means that a person standing 20 feet from a chart sees objects that anyone with normal vision would see at 20 feet. 20/40 vision means that the person needs to be 20 feet away to see things that people with normal vision could see from 40 feet. People who cannot cooperate with reading charts because of age, or developmental level, or due to behavior problems, can be difficult to assess. If your child can sit still and focus on an object a known distance away (such as 20 feet), an ophthalmologist may be able to look into the his eyes through a lens and esti-mate how well the eye works.

Children with Down syndrome have increased risk of vis-ual defects, with the usual spectrum of myopia, hyperopia, and astigmatism, but specific studies vary tremendously re-garding the actual percentages of each type of visual error. A conservative estimate would be that at least half of people with Down syndrome have some kind of visual error.

Fitting children with Down syndrome with glasses can be a frustrating experience, because those who need glasses may still constantly pull them off even when they are of some bene-fit for vision and functioning. There needs to be sufficient nearsightedness, farsightedness, or astigmatism to justify us-ing glasses; otherwise, you may spend a lot of money for spec-tacles that your child will not wear, or you may impose glasses on your child when the need is marginal.

The first question to answer to determine whether your child should wear glasses is whether he really needs glasses. Young preschool children typically have a visual world that is up close, and therefore are usually not bothered by mild near-sightedness. They are not yet in school reading from books and looking at the blackboard, with the rapid shifting of gaze from near to far vision. As children reach school age, the de-mand for optimal vision, and the need to quickly adapt to ob-jects at various distances, may change the need for correction. Because the decision to prescribe glasses is tricky, the more experienced the eye doctor is with children with Down syn-drome the more likely it is that a correct decision about glasses will be made.

Once your child is prescribed glasses, the next question is how to encourage him to wear them. Children with Down syn-drome tend pull glasses off unless they are of significant bene-fit. If your child feels his glasses make a big difference, he will grab for the glasses and not remove them at all. Some parents find it easier to uphold the strict rule of wearing glasses all the time, simply because it becomes a habit. Other parents are selective, requiring glasses only for school work or other visually demanding tasks. Again, this has to be evaluated with your child's eye doctor.

Nystagmus

Nystagmus is the medical term for eyes that seem to jiggle or vibrate (oscillate). It is caused by an abnormality in the nerves controlling the eye muscles, but is not usually associated with other nervous system diseases. Just as an unsteady camera creates a blurry photograph, nystagmus blurs vision.

Nystagmus is more common in children who have strabismus, and the oscillations are about the same in each eye. Thus, visual acuity is similar in each eye. The condition usually first appears sometime within the first year of life. Nystagmus occurs in approximately 10 to 15 percent of children with Down syndrome. A study by a pediatric ophthalmologist found that up to 30 percent of all children with Down syndrome had nystagmus, but this includes children with very fine "shimmering nystagmus" that is not ordinarily noticeable.

Nystagmus takes various forms. Some eye movements are jerky; others are pendular (the horizontal movement from left to right is equal), like the pendulum of a clock. A less common form of nystagmus called *spasmus nutans* is sometimes seen with head bobbing along with a head turn or tilt. In *latent nystagmus,* both eyes are steady until one eye is covered. Then the other eye jerks outward, making visual acuity and testing less accurate.

Nothing can be done to eliminate nystagmus; however, it tends to decrease somewhat by the elementary school or teen years. Nystagmus is not under your child's control, so admonitions to stop it are not helpful. When there is a face turn with nystagmus, an ophthalmologist can perform eye muscle surgery to straighten the head posture.

Nystagmus can also be a sign of an underlying vision problem. For example. if there are congenital cataracts (discussed below) or underdevelopment of the optic nerve, visual ability will be impaired from early in life; this in turn can lead to nystagmus. This is called *sensory nystagmus,* and is by far the least common form of nystagmus in children Down syndrome.

Red Eyes and Eyelids

Blepharitis, a bacterial infection of the eye, occurs when the margin of the eyelid becomes inflamed and the oil secreting glands next to the eyelashes become infected. It gives a pink appearance to the eyelid margins, creating a condition that looks like "raccoon eyes." This red ring around the lid margin may be accompanied by scaling and crusting at the base of the eyelashes. Your child may also feel burning or irritation. Children will often rub their eyes for relief. This can become a vicious cycle, because the more they rub their eyes the more irritated or infected the eyes become. Blepharitis is more common in children with Down syndrome, but the reason for this is unknown.

Blepharitis is a chronic, recurrent problem, but it can be partially prevented. It responds to treatment during acute episodes. Prevention includes keeping the eyelid region washed by using a non-irritating baby shampoo on a clean wash cloth. Cleanse the outside eyelids. Flare-ups of blepharitis with mucous or pus discharge should be treated with a steroid and an antibiotic medication. A physician's prescription is necessary to obtain this medication. The antibiotic kills the bacteria, usually staphylococcus, that causes the irritation. However, when the staph germ is killed, the cell wall and the contents of the bacteria (endotoxin) remain as irritants to the eye. This may cause the eye itself to become red *(conjunctivitis).* It can also irritate and inflame the clear window of the eye (cornea). Steroid or cortisone medication relieves this inflammation. Fortunately, bouts of blepharitis tend to decrease as a child gets older, and require less frequent cleansing of the eyelid margins to prevent recurrence.

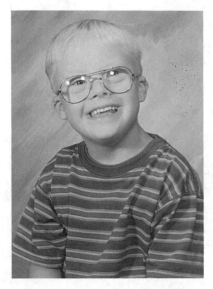

Watery Eyes and Blocked Tear Ducts

Watery eyes are commonly seen in children with Down syndrome. Although tearing can be due to inflammation of the eyelids or of the surface of the eyes, another cause of watery eyes in children with Down syndrome can be obstruction of the tear duct. Like other parts of the middle of the face *(midface),* these ducts may be smaller than usual.

The tear ducts are passageways that connect the eyes to the nose and allow tears to enter the nasal cavity. We know about this connection because, upon crying, the excess lacrimation (tearing) leads to nose sniffles.

During the development of the tear ducts there are thin membranes that usually disappear by the time of birth. Sometimes this does not occur. The resulting obstruction of tear flow leads to watery eyes, mucous accumulation, and crusting of the eyelashes. The mucous and crustiness occurs because tears contain protein in addition to water. The "sleep" that you clean from your child's eyes in the morning is nothing more then dried out tears. When the tear ducts are obstructed, much more mucous accumulates on the eyes. The prevalence of blocked tear ducts is much more common in children with Down syndrome than in other children.

Treatment of blocked tear ducts is somewhat controversial. Persistent and recurrent tearing eventually requires a procedure called probing and irrigation. In this procedure, a small wire-like probe is passed from the eye into the nose, thereby breaking the membrane obstructing tear flow. Historically children have been anesthetized during this procedure. Because probing and irrigation is an elective procedure (that is, not an emergency), doctors usually wait until a child is six months old, at which time a general anesthetic can be given with less risk. Another guideline is to wait until one year of age, because many obstructed tear ducts clear up spontaneously by age 12 months. Thus, there is a body of opinion that recommends waiting until one year of age.

This procedure can be performed in the office by an ophthalmologist. A papoose board is used to immobilize your child, and the ophthalmologist passes the probe from the inner corner of the eyelids into the nose without any anesthetic at all. In adults with chronic infection, this procedure is always performed in the office. Thus, children under the age of six months can be probed in the ophthalmologist's office, if there is bothersome crusting and "gunkiness." Whether or not a general anesthetic and hospitalization are needed depends upon the physician performing the procedure.

If probing and irrigation does not resolve the problem, then a procedure can be performed to enlarge the space under the bones in the nose where the tear ducts enter the nasal cavity. This requires a general anesthetic. Another treatment involves *silicone stent intubation* to widen the tear duct passage. Silicone stents are thin tubes approximately the size of ultra thin spaghetti. They are threaded through the upper and lower openings of the inner eyelids and then passed into the nose. The tubes remain there for 4 to 6 months in hopes of dilating the tear duct. This procedure requires a general anesthetic.

If these treatments fail, a child with blocked tear ducts may then require a dacryocystorhinostomy (DCR). This is an operation in which a skin incision is made along side the eyelid and bone of the nose, and a hole is drilled through the bone into the nasal cavity. This is a major operation requiring stitches, although it is performed on an outpatient basis. It leaves a small scar in the lid crease. Children with Down syndrome tend to have recurrent tear duct difficulty, and there-fore are more likely to need a DCR.

Congenital Eversion of the Upper Lids

Congenital eversion of the upper lids occurs when a baby is born with upper eyelids that are folded upward to expose the moist inner surface of the eyelid. This condition may oc-cur more frequently in children with Down syndrome. There are several possible causes. First, there is generalized "floppi-ness" or low muscle tone in children with Down syndrome. Second, there is a tendency for loose connective tissue, the fi-brous stuff that holds us together such as tendons and liga-ments. This affects the structures in and around the eye. The *tarsal plates,* which are the connective tissues that give firm-ness to the upper and lower eyelids, may be looser than nor-mal, allowing the eyelids to fold. Another theory is that a child's hand may swipe the eyelid while he is still in the uterus, flipping the lid upward. This can happen after birth as well. A third explanation is that the levator muscle of the up-per eyelid, which usually pulls the lid back to its normal posi-tion, does not function properly.

Some ophthalmologists report that congenital eversion of the upper lids can be corrected by eyelid surgery. This is usu-ally unnecessary, however, if the condition is treated early. The easiest treatment is to apply a tight patch to one or both lids for several days just after birth. If patching is not effective, your child's ophthalmologist may recommend temporary su-turing (stitching) of the upper lid to the lower one, or other surgical procedures that straighten out the lids

Keratoconus

Keratoconus is another condition associated with loose connective tissue and with children with Down syndrome, al-though the exact incidence is not known. *Kerato* is the root word from which we get "cornea," the clear window in the front of the eye. *Conus* refers to the conical shape of the cornea. In keratoconus the cornea bulges forward, like the tip of an ice cream cone. This causes the eye to become very nearsighted and often very astigmatic. Your child's ophthalmologist may suspect keratoconus when there is severe nearsightedness or astigmatism. In keratoconus an acute swelling of the cornea (called *acute hydrops*) can occur; it is far more frequent in children with Down syndrome than in other children. The swelling is accompanied by a decrease in vision, and sometimes requires a corneal graft operation, in which a human cornea is transplanted onto the eye to replace the damaged cornea. Fortunately keratoconus does not occur frequently.

One factor that predisposes children with Down syndrome to keratoconus is the looseness of their connective tissue. In addition, frequent eye rubbing may contribute to keratoconus. As explained above, eye rubbing may occur because of watery or crusty secretions that accumulate on the lid margin. However, other young children who frequently rub their eyes almost never develop keratoconus; and keratoconus that occurs after puberty is not always associated with eye-rubbing. Thus, it is unclear whether eye rubbing causes keratoconus.

Keratoconus rarely occurs in young children with or without Down syndrome, but it becomes more frequent in the teenage years. Treatment of keratoconus requires skilled ophthalmologic care. Often surgery is eventually needed, and people with Down syndrome respond to this surgery as well as other people.

Cataracts

Children with Down syndrome are more likely than other children to have cataracts. Cataracts cause the lens of the eye to become cloudy. Whereas the lens is usually transparent, cataracts make the lens opaque, much like dirt on a windshield. Although cataracts are more common in children with Down syndrome, the reason for this is not known. In general cataracts occur infrequently, but the incidence increases into later childhood and young adulthood. A cataract can either be minimal, as is often the case in children with Down syndrome; or it may be sufficiently opaque to cause blindness. Cataracts can appear in one eye (*unilateral*) or in both (*bilateral*), and may or may not worsen with time.

Typical cataracts in children with Down syndrome are "flake-like" or look like a set of tiny dots, like a "snowflake," near the edge of the lens. Sometimes they cannot be seen unless the pupil is dilated. As long as the opacity stays out of the central part of the lens, vision will not become diminished. If a cataract is present within the central visual axis, however, vision may be impaired significantly. Cataracts can appear on both the front and back sides of the lens; cataracts on the lens's inside surface are more difficult to detect with the naked eye.

Because the obstruction of vision in one eye can lead to amblyopia (see above), it is critical to detect cataracts as soon as possible, especially when children are below nine years of age. In young infants, the earliest sign of a unilateral cataract is usually strabismus in one eye (typically crossing inward). Nystagmus is the most common sign of bilateral cataracts in young infants. For both unilateral and bilateral cataracts, the most noticeable and common sign is a cloudy white pupil. In older children, the first symptom of cataracts may be difficulty in seeing. However, do not jump to the conclusion that cataracts are present just because your child with Down syndrome has difficulty seeing; he might simply be inattentive or need glasses for a refractive error. In either case an eye examination is needed.

The decision to remove a cataract depends primarily on the degree of vision loss. In children this usually means an inability to read school material or to see objects across the living room or across the street. In addition, stumbling, falling, and bumping into furniture may also occur. In children with Down syndrome, it is difficult to precisely quantify the loss of visual acuity from cataracts (such as 20/40 or 20/100) because their answers to vision tests can be unreliable. In general, cataracts are usually removed when acuity drops below 20/60 to 20/80. In children under age nine, because of amblyopia, an ophthalmologist who is experienced with patching for amblyopia after surgery should be used for this operation.

Cataract surgery in children requires a general anesthetic. The procedure, known as lensectomy, removes the clouded lens through an incision in the side of the eye. Usually, the clouded lens is removed, and a contact lens is used on the front of the eye to put the eye into clear focus. Sometimes, the lens is replaced with an artificial lens (*intraocular lens,* IOL).

Eye Injuries

Statistics show that children with serious developmental delay are more likely to injure their eyes, either by vigorous rubbing or by self-inflicted trauma. A small percentage of children with Down syndrome have more extensive developmental delay, and can present challenges for both parents and eye care professionals.

Minor injury may result in bruised eyelids or a scratched cornea or other part of the eye. Surface abrasions are treated with a tight patch and heal in one or two days. A more severe blow to the eye can cause *hyphema* (bleeding) within the eye or disrupt the thin fibers (*zonules*) that hold the lens in place. The effect of this is a dislocated lens, which in turn puts the eye out of focus. In young children this may lead to amblyopia. Treatment requires either glasses or replacement of the lens itself. The surgery for this is the same as a cataract extraction.

There are even more serious eye injuries. Injury to the back of the eye can lead to a detached retina and bleeding in the back of the eye. These usually are caused by severe head injury. This injury is far more serious because it involves the retina. Loss of the retina leads to permanent blindness. Chronic injury to the cornea will eventually cause scarring and cloudiness. Damaged corneas can be surgically replaced with transplanted corneas. If the damage was self-inflicted, most corneal transplant specialists are reluctant to perform a graft on children who have struck their own eyes because they may injure themselves again. Some of these children wear football-like helmets to prevent future self-inflicted trauma. As in any case of self-injury, behavior specialists should be consulted to look for the reasons behind the behavior. Most of the time the problem is related to communication, and can be improved with appropriate understanding of the person's needs.

Miscellaneous Conditions

There are several eye conditions that medical reports have linked to Down syndrome. However, it is still not clear whether there is an increased incidence of these conditions in children with Down syndrome. Their diagnosis and treatment is the same as for other children. Each of these diseases is un-common in the general population.

Retinoblastoma is a congenital cancer of the retina, first appearing at birth or in the first year or two of life. With this condition, the eye may have a white pupil or appear crooked. However, these same signs may be symptoms of other condi-tions. Your ophthalmologist can easily make this distinction. Retinoblastoma is rare, and has a strong tendency to run in families. Left untreated it is dangerous. Treatment is radiation or removal of the affected eye.

Congenital glaucoma is disease which causes increased pressure within the eyeball. The eye is filled with fluid that is produced and drained inside the eye. Overproduction or poor drainage causes a buildup of pressure. Glaucoma causes pain. Your child will be irritable and cry readily. He will also have watery tearing and be very sensitive to sunlight. Eventually the eye becomes enlarged from the increased *intraocular* (inside the eye) pressure, and has a cloudy cornea. Each of these signs and symptoms can be seen with other diseases. But with glaucoma, there are all seen together. Treatment depends upon the cause of the pressure increase, and may consist of medicines or surgery or both.

Optic nerve hypoplasia is the underdevelopment of the nerve which connects the eye to the brain, originating in the first few months of pregnancy from unknown causes. It occurs sporadically, but seems more common in people with genetic differences. Infants with optic nerve hypoplasia act blind. A neurologist may suspect the diagnosis, but, in order to obtain a diagnosis, a pediatric ophthalmologist will dilate the pupils and view the back of the eye. The degree to which the nerve is small and poorly functioning does not worsen over time, but this condition has no remedy. It is important to diagnose optic nerve hypoplasia in order to distinguish it from central nervous system (CNS) abnormalities. With optic nerve hypoplasia, the images made by the eyes are not transmitted to the brain.

Summary

A variety of eye conditions can affect your child's vision and, consequently, his ability to learn and get along successfully in day-to-day life. Children with Down syndrome are particularly affected by both serious and by merely cosmetic conditions.

As a parent it is important to be watchful for vision problems. There are effective treatments for most eye conditions your child is likely to have. The sooner they are begun, the less likely he is to have lasting negative effects. Finding an eye doctor experienced in working with children with Down syndrome should therefore be a top priority. Your child's pediatrician usually knows who in your community is best able to deal with the diagnosis and treatment of eye conditions seen in children with Down syndrome.

References

Caputo, A.R., et al. "Down Syndrome: A Clinical Review of Ocular Features." *Clinical Pediatrics,* Vol. 28, 1989, 355–358.

Catalano, R.A. "Down Syndrome." *Survey of Ophthalmology.* Vol. 34, 1990, 385–398.

Fraunfelder, Frederick T. and Roy, F. Hampton. "Down's Syndrome." *Current Ocular Therapy,* (Philadelphia: W.B. Saunders, 1990), 216–218.

Gold, F.H. and Weingeist, T.A. "Down Syndrome," in *The Eye in Systemic Disease* (New York: Lippincott, 1990), 35–37.

Jones, Kenneth L. "Chromosomal Abnormality Syndromes: Down Syndrome," in *Smith's Recognizable Patterns of Human Malformation,* 4th edition (Philadelphia: W.B. Saunders, 1988), 10–15.

Nelson, L.B. et al. "Trisomy 21 (Down Syndrome)," in *Pediatric Ophthalmology* (Philadelphia: W.B. Saunders, 1991). 31–33.

Shapiro, M.B. and France, T.D. "The Ocular Features of Down's Syndrome." *The American Journal of Ophthalmology,* Vol. 99, 1985, 659–663.

7 | Skin Conditions
Elaine M. Siegfried, M.D.

Introduction

There are a great number of skin and nail problems that can affect any child. Children with Down syndrome, however, are more likely than other children to have certain skin, nail, hair, and scalp problems. This chapter explains these conditions and their treatment.

There are no disorders of the skin or nails that occur only in people with Down syndrome. However, several conditions of skin and hair are seen much more commonly in people with Down syndrome than in other people. These conditions can be classified into two groups: 1) conditions that may prompt concern but require only observation or preventative care, and 2) conditions that can and should be treated. In each category, some conditions are very common while others are unusual. Table 1 displays the different skin conditions that can affect children with Down syndrome.

Conditions Not Requiring Treatment

There are several skin conditions children with Down syndrome may have that do not require treatment or do not respond to treatment. This is because they pose no serious health risks, are not contagious or unsightly, and cannot be "cured."

Morphological Conditions

There are a few skin-related conditions that are present in so many newborn children with Down syndrome that doctors

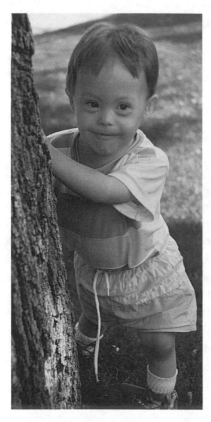

look for these features in trying to diagnose Down syndrome. Many of these are called *morphological* because they involve a difference in shape or structure. The morphological skin conditions seen in children with Down syndrome are loose skin at the back of the neck and fissures of the tongue. These conditions generally do not cause discomfort or infection and do not require treatment.

Loose skin at the back of the neck is found in 80 percent of children with Down syndrome. In most children who have loose skin, it is possible to gather it in your hand. Loose skin alone does not call for treatment, but extra fluid beneath this skin may be a sign of a condition called *cystic hygroma*, and this may require treatment. Cystic hygroma can be associated with heart defects. Evaluation for heart defects should be done for all infants with Down syndrome, and special attention should be given to children with cystic hygroma. Chapter 3 discusses heart conditions in detail.

Another common morphological difference in children with Down syndrome are differences in the tongue. Often the tongues of children with Down syndrome have a pebbled or grooved appearance to the surface, and have intersecting fissures. This occurs in 3 to 5 percent of the general population, but in almost everyone with Down syndrome. The condition has several names, including *fissured*, *scrotal*, and *furrowed* tongue. These surface changes alone do not cause discomfort and do not affect taste. However, they may collect food particles and become irritated. This is called a secondary inflammation. Routine brushing of the tongue with a soft toothbrush and warm mouthwash prevents excess food build-up and secondary inflammation.

Vascular Patterning

Children with Down syndrome can have other non-harmful skin conditions that change the color and general appearance of their skin. These conditions, called *cutis marmorata* and *acrocyanosis,* occur when the nerves and small blood vessels of the skin over-respond to cold temperature. With cutis marmorata the skin takes on a mottled bluish-red discoloration, especially on the trunk and the arms and legs. It is very common in all newborns, but with most children usually disappears early in infancy. Acrocyanosis is a bluish discoloration of the hands and feet that can occur in any newborn. In children with Down syndrome, especially those with heart disease, acrocyanosis may persist further into infancy. Both conditions persist for several years in children with Down syndrome. The discoloration usually disappears when your child is warm and reappears when she is chilled. This skin condition requires no treatment. Again, because acrocyanosis can indicate that your child has a heart problem, you should consult your doctor if you see it. Chapter 3 discusses heart problems.

Accelerated Aging

Some of the physical characteristics of Down syndrome (as well as those of a few other types of genetic conditions) are believed to result from accelerated aging. One of these, early aging, may appear in the form of age spots, wrinkles, and gray hair in adults with Down syndrome, beginning around age 20 to 30. In addition, dry and coarse skin (discussed below) may also be signs of aging.

Sun exposure contributes to skin aging. Protection against excessive sun exposure is even more important to infants and children with Down syndrome. This protection should include:

- using a waterproof sunscreen with a SPF (sun protective factor) of 15 or more;
- avoiding outdoor activity between 10 a.m. and 3 p.m.; and
- wearing wide-brimmed hats, tightly woven and long-sleeved clothing, and sunglasses to block or shade ultraviolet (UV) light.

More research about the effects of sun on the skin of children with Down syndrome is needed, but it is best to be safe for now.

Conditions That Are Treatable

Children and adults who have Down syndrome may also develop skin conditions that are contagious, cause discomfort, or are unsightly. Most of these conditions benefit from treatment. Doctors have only a limited understanding of exactly what causes these diseases or why they occur more often in people with Down syndrome. Many of these conditions are believed to result from abnormal responses of the immune system. This can cause an increased susceptibility to skin infection as well as a variety of noninfectious disorders called *autoimmune* diseases. Immune system conditions are discussed in detail in Chapter 4.

Disorders that are not related to immune system problems respond better to medical care than do autoimmune conditions (see Table 1). Although most conditions can be effectively controlled with the appropriate treatment, few can be permanently cured. It is important to promptly recognize and treat these conditions because it is much easier to treat

Table 1: Skin conditions seen in people with Down syndrome.					
	Conditions requiring only observation and/or preventative treatment		Conditions responsive to therapy		
Common (seen in more than half)	Morphologic	Accelerated Aging	Miscellaneous	Infections	Autoimmune Disorders
	Loose skin at the back of the neck	Premature wrinkling	Xerosis	Fungus	
		Gray hair	Thickened skin	Yeast	
			Atopic dermatitis	Bacterial	
	Fissured tongue		Cheilitis	folliculitis	
		Age spots		Impetigo	
Less Common (seen in less than half)	**Vascular Patterning**		Icthyosis vulgaris	Seborrheic dermatitis	Alopecia areata
	Cutis marmorata		Syringomas		
				Norweigan	
	Acrocyanosis		Elastosis perforans serpiginosa	scabies	Vitiligo

early, mild skin disease than more advanced, severe disease. Early treatment may also prevent other complications. This section explains the different types of skin conditions that can be treated in children with Down syndrome.

Miscellaneous Skin Conditions

Infants with Down syndrome have skin that is often called "thin, soft, and velvety." During childhood, this texture changes and the skin may become dry, coarse, thickened, and scaly. The common treatable skin conditions that children with Down syndrome may have may be related to a subtle, progressive skin abnormality that has not been well studied. These specific skin changes can also occur in people who don't have Down syndrome, but occur much less often. This section reviews the skin conditions of children with Down syndrome that do not result from either infection or autoimmune disease.

Dry Skin and Atopic Eczema. Dry skin (*xerosis*) occurs in almost everyone with Down syndrome. Left untreated, dry skin can cause itching and scaling as well as impair the important "barrier function" of the skin. This leaves the skin more susceptible to injury and infection, and slows healing. In se-

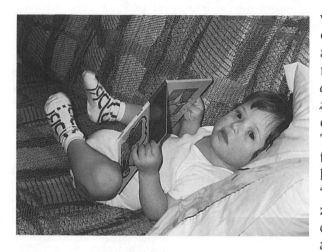

vere cases of dry skin a severe rash called *asteotic eczema* may develop. This condition is also known as "winter eczema" because drier air during the winter months contributes to the eczema.

Another form of eczema that is common in children with Down syndrome is called *atopic eczema,* or *atopic dermatitis* (inflammation of the skin). In the general population, this condition occurs in families with asthma and hay fever, and affects up to 10 percent of all children. It is more common in people with Down syndrome, but no one knows why it is more common.

Atopic dermatitis usually appears during early childhood. The condition is characterized by very dry skin and a red, scaly, often weepy rash that is usually very itchy. In infants the rash is more prominent on the cheeks, trunk, and over the arms and legs. However, it usually does not affect the area under the diaper. In older children, the rash typically occurs on the wrists, inner elbows, and behind the knees. In some case, it can also affect the scalp.

No permanent cure for atopic dermatitis is known, but the condition usually can be well controlled. The best way to control dry skin as well as atopic eczema is by adding layers of oil to the skin to prevent evaporation of skin moisture. Bathing need not be severely restricted. In fact, daily or even twice daily bathing may help moisturize the skin, especially during dry seasons (such as winter) and in locations where the air is very dry. Bathing should be limited to short periods in warm rather than hot water. Soap should be used as little as possible, only at skin folds or on dirty areas. This is because soaps and hot water strip the skin of its protective oily layer. Mild soap or soap-free cleansers are best. One soap free cleanser available is Cetaphil, from Galderma Laboratories.

Immediately after bathing, your child should be gently patted dry, not rubbed vigorously. Within 3 minutes a thick emollient should be applied, before the skin has a chance to dry out. The best emollients are thick and greasy, and are usually more effective than ointments, such as Vaseline. Ointments are more effective than creams, such as Eucerin. Creams are more effective than lotions. Some children do not like the feel of heavy greasy ointments, which also take longer to apply. Select the thickest type of emollient that your child will tolerate. Try a wide variety of ointments, emollients, creams, and lotions to see what works best.

Bath oils add little to the treatment and will make the bathtub slippery, a potential cause of accidents. In the past, bath oil was thought to help moisturize and protect the skin. Later, it was thought that it merely sealed the skin and prevented bath water from touching the skin. The facts now appear to be that bath oil is too thin to seal the skin, but is also useless in helping to moisturize skin.

Sometimes children with Down syndrome develop very dry and cracked fingertips. One solution is to apply an ointment or heavy cream to the hands and fingers at bedtime and then wrap the hands in an air tight wrapping or put rubber gloves on them. This bathes the fingertips in moisture all night and generally helps relieve the cracking.

More severe cases of xerosis or atopic dermatitis should be treated by a dermatologist, a physician with special knowledge of skin disorders and their treatment. Itching can be controlled with over-the-counter antihistamines or topical anti-itch preparations (a *topical* medication is one that is applied to the skin)(see the section below on Norwegian scabies). Antihistamines will also promote more restful sleep, which is very important for children with atopic dermatitis because it prevents them from scratching. Treatment of moderate to severe eczema requires topical corticosteroids, an anti-inflammatory cream, which turns off the inflammation process in cells. The strength and type of preparation is best determined by a physician. Corticosteroids can cause the skin to thin and become fragile if they are used for more than 1 to 2 months. In addition, an antibiotic may be necessary to control secondary infections that can occur when skin breaks open allowing bacteria in.

Thickened Skin. Children with Down syndrome may have thickened (*hyperkeratotic*) skin on their palms, soles, knees, and elbows. These patches of skin can feel scaly (like the skin on most elbows). Occasionally the skin may become so thickened and stiff that it cracks. These cracks, or fissures, can be very painful and may become infected. Hyperkeratosis may be prevented by daily application of a topical medication that helps dissolve the scales. Creams which have 10 percent urea or 5 percent ammonium lactate as active ingredients are available over-the-counter. If these are not effective, stronger preparations are available by prescription. If painful cracks develop, petroleum jelly or an antibiotic ointment (prescription or over-the-counter) should be applied frequently.

Cheilitis. *Cheilitis*—redness, scaling, and crusting around the lips—is common in children with Down syndrome. It can occur with atopic dermatitis, or as a result of lip licking, allergies, or infections (including impetigo, thrush, or cold sores). More rarely, it is caused by nutritional deficiencies, including deficiencies of riboflavin, pyridoxine, zinc, and biotin.

The most frequent cause of cheilitis is excessively dry, irritated skin. The easiest therapy is moisturization and protection of the lips with white petrolatum or zinc oxide ointment. If the condition does not improve or worsens, evaluation by a your child's pediatrician is necessary to rule out other causes. He or she can refer you to a dermatologist if necessary.

Ichthyosis Vulgaris. *Ichthyosis vulgaris* is a skin condition characterized by rough, white, "fish-like" scales, most prominent on the arms and legs. It is not an uncommon problem in the general population, but is more common in people with Down syndrome, occurring in as many as 90 percent of them. Ichthyosis vulgaris runs in families; about one person in every 300 has this condition. It can be thought of as a more severe form of dry skin and is treated in a similar way. If daily bathing followed by liberal use of emollients is not effective, compounds containing urea or ammonium lactate may be used. These include Lacti-Care and Lact-Five (which are available over-the-counter) and Lac-hydrin (Westwood) (available by prescription). These are soothing topical preparations. In addition, over-the-counter antihistamines can help control itching and promote restful sleep.

Syringoma and Elastosis Perforans Serpiginosum. Two other relatively rare conditions, *syringoma* and *elastosis perforans serpiginosum* (EPS), also occur more often in people with Down syndrome. Once again, however, doctors do not know why.

A syringoma is a noncancerous tumor of the sweat glands. Sweat glands are located all over the body (especially on the face and in the armpits) and secrete sweat for cooling and lubrication. Syringomas appear suddenly as multiple small, flesh colored or yellowish, soft bumps, often on the lower eyelids and cheeks, but can also appear on the neck, armpits, and abdomen. Syringomas almost never appear before puberty. They occur in females twice as often as males. Up to 60 percent of females with Down syndrome will develop these tumors. Syringomas do not grow; they do not become cancerous. But they do not go away, either.

No ideal way has been found to permanently remove syringomas. They can be surgically removed using different techniques, but each method carries with it the risk of pain, infection, and scarring. Moreover, there is a high risk that the tumor will reappear. Surgical removal can be performed under local anesthesia only with a very cooperative patient. Treatment should be undertaken only in the very rare cases where the condition causes psychological distress.

EPS is a rare skin condition that appears as small red bumps with firm central plugs. Often the bumps appear in a snake-like pattern on the face, arms, or back of the neck. EPS typically erupts in childhood or early adolescence. It does not hurt or itch, but if the central plug is scratched off, it will bleed. EPS results from a build-up of fibers in the connective tissue of the skin. These fibers are then pushed through the skin surface, resulting in the thickened plug.

EPS does not run in families. In the general population, 75 percent of people with EPS do not have other conditions. For the other 25 percent, EPS is a marker for a variety of medical problems, including certain rare disorders. The relationship between EPS and these disorders is not well understood. It is seen more often in children with Down syndrome (about 1 percent of people with Down syndrome) than in other children. In addition, the problem can be more widespread and persistent than in other children.

EPS can resemble other skin problems, and often, a skin biopsy is necessary to confirm the diagnosis. Unlike syringomas, the lesions of EPS will flatten over time and eventually leave a depressed scar, but in people with Down syndrome this may take up to 10 years. Treatment is recommended only for children who repeatedly pick at the bumps, leaving them open to bleeding or infection. Treatment may also be recommended for children who find the condition psychologically traumatic.

There are several treatments for EPS. The simplest treatments involve repeated application and removal of scotch tape ("tape stripping") to pull off the skin plugs, or frequent application of creams containing urea or ammonium lactate, which help dissolve the scaly plugs. If this is ineffective, a dermatologist can use liquid nitrogen (cryosurgery) to freeze and remove the bumps.

Infections

A few types of skin infections are more common in people with Down syndrome than in the general population. These include fungus infections, bacterial infections (*impetigo* and *folliculitis*), seborrheic dermatitis, and Norwegian scabies. These disorders probably occur more frequently in people with Down syndrome because their immunity is lower and their skin is not as effective in acting as a barrier to disease (see the section on dry skin).

Fungal and Yeast Infections. Many types of fungus and yeast can affect the skin. Fungi and yeast are similar kinds of organisms and cause similar kinds of problems. Yeast thrive in moist areas while fungi prefer drier areas. Fungal and yeast infections of the skin can cause the following symptoms:

- dandruff;
- diaper rash;
- hair loss;
- painful cracks at the corners of the mouth;
- scaling skin on the palms and soles;
- scaly patches on the body;
- tender white patches in the mouth; and
- thickened discolored nails.

The infections that cause these symptoms are common in the general population, but even more common in both adults and children with Down syndrome, affecting up to three of every four persons. Specific fungal infections appear more often in certain age groups. Infants are more susceptible to yeast *(Candida)* infections of the mouth (thrush) and diaper area, especially when they are receiving antibiotics. Young children most often develop fungal infections of the scalp (*tinea capitis*), face (*tinea faciale*), and body (*tinea corporis*). Adolescents and adults have problems with fungal infections of the feet (athlete's foot or *tinea pedis*) and nails (*onychomycosis*) that can spread to one hand (*two-foot-one-hand tinea*).

These infections can resemble other skin problems. For example, a diaper rash may be caused by simple irritation, allergic reaction, *or* Candida yeast. Dandruff or hair loss may be caused by *seborrheic dermatitis* (discussed below) *or* fungus. Similar appearing rashes on the face or body can be due to eczema *or* fungus. For effective treatment, it is important to identify the exact cause of the skin condition. For any new rash, it is best to consult a dermatologist to make a diagnosis. Often, it will be necessary to take a skin scraping, hair sample, or nail sample to examine under a microscope for evidence of yeast or fungus. For better identification and more precise diagnosis, samples may be taken to grow in the laboratory, a process that can take up to a month.

For fungal infections of the skin, a number of effective topical medications are available, some without prescription (such as the over-the-counter cream, Tinactin). Infections with yeast, however, will respond only to some of these prescription topical preparations (miconazole, clotrimazole, econazole, and ketoconazole). Even after treatment, fungal infections, especially athlete's foot, may recur. Regular daily application of a topical antifungal cream can help control spreading, increased scaling, cracking, and itching.

Widespread or stubborn fungal infections of the skin, and infections of the hair, scalp, and nails require more prolonged treatment with an oral antifungal medication. The drug most often used is griseofulvin. This medication disrupts the growth process of fungus cells, and allows tissue to grow normally. This medication must always be taken with fatty foods such as whole milk, ice cream, or cheese, in order to improve its absorption in the stomach. Griseofulvin must be continued for at least 6 to 8 weeks for scalp infections and 6 to 12 months for nail infections. If the condition persists, the dose may need to be increased. Newer oral antifungal drugs (fluconazole, terconazole, and itraconazole) may be more effective in the treatment of fungal infections, especially nail infections, but they have not yet been used extensively in children. Griseofulvin is not effective against Candida yeast. For widespread Candida infections, oral ketoconazole is used.

Bacterial Skin Infections. Bacteria are a common cause of skin infections in all children. Children with Down syndrome are particularly susceptible to these infections, probably because they tend to have dry skin and eczema. Two types of bacteria, *staphylococcus aureus* and *streptococcus*, are chiefly responsible for these infections, which take on a variety of appearances.

The most common infection caused by staphylococcus aureus or streptococcus bacteria is *impetigo*. Impetigo appears as tiny grouped pustules (pus-filled bumps) that spread to become weepy, honey-colored areas of crusting, or as much larger blisters or pustules that break easily. Impetigo often begins around the nose and on skin that is broken due to injury, bug bites, or eczema. It can spread rapidly to adjacent skin, or to the skin of another person.

Impetigo is a serious health condition. It is very important to treat it promptly, because it can spread rapidly and it is contagious. Occasionally the infection moves deeper under the skin, resulting in *cellulitis*, with redness, warmth, swelling, and tenderness; or it can cause a pus-filled boil called a *furuncle*. Rarely, certain strains of bacteria can also cause systemic diseases, such as *staphylococcal scalded skin syndrome, scarlet fever,* or a kidney disorder called *acute glomerulonephritis*.

Impetigo that is confined to a very small area may be easily treated by cleansing with soap and a topical antibiotic ointment (Polysporin or Bacitracin™), available over-the-counter. Widespread impetigo or impetigo that does not respond to over-the-counter medications require prescription medications. A very effective topical prescription ointment, mupirocin, may work as well as oral medication. Oral antibiotics are more easily administered and are more cost-effective for chil-

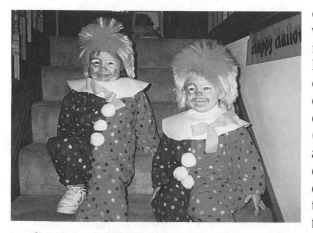

dren with widespread impetigo. Erythromycin, cephalexin, and dicloxacillin (which has a taste children often dislike) are the preferred oral medications. Erythromycin is the least expensive and is available in chewable tablets. However, it may cause stomach upset and diarrhea. In some areas, strains of bacteria exist that are resistant to erythromycin and another antibiotic such as dicloxacillin or Augmentin must be used.

Another form of bacterial skin infection is called *folliculitis* because it affects hair follicles. It is sometimes called "infected hair." Folliculitis usually occurs in adolescents and adults when the bacteria that always covers the skin gets inside as a result of a local inflammation or crack. Folliculitis is characterized by patches of small pustules and red bumps. These are evenly distributed over the affected areas, often the thighs, buttocks, back, and arm pits. On close inspection, a hair can be seen in the center of most of the pustules. It is sometimes itchy. Folliculitis is a less serious but more bothersome problem than impetigo. Left untreated a secondary infection may occur. It is not as contagious and does not spread as easily; only those in close contact such as family members may contract this disorder.

Folliculitis can be difficult to eradicate. Treatment should include routine cleansing with antibacterial products like Visohex (chlorhexidine gluconate and hexachlorophene) or other over-the-counter antibacterial soaps. In children prone to dry skin and eczema, this may be too painful. For these children, or for those with widespread itchy folliculitis that does not improve, treatment with oral antibiotics for a minimum of 4 to 6 weeks may be effective. Often the condition will reappear after the medication is discontinued. If folliculitis becomes worse while on oral medication, testing should be done to identify the specific type of bacteria causing the problem in order to choose the most effective antibiotic.

Seborrheic Dermatitis. Seborrheic dermatitis is a chronic skin condition that causes reddened skin with greasy yellow scales. It usually affects areas around the nose, eyebrows, ears, and scalp of adolescents and adults. Another form, common in infants, affects the scalp with waxy scales (called cradle cap) and the diaper area with a sharply defined orange rash. For reasons that are not clear, seborrheic dermatitis is more common in both adults and children with Down syndrome, affecting up to 33 percent.

The cause of seborrheic dermatitis is unknown, but it has been associated with the overgrowth of a yeast called *pityrosporum ovale*. In severe cases, seborrheic dermatitis can affect the entire body. It can also cause a change in skin pigmentation that is similar to vitiligo (see below).

In most people, seborrheic dermatitis can be easily controlled. However, when treatment ends the condition often reappears. Initial therapy should include antiseborrheic shampoos (such as Selsin Blue, Head & Shoulders, and Denorex) containing zinc pyrithione, selenium sulfide, or sulfur and salicylic acid, all available over-the-counter. For best results, the shampoo should be used 3 to 7 times a week, and left on for 5 to 10 minutes before rinsing. If redness or scales remain, a mild topical corticosteroid (available over-the-counter) may be used. Hydrocortisone (0.5%-1.0%) lotion is also available over-the-counter, but there are risks associated with its long-term use such as thinning of the skin.

If nonprescription treatment is ineffective over a long period of time (more than one month), a physician should be consulted about treatment. Topical ketoconazole, an antiyeast medication, has lately been shown to be effective against seborrheic dermatitis. Ketoconazole is available as a shampoo and a cream, by prescription. It is more expensive than hydrocortisone and can cause irritation in some people, but its use does not carry the same risk of complications as does the long-term use of topical steroids.

Norwegian Scabies. Scabies is a skin condition caused by a tiny insect called a mite (*Sarcoptes scabei*). Everyone can have these mites. People with a scabies infection usually harbor 5 to 10 mites on the body; a person with *Norwegian or crusted scabies* is infected with ten to one hundred thousand times more. Prompt diagnosis and treatment is very important, because scabies is contagious and can cause secondary infections. Because the condition often goes unrecognized for a long time, a single patient may infect hundreds of other people.

In the past, Norwegian scabies were thought to be linked with people with Down syndrome. We now know that this higher incidence in people with Down syndrome was related to excessively dry skin, communal living (in institutions), poor hygiene, and longer periods of infestation (because children with Down syndrome received poor medical care). Today, Norwegian scabies is more often seen in people with severe immune deficiency disorders due to leukemia, AIDS, or high dose steroid therapy. In general, Norwegian scabies occur in people who have an immune system deficiency. Because children and adults with Down syndrome are more likely to have these problems, Norwegian scabies are more common among people with Down syndrome.

The skin of individuals who have Norwegian scabies will have widespread thickened scaling with fissures, especially on the scalp, the arms and legs, and over the joints. It may be mistaken for eczema or psoriasis. Nails may be thickened, and a secondary infection may be present, but there is typically little or no itching. Paradoxically, other family members who catch the mites may have more typical but less apparent skin lesions and much more itching.

Many treatments exist for scabies. Cost, side effects, and efficacy should be considered in picking the appropriate therapy. Although topical lindane is often used for the treatment of scabies, the recommended treatment for children with Down syndrome is topical permethrin. Elimite, a 5 percent permethrin cream, is a newer medication made of a chemical related to a compound gotten from the chrysanthemum flower. Although it is more costly than lindane, it is recommended for the treatment of Norwegian scabies in people with Down syndrome. It is more effective than lindane, and has fewer side effects than lindane (which can include excema and alopecia). To date, no scabies have developed resistance to permethrin. Treatment with permethrin kills the mites, so that a single treatment is generally effective. It is a cream, applied to the entire body and left on overnight.

In any case of scabies, all people who have had contact with the patient must be treated. All sheets and bedclothes should be laundered after each treatment. Nonwashable items that have been in close, frequent contact with the child, such as a favorite blanket or stuffed animal, can be put in a dryer and dried on high heat for 45 minutes.

Following any treatment for scabies, a skin rash and itching may persist for 4 to 6 weeks. This is because the skin may react to mite parts remaining in the skin. Antihistamines such as diphenhydramine (Benydryl) or a topical anti-itch cream may help control these symptoms. The most effective creams contain the topical anesthetic pramoxine, or other ingredients such as camphor or menthol that can mask the itch by creating a distracting tingling or warm sensation. Over-the-counter choices include Prax, Anti-Itch, and Aveeno baths, while prescription choices include Pramosone and Zonalon. Another topical anesthetic, benzocaine, frequently causes rashes and should be avoided. Topical corticosteroids such as hydrocortisone may be used for a short period of time to help relieve itching, but remember that prolonged or excessive use of corticosteroids may encourage scabies infection or cause thinning of the skin. If the itching or rash persists for more than two months, a dermatologist should examine your child to look for persistent or recurrent infection.

Autoimmune Diseases

Autoimmune diseases are believed to result from an immunologic reaction of the body against its own normal tissues. It is thought that the body mistakenly identifies normal skin cells as foreign and attacks them. Autoimmune diseases are discussed in detail in Chapter 4. Many different autoimmune diseases have been identified. They tend to run in families. Specific autoimmune diseases involving the hair and nails (*alopecia areata*) and skin pigment (*vitiligo*) are seen in people with Down syndrome. The exact cause of these diseases, their relationship with each other, and with Down syndrome, is not well understood. Furthermore, alopecia areata and vitiligo may rapidly worsen or spontaneously disappear, so the effectiveness of any treatment is difficult to judge. No specific or universally effective treatments for these conditions have been found.

Alopecia Areata. Alopecia areata (AA) is a specific type of hair loss characterized by the sudden appearance of well-defined bald spots on a normal-appearing scalp. The more unusual symptoms of AA include generalized hair thinning, total loss of all hair on the face and scalp (*alopecia totalis*), or total loss of all scalp and body hair (*Alopecia universalis*). Often, hair from areas surrounding the bald spots can be pulled out easily. Short, stubby broken hairs (called "exclamation point hairs") are often present. Pitting in the nails may also appear in some children. AA is diagnosed by physical examination and confirmed by a scalp biopsy if there is any doubt. The cause of AA is not well understood, but it is believed to be an immune reaction affecting hair follicles.

Up to 10 percent of people with Down syndrome may develop AA at any point throughout their lives. It is more common in people with Down syndrome than other people. Most children with AA have only a few small bald patches. In these cases, the hair will usually regrow without any treatment, usually within one year. However, with more extensive or long-standing hair loss, regrowth is less likely. The decision to treat children with Down syndrome and AA should be based on the duration and extent of the hair loss, and how much the problem bothers the child. Treatment must be continued for 4 to 6 weeks before you judge it a success or a failure.

Many different treatments have been proposed for AA. The ideal treatment would be effective, easy to apply, painless, free of side effects, and inexpensive. In selecting the appropriate therapy, you should start with a treatment that fulfills as many of these criteria as possible. Choose a different treatment only after an unsuccessful 4–to–6 week trial, or the development significant side effects. Treatment should always be done under the supervision of a dermatologist or a physician with experience in the treatment of children with AA.

In children with Down syndrome, appropriate initial therapies include potent topical steroids, or *anthralin*, a topical irritant, which causes the body to shed the affected skin. Topical steroids are easy to apply and nonirritating. Anthralin, a tar-like compound, must be applied according to a specific schedule that gradually increases both the amount of time the compound is left on and its strength. Anthralin will stain the scalp brown, which may help hide the bald spots in dark-haired people. However, it also stains sheets, clothing, and normal skin, and it can be very irritating.

Steroids may also be injected locally, at 1 to 2 month intervals. This treatment is too painful for most children, and it is not practical for widespread AA. Some physicians recommend use of oral systemic steroids for people with AA. This treatment can be temporarily effective but must be weighed against the very significant and serious side effects (such as appetite suppression, puffiness, and changes in bone metabolism), especially when therapy is continued for more than a few weeks.

As more is learned about the specific cause of AA, better treatments will be designed. For long-standing, widespread AA, many people prefer to wear a wig. Several companies specialize in custom-fitted, long-wearing, comfortable wigs for people with AA. Further information may be obtained from a dermatologist or from the Alopecia Areata Foundation, listed at the end of this chapter. The Alopecia Areata Foundation provides support as well as the newest information for patients with AA and their families. It also funds important research.

Vitiligo. Vitiligo is a disease characterized by sharply outlined patches of completely white skin. These patches are usually symmetrically arranged on the body. In *generalized* vitiligo, they will be found around the eyes, nose, mouth, hands, elbows, and feet. In the less common *segmental* form, the patches can appear anywhere on the body. Vitiligo also has a tendency to occur at sites of injury such as old scars, burns, and scrapes. Often the affected areas will initially increase in size over a period of one to two years, and then remain stable. Spontaneous repigmentation can occur but is not common.

Vitiligo occurs in about one percent of the general population, and at least half of all cases occur in childhood. The condition is somewhat more common in people with Down syndrome, corresponding to the increased incidence of AA and thyroid disease. Vitiligo results from an immune reaction against the skin cells that produce pigment. As a result, the affected skin will not tan, and will sunburn very easily. It is important for people who have vitiligo to protect affected areas against sun exposure by using a waterproof sunscreen of the highest SPF available. The safest and easiest therapeutic approach for fair-skinned people is to avoid exposure to the sun. This not only protects against sun burn and skin cancer, it also camouflages the difference between affected and unaffected skin. For darker skinned people, cosmetics can be used to mask prominent white spots. Cosmetic companies such as Covermark and Dermablend produce waterproof cosmetics that come in a wide variety of shades. Trained dermatologic nurses or company representatives can provide instruction in the proper application of these cosmetics.

For children, few treatment alternatives are available. All treatments should be carried out under the supervision of a dermatologist or physician that is experienced in treating childhood vitiligo. Topical steroids may help prevent enlargement of the patches when used very early in the course of the disease. Prolonged or excessive use of topical steroids, especially on thin facial skin, may cause more thinning and the appearance of "broken blood vessels" or stretch marks. As with AA, an ideal treatment is not available. The decision to treat should be based on the duration and the extent of the disease, as well as its effect on your child's self esteem and social development.

A widely used and often successful treatment for adults involves topical or oral use of a medication called psoralen, followed by exposure to ultraviolet light. This treatment is complex, costly, and time consuming. It is not recommended for children because of the risk of serious side effects, including severe sunburn, cataracts, and skin cancer. Research continues into the treatment of vitiligo. The Vitiligo Foundation is an excellent source of support and up to date information for patients with vitiligo and their families. It is listed in the resources section of this chapter.

Summary

Children with Down syndrome may develop a variety of skin conditions. Some morphological conditions, such as loose skin at the back of the neck, fissured tongue, and changes in skin color due to cutis marmorata and acrocyanosis, can be seen in infants. They are looked for in diagnosing Down syndrome. Others, such as fungal infections, bacterial infections, seborrheic dermatitis, cheilitis, and xerosis, are common problems that can be easily identified and treated with over-the-counter topical skin care products. Less common conditions, including alopecia areata, vitiligo, Norwegian scabies, syringoma, ichthyosis vulgaris, and severe atopic dermatitis, are sometimes the cause of significant physical or psychological discomfort. These typically require the care of a qualified dermatologist or physician.

Each of the skin conditions listed above occur more often in children with Down syndrome. None occur just in people with Down syndrome. Doctors do not know why they occur more often in children with Down syndrome. As knowledge increases about Down syndrome, the immune system, and skin disorders, there will be a better understanding of the cause and treatments of these skin disorders.

Resources

Eczema Association for Science and Education
1221 Southwest Wamhill Street
Suite 303
Portland, OR 97205
503/228–4430

National Psoriasis Foundation
6600 Southwest 92nd Avenue
Suite 3000
Portland, OR 97223
503/244–7404

The Alopecia Areata Foundation
Suite 202, 714 C Street
San Rafael, CA 94901
415/456–4644

The National Vitiligo Foundation
P.O. Box 6337

Tyler, TX, 75711
903/534–2925

References

Du Vivier, A. and Munro, D.D. "Alopecia Areata, Auto-immunity and Down's Syndrome." *British Medical Journal*, Vol. 1, 1975, 191–192.

A number of good articles can be found in *Pediatric Clinics of North America*, Vol. 38, No. 4, 1991, including:

> Hanifin, J.M. "Atopic Dermatitis in Infants and Children." 763–788.

> Levy, M. "Disorders of the Hair and Scalp in Children." 905–919.

> Hogan, D.J., et. al. "Diagnosis and Treatment of Childhood Scabies and Pediculosis." 941–957.

> Pinto, F.J and Bolognia, J.L. "Disorders of Hypopigmentation in Children." 991–1016 .

> Shwayder, T. and Oh, F. "All about Ichthyosis." 835–857.

Hebert, A.A. and Esterly, N.B. "Mucous Membrane Disorders." in Schachner, L.A and Hansen, R.C., eds. *Pediatric Dermatology*. (New York: Churchill Livingstone, 1988) 462–463.

8 | Ear, Nose, and Sinus Conditions of Children with Down Syndrome

Kevin T. Kavanagh, M.D.

Introduction

Children with Down syndrome may have a variety of ear, nose, and throat problems. Many of these problems are easily detected and may worry parents, but they typically correct themselves as children grow older. These conditions include sinus drainage, drooling, mild blockage of the nasal airways, and tongue protrusion.

Other conditions may be less apparent and commonly go unnoticed by the family. Unfortunately, these problems are often more serious. They may include hearing loss and more serious blockage of the nasal airways. When any of these conditions are detected, they should be promptly treated.

Though the above list may seem long, not all children with Down syndrome will have these conditions. If your child has one of these conditions, talk with your primary health care provider such as a nurse practitioner, pediatrician, or family practitioner. They can refer you to an ENT physician if necessary. For typical ear, nose, and throat conditions, treatment for children with Down syndrome is the same as for other children. However, some circumstances that call for special considerations do exist, and these are discussed below.

Your Child's Ears and Hearing

Your child needs to hear in order to learn to speak. First he learns to listen, then to talk, read, and write. These skills are usually learned in this order. If your child has a hearing loss, he will have difficulty learning to speak, and later, will find school more difficult. Unfortunately, more than half of all children with Down syndrome have a hearing loss. When hearing problems are detected early, however, steps can be taken to minimize their impact on learning.

Children with Down syndrome should have their hearing tested soon after birth, preferably in the first six to twelve months of life. This can be done by your primary health care provider, through public health clinics, or through your school district if there are school personnel qualified to do hearing screens. Detailed audiological evaluations need to be done by an audiologist who is specially trained to test hearing in children.

A test that is commonly done is called a *brainstem auditory evoked response* and can be performed in the newborn nursery as a screening test. Brain stem audiometry is a sophisticated test of hearing done by measuring the electrical activity of the brain when it is stimulated by sound. In this test, electrodes are glued to the skin (as is done with EEGs—a test that measures brain electrical activity). Then the brain's response to sound is measured. If hearing is impaired, the electrical activity will be absent or abnormal. If a hearing loss is detected, treatment can start when your child is as young as three to six months of age.

Looking into the ears of a small child is not easy. Infants have very small ear canals. They squirm and move around a lot, and, when they strain, everything—including the ear drums—turns red. To further complicate matters, children with Down syndrome usually have small ear canals and lots of wax. For these reasons, it can be very difficult to see the eardrums. Restraining your child and using special techniques may be necessary. One of these techniques involves the use of a restraining board called a *papoose board* to prevent him from moving. In rare situations, a mild sedative may be prescribed. In both cases, the goal is to limit sudden movements that make the exam difficult and that might result in pain or injury to your child. It is a good idea to talk with your doctor before the examination so he or she is aware of your concerns.

Sometimes, if your child becomes upset and struggles during an exam, small red spots may later appear on his face. These are called *petechiae,* and they are caused by the breaking of tiny blood vessels just under the surface of the skin. Petechiae do not hurt, and go away by themselves in a few days.

If no hearing problem is detected during your child's first screening, do not assume he will never have a hearing problem. Because hearing problems in children with Down syndrome frequently develop over time, you should have your child, adolescent, and young adult tested periodically. The schedule for testing is found on the preventive care checklist in Chapter 2. You should also keep your eyes open to notice possible hearing problems. Lack of response to sound, poor language and communication development, and problems with articulation are all signs of potential hearing problems. Even without symptoms, your child's hearing should be checked regularly; recent studies have found that a significant percentage of children with Down syndrome who show no symptoms of hearing loss had abnormal hearing. Therefore, regardless of what your child's last hearing test showed, have his hearing tested again.

How Hearing Impairments are Classified

Hearing loss may be classified in a number of different ways, including degree of impairment, severity of the hearing loss, age when the hearing loss began, and the cause of the hearing loss. Functionally, hearing is the ability to perceive and understand speech; hearing loss reduces (or eliminates) that ability.

Degree or severity of hearing loss is the most common and most functional method of describing hearing impairment. Hearing loss is usually described both as specific fre-

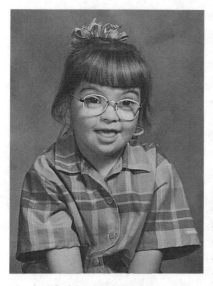

quencies of sound lost and as the degree of loss in decibels. That is, hearing and hearing loss are measured both by how well your child can hear over the full range of frequencies (high and low pitch) and decibels (loudness). The normal range of frequencies humans can hear is 250 to 8000 Hertz. The range of sound intensity humans can hear is approximately 5 decibels (softer than a whisper) to 130 decibels (jet engine). Children who have a moderate hearing loss usually cannot hear less than 40 to 70 decibels across a critical range of frequency needed for normal hearing. These sounds include quiet office noise and normal conversation. Children with moderate hearing loss usually require hearing aids or other forms of amplification. They often require some special support in school. Children with a severe hearing loss (also called "partial hearing") cannot hear lower than 70 to 90 decibels, roughly the sound of heavy traffic. These children often require special education and prolonged auditory training to learn special communication and language skills. These children often benefit from hearing aids and amplification systems. Children who are deaf usually have profound hearing loss in both ears; typically they cannot hear sound of an intensity of less than 90 decibels (the sound of heavy machinery) or cannot hear sound at all. These children are totally dependent on visual sources for language and communication. Hearing aids and amplification are usually not very helpful.

Other classifications of hearing loss depends on the degree of difficulty in learning speech and language. In this classification system, levels of impaired hearing are based on the level of hearing in the better ear. The classifications are arranged as follows:

- Children with Level I hearing have a 26 to 54 decibel loss;
- Children with Level II hearing have a 55 to 69 decibel loss;
- Children with Level III hearing have a 70 to 89 decibel loss; and
- Children with Level IV hearing have a loss of 90 decibels and above.

Another classification of hearing loss is made by age of onset, or when the hearing loss began. The three categories usually used are:

- *Prelingual hearing loss*—Hearing loss that occurs before the development of speech and language;
- *Prevocational hearing loss*—Hearing loss that occurs between ages 2 to 3 and 18 to 19; and
- *Late Onset*—Hearing loss that occurs after age 19.

A final classification is based on *etiology,* or the cause of the hearing loss. The different causes of hearing loss are discussed in the following section.

Causes of Hearing Loss

If your child is found to have a hearing loss, treatment will depend on the cause of his hearing loss, The doctor will therefore examine the various parts of your child's ear for any abnormalities in structure or function. These parts include:

- The ear canal, which transmits sound to the middle ear;
- The middle ear, which contains the eardrum and three small bones (malleus, incus, and stapes) which also transmit sound; and
- The inner ear, made up of the cochlea and semicircular canals, which changes sound energy

into nerve impulses and sends them to the brain via the auditory nerves. Figure 1 is an illustration of the structure of the inner ear.

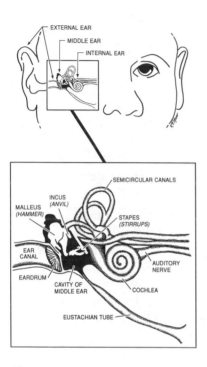

Figure 1

There are two types of hearing loss, although both types can be present at the same time. Most hearing loss in children with Down syndrome results from what is called a *conductive* hearing loss. It is called conductive because a problem with the ear itself prevents it from properly converting sound into nerve signals. Conductive hearing loss can result from many causes, but most commonly, it is due to fluid build-up behind the eardrums, called *serous otitis media*. Fluid behind the eardrum dampens or muffles sound—it's like trying to hear a conversation while you are swimming underwater. It is not clear exactly why fluid builds up behind the eardrum. It may result from inflammation, infection, or anatomical differences that lead to poor ventilation of the middle ear. Often, all three of these factors play a role in producing fluid. It is also not clearly known how many children with Down syndrome suffer hearing loss from fluid buildup. Some studies indicate that 60 to 90 percent of people with Down syndrome have a hearing loss from chronic middle ear fluid.

Conductive hearing losses can come and go, depending on the cause of the fluid. If the fluid in the middle ear remains, the loss can be chronic. Chronic or acute ear infections can damage the *tympanic membrane* (eardrum) the small thin piece of skin that acts like the head of a drum, transmitting sound into the middle ear. The membrane can become thickened or a hole, called a perforation, can develop. Thickening or perforation can lead to damage of the small bones of the middle ear. They may become fused together, and lose the flexibility needed to transmit sound vibrations to the inner ear. This can significantly reduce hearing.

Hearing loss can also have other causes. Earwax (*cerumen*) can build up and become impacted on the eardrum. This can also dampen the eardrum and hinder hearing. Because children with Down syndrome have very small ear canals, the ear may become blocked by ear wax. If this happens, have your doctor remove the wax. You should never stick anything into the ear canal yourself because you might accidentally damage the eardrum or ear bones.

Conductive hearing loss may also be due to problems with the middle ear bones. In some cases, the innermost ear bone, the stapes or "stirrup," may be malformed or cannot work properly because it is held down by tissue.

Less often, children with Down syndrome may have sensorineural hearing loss, which occurs in the inner ear, where sound energy is translated into nerve impulses that are then sent to the brain. In this type of hearing loss, the eardrum and inner ear bones work properly, but there are problems with the *cochlea* (the spiral inner organ that converts sound into nerve impulses) or the auditory nerve. In addition, some children may have "central deafness," a condition in which all the hearing organs function properly, but the brain, due to injury, cannot receive or process auditory information. It is not known what causes the problems that lead to sensorineural hearing loss. Sensorineural loss is usually permanent. It is estimated that approximately ten percent of children with Down syndrome have this type of hearing loss.

Table 1

64% of patients with Down syndrome have a hearing loss greater than 15 decibels

87% have a conductive hearing loss (middle ear)

60% have middle ear fluid or eardrum perforations

52% have abnormal or fixed middle ear bones

35% have sensorineural hearing loss (inner ear)

Hearing loss can be both conductive and sensorineural. Because conductive loss can mask a sensorineural loss, it is important to treat the conductive loss first. Once the conductive loss is eliminated, the sensorineural loss can be measured.

Table 1 shows how frequent the different types of hearing loss are in children with Down syndrome.

Treatment of Hearing Loss

Your child's doctor may try a variety of treatments to improve your child's hearing. Fluid in the middle ear—the most common cause of hearing loss in children with Down syndrome—can often be treated with antibiotics. These drugs kill the bacteria that may be causing the infection producing middle ear fluid. If antibiotics do not solve the problem, ear *(myringotomy)* tubes can be inserted in the eardrum to allow the fluid to drain away. These tubes allow the fluid to drain into the outer ear, and also ventilate the middle ear so that the tissue in the middle ear can absorb the remaining fluid (if there are no recurring infections). Draining the fluid may improve hearing, and may also reduce recurrent ear infections, because bacteria no longer have a medium in which to grow.

The use of ear tubes is somewhat controversial. Some studies question their effectiveness in the large number of children who have them. Parents report differing results. It can be confusing making a decision. As a general rule, tubes are used as a last resort for children who have failed other kinds of medical treatment. In addition, for some children with Down syndrome who have cleft palate or other disorders that cause recurrent ear infections, tubes are a prudent choice because other medical treatment may be ineffective. For other children with Down syndrome, you should work closely with your child's ENT physician to assess the usefulness of ear tubes.

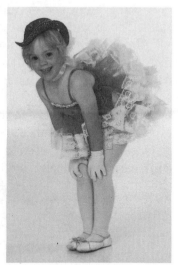

When a child has tubes placed in his ears, surgery is required. A general (rather than local) anesthetic is used to sedate your child for a short while. A small incision is made in the eardrum, and tiny drainage tubes are inserted. Usually, this surgery is done as day, or "outpatient," surgery. Sometimes the small size of the ear canal can make placement of an ear tube difficult. Once a tube is in place, your child needs to see the doctor regularly for monitoring. Ear tubes stay in for varying lengths of time, usually for several months to years, depending in part upon the type of tube inserted. Your child's body will slowly work the tube out of the eardrum, and then the eardrum usually heals by itself. Sometimes tubes need to be reinserted if they fall out or become blocked. In general, tubes that are designed to stay in the ear for a long time are more likely to leave a hole in the eardrum when they work their way out. This hole may need to be surgically repaired if it does not heal.

Water (particularly water from wading pools, creeks, and ponds) should be kept from entering the tube because it can bring bacteria into the middle ear, increasing the chance of infection. Your child should wear ear plugs when shampooing or bathing. Some doctors allow their patients to swim in chlorinated pools with ear plugs; some do not.

Abnormalities in the middle ear bones are sometimes corrected with surgery to remove the tissue that holds the stapes down or to remove the malformed bone. However, this type of surgery is often unsuccessful, and should only be attempted by an experienced otologic surgeon. Otologic surgeons with experience with ear tubes are usually ENT physicians.

Hearing aids are used to treat sensorineural hearing loss and hearing loss due to abnormal inner ear bones. Hearing aids amplify the sounds needed for normal hearing, although they cannot restore perfect quality hearing. They are usually prescribed by an ENT and fitted by an audiologist. Good fit is important; if the hearing aid is uncomfortable to wear or works poorly, your child will not want to wear it. Some children with Down syndrome are very sensitive to touch around their head, and may need extra help getting comfortable with hearing aids. Your child's occupational therapist can help you with this. It is also very important to regularly monitor your child's hearing aids to make sure they are working properly.

Neck Instability

Children with Down syndrome should be screened for *atlanto-axial instability* before they participate in gymnastics or contact sports or before they undergo surgery. In surgery, the neck is often extended backwards in order to insert a breathing tube. This maneuver may cause significant damage to the spinal cord. Atlanto-axial instability is discussed in detail in Chapter 10.

Breathing Concerns

Children with Down syndrome often have difficulty breathing because airways in the nose and mouth are smaller than normal. Breathing can become even more difficult when

health conditions narrow the airways further. Some problems
that frequently lead to narrowed airways are colds, influenza,
allergies, and enlarged tonsils and adenoids. As a result of narrowed airways, children with Down syndrome may have a
number of breathing problems, most of which occur during
sleep.

- Mouth breathing may be a habit or a sign of airway
  obstruction. Chronic mouth breathing may lead to
  poor dental occlusion (how the teeth fit together
  when the mouth is closed), drooling, and abnormal
  swallowing.
- Snoring is one of the initial signs of airway
  obstruction; if severe, episodes of sleep apnea may
  result.
- Obstructive sleep apnea, or abnormal delays in
  breathing while asleep. Dangerous episodes last
  for 10 seconds or longer. If these episodes occur,
  the oxygen levels in the blood can fall, leading to
  periods of chronic *hypoxia,* or lack of oxygen in
  the blood.

Sleep apnea in children with Down syndrome can have
several different causes, including small airways, enlarged tonsils and adenoids, and hypotonia of the muscles of the mouth
and throat. Periods of falling oxygen levels in the blood can
lead to pulmonary hypertension (discussed in detail in Chapter 3), the fatal thickening of the arteries in the lungs. Sleep
apnea may also make children with Down syndrome more
likely to snore excessively and to have attention, behavioral,
and growth problems.

The initial evaluation of sleep apnea problems should be
by your child's primary care doctor in consultation with an
ENT specialist. There are major medical centers that can
evaluate sleep disorders in the United States, and a few of
them have the ability to evaluate children. Children with severe sleep disorders may need to be referred to a center for a
sleep study.

In a sleep study, your child's brain waves, oxygen levels, muscle movement, and a variety of physiologic signs are monitored while your child is asleep overnight. Sleep centers have specially equipped rooms resembling bedrooms and can allow you to stay in the room with your child. Monitoring is done by electrodes, similar to those used for EKGs or EEGs which are taped or glued to the head and body (they are easily removed after the test).

If your child's sleep study shows normal breathing and normal sleep patterns, no treatment may be needed. If your child's sleep study is abnormal, and he is breathing at his best, treatment may be needed. However, a sleep study is not always reliable, because it only measures the sleep pattern for one night and your child's airway may change frequently. As a parent, you can provide vital information about your child's breathing during sleep, and this will be a key part of any evaluation.

Tonsillectomy

If your child is having breathing problems, you may be asked to consider surgery to remove the tonsils and adenoids— a "T & A," or *tonsillectomy and adenoidectomy.*

Many children with Down syndrome have enlarged tonsils and adenoids. The tonsils are mounds of lymphoid tissue located in the back of the mouth on both the right and left sides. The adenoids are located directly behind the nose. You can see the tonsils but not the adenoids. Tonsils can become enlarged from recurrent infections. Symptoms of large tonsils include snoring, noisy breathing, drooling, and sleep apnea. It is also possible to see the enlarged tonsils. Tonsils can become inflamed (*tonsillitis*); this can be caused by viral and bacterial infections and chronic irritation.

Removing the tonsils and adenoids (T & A) in a child with Down syndrome carries certain risks. First, there is the concern that swelling due to surgery may temporarily make breathing difficult because the airways of children with Down syndrome are already quite small. This swelling can last for seven to ten days. For this reason, children with Down syndrome should be admitted to the hospital as "inpatients" for T & A surgery. They should seldom have T & A surgery in an "outpatient" clinic, where they will be sent home the day of the surgery. They need to be monitored so that the medical staff can immediately insert a breathing tube if serious breathing problems arise. The risks of surgery and anesthesia are discussed in more detail in Chapter 16.

It is hard to predict whether, or how much, a child's breathing will improve following a T & A. Research suggests that T & A surgery is not as likely to produce improved breathing in children with Down syndrome as it would in other children. Snoring and apnea will improve in approximately 80 percent of patients with Down syndrome. However, in some children breathing may not improve because of very small breathing passages. Mouth breathing may take a long time to go away. If your child has been breathing through his mouth for many years, opening the nasal airway will not necessarily lead him to breath through his nose. Remember, a long-time habit has to be broken and a new way of breathing has to be learned.

In deciding whether or not your child should have a T & A, you should also consider the possible effect on speech development. Children with Down syndrome may find speaking more difficult following a T & A. Why is this? When a person talks, the muscle at the back of the throat, called the soft palate, moves sealing off the air passage that links the throat and the nostrils. The muscle does this by pressing against the adenoid pad, usually creating a airtight seal. When the adenoid is removed, your child must move this muscle farther in order to close the passage to the nose, For children with Down syndrome, who often have weakness (hypotonia) in their throat muscles as well as slow motor development, this can be difficult. If the passage is not completely closed, it causes air to leak. This medical term for this condition is *velopharyngeal incompetence.* The speech disorder that results—called *hyper-nasality*—sounds like your child is "talking through his nose."

Usually hypernasality can be slowly corrected through speech therapy. To avoid this complication, a surgeon will try to remove only the front part of the adenoid. The other most common risk of T & A surgery is excessive bleeding. About one of every thirty to fifty patients who have T & A surgery have bleeding that is severe enough to require a return to the operating room for treatment.

Because of the uncertainties with T & A surgery and its outcomes, it should only be performed to correct airway obstruction associated with apnea or recurrent, severe infections. In mild airway obstruction, there is a good chance that your child will eventually outgrow breathing problems as his airway becomes larger in relation to his adenoids and tonsils.

Other Treatments

If severe breathing difficulties and apnea persist after surgery, further treatment may be necessary. Tongue reduction surgery on the back of the tongue may be suggested to further open the airway. The results of this procedure are unpredictable and temporary swelling after the operation may cause further airway obstruction. Tongue protrusion and tongue reduction surgery are discussed below.

Sometimes surgery fails to correct a severe, ongoing breathing problem. In these instances, a tracheostomy may be the final resort. This is an operation where a small breathing tube is inserted through a hole in the neck at the base of the throat. This is usually a temporary measure, although sometimes tracheostomies are long-term or permanent. People with permanent tracheostomies need to work with a speech pathologist specially trained to help re-establish speech. Fortunately, tongue reduction surgery and tracheostomies are rarely necessary.

Sinusitis

Sinuses are the small cavities in the cranial bone located behind the nose. They serve as air passages that open off the main nasal airway. They act like a sounding board, and effect the quality of speech greatly. When sinuses become filled with fluid, as they do when there is an infection, the quality of speech changes.

Because of the relatively small size of the nasal cavities in children with Down syndrome, *sinusitis* (sinus infection or inflammation) is common. So, too, is drainage from the nose (runny nose), because nasal drainage is often due to infection or inflammation of the sinuses. Eight out of ten children with Down syndrome have persistent nasal drainage. Although most children have runny noses occasionally, children with Down syndrome can have this problem much more frequently and for longer. For most children with Down syndrome, the problem decreases as they reach adulthood.

If nasal drainage is thick and yellow-green in color, this suggests a possible bacterial infection. Initial treatment may be with antibiotics. If the drainage starts up again soon after you stop giving your child antibiotics, your primary care health provider may prescribe a low dose antibiotic to be given over a long period of time (months to years) to prevent a return of the infection. The side effects are usually minimal; however, in some children, the antibiotic can alter the bacteria that live in the GI system, and result in diarrhea, allergic reactions, and failure to kill the targeted bacteria.

Sometimes it is suggested that modifying your child's diet can reduce sinus infections, but there has been no scientific evidence that this works. Some allergists prescribe nutritional modifications for children who have shown an allergy to some specific food and who have persistent sinus infections.

If your child's drainage is clear, your child may have allergies. In this case your doctor may prescribe antihistamines or decongestants. In a formal survey, six of ten patients with Down syndrome obtained relief from drainage and other

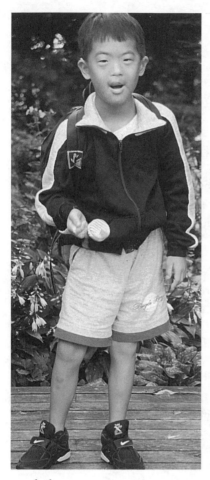

allergy symptoms when they used antihistamines or decongestants. However, those medicines make some children sleepy. In other children, they may cause increased activity. These symptoms usually go away in about two weeks. There are no studies showing that children with Down syndrome are more prone to allergies than other children.

If your doctor suspects that your child has a serious sinus infection or inflammation he or she will usually ask for x-rays of the sinuses. In some cases the doctor may order a CT scan of the sinuses. A CT or *computerized tomography* is a special x-ray test that will give a clearer view of the sinuses and can be helpful in making a decision about whether or not surgery is needed.

As a last resort, surgery to promote sinus drainage is an option. This should only be performed if the drainage is excessive or your child has recurrent sinusitis with fever. The most common sinus surgery is the placement of a drainage hole or "window" in the sinus located in the upper jaw (*maxilla*). This surgery is done under general anesthesia. More extensive sinus surgery is only done as a last resort in children under age 8 to 10. In these children, the sinus cavities are small, the operation is technically more difficult, and results are often unpredictable.

Tongue Protrusion

Tongue protrusion—not keeping the tongue inside the mouth—is common in children with Down syndrome. There are no studies measuring exactly how common this is in children with Down syndrome or exactly why it occurs. Suspected reasons include differences in the structure of the mid-face and possibly a smaller oral cavity.

Your child's tongue may protrude all the time, it may protrude only when your child swallows, or only when your child is concentrating. This last situation—tongue protrusion while concentrating—is seen in many young children, with and without Down syndrome, especially while they are drawing. In fact, it sometimes seems as if all youngsters cannot draw without sticking out their tongues! As children get older, this "aid to concentration" usually disappears. Likewise, tongue protrusion while swallowing (tongue thrust) is also fairly common among all young children.

Because tongue protrusion can lead to drooling and contribute to uneven or protruding front teeth, it is important to determine its cause. Often, the reason is that your child needs to extend his tongue in order to breathe, due to small airways. The first step in assessment should be to check the airways for any of the obstructions described above. Once the obstruction is removed, tongue protrusion may gradually disappear. Then again, as with chronic mouth breathing, tongue protrusion is a learned behavior and may not go away even after an obstruction is corrected.

The first step in the treatment of tongue protrusion should always be speech or occupational therapy to increase motor control and promote a normal swallowing pattern. As children grow older, this problem usually becomes minor or disappears.

Some professionals advocate reducing the size of the tongue through a surgery called tongue reduction. The goal of this surgery is to lessen the size the tongue by about fifty percent. In this procedure, a surgeon removes a V-shaped wedge of tongue from the tongue's tip and the edges are then sewn together.

The operation often lessens tongue protrusion and drooling. Typically, however, speech is *not* easier to understand following this treatment. This operation is controversial in part because it is not done to treat an illness, but to improve appearance—to reduce tongue protrusion because it can call up stereotypes of people with mental handicaps. This operation should only be tried as a last resort if significant problems are present and other treatments do not work.

Drooling

Drooling is a problem for about forty percent of all children with Down syndrome, and is often a major concern to parents. Like many other concerns, drooling usually lessens as children grow older. Like tongue protrusion, drooling is often more common when children are concentrating.

There are many underlying causes of drooling—chronic mouth breathing due to airway obstruction; tongue thrusting; and inability to close the mouth due to crooked or protruding teeth. The first step in treating this problem is to correct any airway obstruction. Next, the teeth should be examined by your child's dentist. If there are problems, an orthodontist should be consulted to oversee proper repositioning.

Often, delayed motor learning and weak muscles are the underlying cause of drooling. In these cases, swallowing and behavior therapies should be tried by a speech therapist. A common way to increase the muscle tone and control of the lips is to "ice the lips." To do this, you circle your child's lips with an ice pack. This will usually make your child purse his lips. With repetition, this exercise increases strength and motor control.

Oral sensory problems may be another cause of drooling. Some children with Down syndrome are very sensitive in their mouths, and do not like the feel of food on their tongues. They may spit out the food. They may also not swallow as frequently as necessary, resulting in drooling. Children who have oral sensory problems should work with a speech or occupational therapist specially trained to handle these problems.

Sometimes drooling is severe enough to cause chronic irritation of the skin around the mouth, yeast infections, or other serious health concerns. If this happens, you may want to consider surgery aimed at lessening the production of saliva. Operations to reduce salivation may involve:

- The removal of major salivary glands;
- Cutting the nerves to the salivary glands; or
- Re-routing the ducts of the salivary glands toward the back of the mouth so that more saliva will run down the throat and not out of the mouth.

At best, these surgeries produce satisfactory results for only 50 to 60 percent of children. It is important to understand that drooling is not the result of your child producing too much saliva. Surgery to decrease the production of saliva in order to limit drooling may result in a dry mouth later in life, when your child's motor control improves and drooling stops. Remember, operations that remove salivary glands or cut nerves are irreversible.

Conclusion

Like all children, children with Down syndrome can have a variety of ear, nose, throat, and sinus problems. Some of these problems, particularly hearing impairments, can contribute to further delays in learning if not promptly and effectively treated. Other problems, such as breathing difficulties, can affect your child's health. And still others, such as mouth breathing, tongue protrusion, and drooling, can make it harder for your child to be accepted socially. Often there are a number of different treatments available for these conditions—some more conservative, but tried-and-true; others more radical and controversial. To ensure that your child receives the best possible treatment, it is important to consult frequently and frankly with competent, caring professionals experienced in working with children with Down syndrome who have ear, nose, and throat problems.

References

Balkany, T.J., et al. "Ossicular Abnormalities in Down's Syndrome." *Otolaryngology and Head Surgery,* Vol. 87, 1979, 372–384.

Kavanagh, K.T., et al. "Risks and Benefits of Adenotonsillectomy Children with Down Syndrome." *American Journal of Mental Deficiency,* Vol. 91, 1986, 22–29.

Klaiman, P., et al. "Changes in Aesthetic Appearance and Intelligibility of Speech after Partial Glossectomy in Patients with Down Syndrome." *Plastic and Reconstructive Surgery,* Vol. 82, 1988, 403–408.

Lemperle, G. "Discussion: Rehabilitation of the Face in Patients with Down's Syndrome." *Plastic and Reconstructive Surgery,* Vol. 77, No. 3, 1986, 392–393.

Margar-Bacal, F., et al. "Speech Intelligibility after Partial Glossectomy in Children with Down's Syndrome." *Plastic and Reconstructive Surgery,* Vol. 79, 1987, 44–49.

Parsons C.L. and Rozner L. "Effect of Tongue Reduction on Articulation in Children with Down Syndrome." *American Journal of Mental Deficiency,* Vol. 91, 1987, 328–332.

Pueschel, S.M. "Facial Plastic Surgery for Children with Down Syndrome." *Developmental Medicine and Child Neurology,* Vol. 30, 1988, 536–549.

Rozner, L. "Postglossectomy Speech." *Plastic and Reconstructive Surgery,* Vol. 80, 1987, 756.

9 | Down Syndrome and the Gastrointestinal Tract

Timothy M. Buie, M.D.
Alejandro F. Flores Sandoval, M.D.

Introduction

The gastrointestinal (GI) tract consists of the body parts and organs that take in food, extract the nutrients, and get rid of the leftover waste. This includes the mouth and throat as well as the esophagus, stomach, small and large intestines, and rectum. The salivary glands, pancreas, and liver add enzymes and other substances to help the GI tract digest and absorb the nutrients.

Children with Down syndrome may have certain conditions that affect the stomach and intestines, or GI tract (see Figure 1). These conditions are most often characterized by:

- Anatomical anomalies—the structure of the organ is abnormal;
- Functional disorders—the organs don't work as they should; and
- Nutrition-linked conditions that prevent the absorption or efficient use of particular nutrients.

Most of these conditions are relatively rare. Some are very obvious right from birth, like *duodenal atresia* (discussed below). Others may be more difficult to identify, because they do not cause problems all of the time. Many babies with Down syndrome have problems feeding, especially in the first few months of life, but most do not have anything wrong with their GI system. Most of the time the problem is the baby's

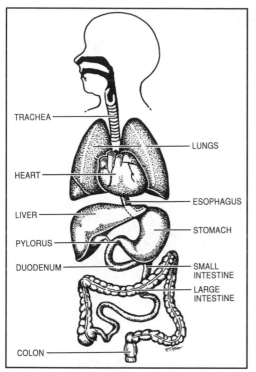

TRACHEA

LUNGS

HEART

ESOPHAGUS

LIVER

STOMACH

PYLORUS

DUODENUM

SMALL
INTESTINE

LARGE
INTESTINE

COLON

Figure 1. The Gastrointestinal (GI) system.

poor ability to suck because of low muscle tone. By the time the infant is a few months old, feeding usually goes much better. Constipation is also common for children with Down syndrome, but is usually not a sign of major GI problems.

There are no good screening tests to look for GI problems ahead of time. You do need to be aware of some of the possibilities, and watch for signs and symptoms that go on too long, or can't be explained some other way. Some of these signs and symptoms include feeding problems like vomiting or coughing with feeding, frequent diarrhea or constipation, or failure to gain weight adequately. Constipation that continues in spite of careful diet, lots of fluids, and exercise may also indicate a need to look further. Your primary health care provider is the best place to start, to decide if there might be a problem that needs more testing. If you do need the help of a specialist, your local doctor can help you find one. Other parents of children who have had problems are also helpful in sorting out places to go for specialized medical services.

This chapter reviews the most common and serious GI problems, and explains their symptoms and treatment.

Anatomical Anomalies

About 10 to 18 percent of all children with Down syndrome are born with anatomical differences in their stomachs or intestines. Researchers have yet to discover what causes these differences. But new research into very early fetal development has found clues at the molecular level. Someday this research may shed light on the exact causes of these anomalies.

The most common anatomical anomalies in children with Down syndrome include *aganglionic megacolon* (abnormal nerves in the bowel), *annular pancreas* (ring-shaped pancreas), *duodenal atresia* and *duodenal stenosis* (blockage or narrowing of the small intestine), *imperforate anus* (no anal opening), and *tracheo-esophageal fistula* (an opening between the windpipe and the throat). *Pyloric stenosis* (narrowing of the point where the stomach empties into the small intestine) is also more common in children with Down syndrome. Each of these conditions is explained below.

Aganglionic Megacolon (Hirschsprung's Disease)

The colon, or large intestine, is the last part of the GI tract immediately before the rectum and anus. It works to save nutrients and absorb water from the stool as it passes through, and it stores the stool until it is passed in a bowel movement. In children with aganglionic megacolon, however, the colon does not work properly because of a lack of nerve cells (called *ganglia*). As the stool collects, the colon enlarges (thus the name megacolon, or unusually large colon).

Children with this condition become very constipated, with a swollen abdomen and, in many instances, vomiting. If this condition is not treated, the growth is delayed, and there will be chronic constipation. The length of colon affected by Hirschsprung's disease can vary. If a very long section is missing the nerve cells, constipation usually happens very early

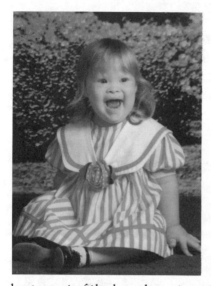

and is hard to miss. When the part without nerves is very short, the problem can be harder to spot. As mentioned above, many children with Down syndrome can have constipation from time to time. The trick is to be able to identify which ones need the special testing to look for this condition. Severe aganglionic megacolon requires immediate medical attention. Otherwise, it can result in bowel obstruction, gross enlargement of the bowel, rupture, infection, and in extreme cases, death.

The most common treatment for Hirschsprung's disease is surgery to remove the part of the bowel that does not function properly. Usually this procedure includes the creation of a temporary opening through the abdominal wall called a *stoma,* which is hooked up to the remaining good bowel. The colostomy that is created allows the remaining bowel to heal well with a low risk of infection. While the colostomy is in use, stool is passed into a bag attached to the stoma. After several months, the intestines are usually healed well enough to allow the colostomy to be removed and the colon to be hooked up to the rectum. How well things work out depends in part on how much bowel remains after the surgery.

Annular Pancreas

The pancreas is the organ that makes insulin and many of the enzymes that help to digest food. It is a long thin organ that attaches to the intestines next to the stomach. An annular pancreas, on the other hand, forms a ring that completely encircles the duodenum, which is the first segment of the small intestine after the stomach. This can result in the narrowing or blockage of the small intestine. The narrowness does not always cause blockage; sometimes the child can eat and grow for years before the tightness causes enough problems to be recognized.

If bowel obstruction occurs, food and liquids will not be able to pass, with vomiting and severe abdominal pain as the result. This is considered a medical emergency. Surgery will need to be performed by a pediatric surgeon, or by a general surgeon with experience working with children. He or she will remove the part of the pancreas that surrounds the duodenum, in order to relieve the blockage. How well your child does after the procedure depends upon how much of the pancreas is removed, and whether the surgery has other complications. Bowel function usually returns to normal, especially if no sections of intestine need to be removed.

Duodenal Atresia and Duodenal Stenosis

Atresia means the failure of an organ to develop properly; if that organ happens to be a tube, like a section of intestine, the middle can be very small or entirely blocked. In duodenal atresia, the duodenum, the first segment of the small intestine which attaches to the stomach, is closed off. This prevents the contents of the stomach from passing into the lower sections of the GI tract.

Overall, duodenal atresia is found in about one newborn out of every 1,500. However, it is much more common in babies with Down syndrome. In one review in 1986, 17 out of 47 children with duodenal atresia were children who had Down syndrome. Another study found that in a group of 503 people with duodenal atresia, 151—about 30 percent—had Down syndrome. Of these patients, 20 percent also had annular pancreas. The number of people with Down syndrome who are born with this problem is not known for sure, but may be between 5 percent and 8 percent of all babies born.

The first symptom of duodenal atresia is usually vomiting. This often appears within a few hours of birth. A child will have no stools after about the third day, and her upper abdomen will become swollen (this is called *distention* of the *epigastrium*).

Duodenal atresia is treated by surgically removing the blocked or narrow segment, and then reconnecting the bowel. The repair is done as soon as the problem is discovered, usually before your baby has gone home from the hospital. Like any major surgery in newborns, these operations have a high risk of complications, but babies with Down syndrome do not seem to have more trouble than other babies who have the same condition.

A related condition, in which the duodenum is unusually narrow, is called duodenal stenosis. Sometimes duodenal stenosis is hard to detect, depending on how tight the narrowness is. In general, children who have problems with frequent vomiting, who do not eat well, or who have abdominal swelling should be carefully examined, preferably by a physician who knows them well. Again, treatment of duodenal stenosis often involves removing the narrowed segment and reconnecting the bowel. Because these repairs are often done when the child is older, there are fewer complications than in newborn babies.

When narrowing is less severe and obstruction of the bowel is less likely, surgery may not be necessary. Instead, the condition may be managed with a low fiber/residue diet, which limits the amount of stool production. This kind of diet may include special formulas and careful attention to solids to reduce the amount of fiber while not leaving out vitamins and other nutrients. The help of a dietician or nutritionist is important for success. Careful medical monitoring by a team including a GI specialist is also essential.

Imperforate Anus

In some children with Down syndrome, the anus—the external opening of the colon—is blocked. This is called *imperforate* (having no opening) anus. If the anus is not completely blocked, your child may have small stools and problems with constipation. When the blockage is complete, the anus will appear as a small dimple (called a *proctodeal pit*). Often this condition is accompanied by blockage (atresia) of the lower rectum, which makes the repair more complicated.

Imperforate anus occurs in about two out of every 100 children with Down syndrome. Children with Down syndrome have this condition about fifteen times more often than other children.

An imperforate anus is typically treated in the newborn period by a procedure called *perineal anoplasty,* in which an anal opening is created or widened surgically. In cases of greater malformation, a more complicated surgical procedure may be used. In this procedure, the blocked or absent part of the bowel is removed and the remaining normal bowel is pulled down through the pelvis to make an opening. The success of the surgery can vary, depending 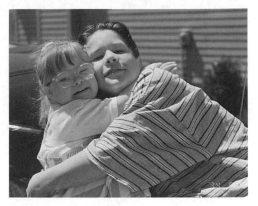 on what needs to be done. It can be difficult to get perfect function of stooling and continence if there have to be a lot of changes made.

Pyloric Stenosis

The *pylorus* is the junction where the stomach empties into the small intestine. If this junction is too narrow, the condition is called pyloric stenosis. It is usually caused by an increase in the muscles that surround the pylorus. In time (usually at one to three months of age), a baby with pyloric stenosis will begin to vomit, and her stomach will become swollen. The vomiting usually begins after eating, and is often described as "projectile vomiting," because the stomach contents shoot out forcefully. Exactly how often this occurs in children with Down syndrome is not known.

A type of surgery called the Ramsted procedure is the usual treatment. During this procedure, some of the muscles surrounding the pylorus are cut to enlarge the outlet from the stomach to the duodenum. This is a simple operation that usually works very well.

Tracheo-esophageal Fistula

The word *fistula* means "pipe," and in medicine it refers to an enclosed passage between two parts of the body that would not normally be connected. With tracheo-esophageal fistula, there is an abnormal passage between the trachea (windpipe), and the esophagus (throat). This abnormality is present at birth, and occurs because of unusual fetal development.

Some children with this type of fistula have no problems, and the defect may go undetected for years. The main risk is that food or fluid from the mouth will find its way into the lungs, and cause pneumonia or severe respiratory distress. With pneumonia, which is an infection of the lungs, your child will usually cough a lot, and may breathe faster than usual. Respiratory distress means that breathing has become very hard, and your child is having trouble getting enough air. With symptoms like these, the doctors will first help your child to breathe, and then try to find the cause. Ordinary chest X-rays can help, but sometimes special x-rays or other tests are needed to find the fistula.

Once a fistula is discovered, surgery may be needed to close it. The location and size of the fistula will determine how difficult it will be to mend the trachea and esophagus. The more complicated the surgery, the more possibility of complications, and the longer recovery may take.

Making Treatment Decisions

In the past, children with Down syndrome who had intestinal blockages frequently died from dehydration, poor caloric intake, or complications of surgery. Their GI tracts simply could not digest and absorb enough nutrients to keep them alive. Improved medical care and advances in surgical procedures have lowered the mortality rate, so that today it is about 10 per cent. One reason that the mortality rate continues to be high is that these disorders are often associated with congenital heart conditions that make surgery even riskier for the newborn or very young infant. Unless it is a medical emergency, you should gather all the information possible before making decisions about treatment for your child's gastrointestinal problems. Talk with your pediatrician or pediatric surgeon about treatment options, and learn all you can about the possible risks and benefits. Do not hesitate to get a second opinion if your child's doctor does not answer all your questions to your satisfaction.

Functional Disorders

Functional disorders of the gastrointestinal tract occur when certain muscles or organs do not function as they should, although there are no anatomical anomalies. In children with Down syndrome, the most common functional disorders include disorders of *esophageal motility* and *gastro-esophageal reflux*.

Esophageal Motility Disorders and Gastro-esophageal Reflux

When the contents of the stomach and the duodenum are allowed to flow back into the throat and esophagus, it is called gastro-esophageal reflux. In the past, some doctors have thought that reflux was a deliberate "behavior problem" in children with Down syndrome. However, recent research has shown that some children with Down syndrome have problems with the way muscles in the esophagus propel food to the stomach (esophageal motility). Often, too, the stomach and duodenum may empty more slowly than usual. In addition, many doctors now believe that children with Down syndrome may have a general malfunctioning of the nervous system that controls the GI tract, which results in reflux and esophageal motility problems. This malfunctioning may be the result of abnormal fetal development.

Gastroesophageal reflux is actually a fairly common event for most people, especially in infancy and early childhood. However, frequent or recurrent reflux is not normal, and is usually a sign of a problem with the way the stomach and esophagus work. Babies who spit up during or after feedings are usually not refluxing, and may just be swallowing a lot of air. Carefully burping babies may help cut down on that kind of spitting. Sometimes your baby's position after feeding is important. Keeping her upright in a infant seat for a short time (30–45 minutes) after eating may help. Avoiding active play right after feeding is always a good idea.

If, in spite of careful feeding, your child is spitting up regularly (several-to-many times a day), you should talk to your doctor about possible problems. Stomach juices are acidic and may damage the esophagus if reflux is frequent. Most children do not aspirate, or swallow things down their windpipe, because they are able to protect their airway by coughing. If your child often coughs or gags during or just after feeding, this may also be a sign of trouble that should be discussed with your doctor. Persistent reflux is sometimes the only indication of the partially obstructing conditions mentioned above (annular pancreas or duodenal stenosis).

When the problem persists, medicines may help to move food through the stomach faster to make reflux less likely. Sometimes surgery is needed to tighten the esophagus where it joins up with the stomach; frequently a feeding tube (gastrostomy) is added at that time, especially if the child also has had a lot of trouble with swallowing.

Nutrition-linked Disorders

Much fascinating research is currently being done in the area of nutrition-linked disorders—that is, conditions caused by the way the body digests and uses food, vitamins, and minerals. We are learning about ways in which nutrition affects such things as the immune system and growth and development. Some nutrition-linked disorders of particular concern for children with Down syndrome are malabsorption syndromes and trace element deficiencies.

Malabsorption Syndromes

When the intestines do not take the nutrients that the body needs from the food that is being digested, it is called malabsorption. Recent research has suggested that children with Down syndrome may be more likely to have problems with malabsorption. In fact, one study found that individuals with Down syndrome are 20 times more likely than others to have a particular malabsorption syndrome known as *celiac disease*.

In celiac disease, the inside surface of the intestines changes so that it can no longer absorb the nutrients the body needs. The disease begins slowly, and often is not recognized at first. In children, its symptoms eventually include frothy, bad-smelling stools, swollen stomach, gas, loss of appetite, irritability, weight loss, delayed growth, fatigue, low levels of vitamins B, D, and K, and electrolyte imbalance. Celiac disease

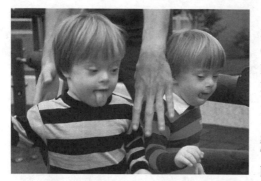

is usually treated by following a special diet which avoids exposure to *gluten,* a protein in grains like wheat, oats, barley, and rye that triggers the reaction. This kind of diet can be hard to manage, and it is often helpful to have a dietician or nutritionist help in planning for alternatives.

There are other causes of malabsorption syndrome that are not more common in Down syndrome. If your child doesn't gain weight well in spite of eating enough food, especially if diarrhea is a frequent problem, you should ask your physician about this group of conditions.

Malabsorption of some vitamins or other essential substances may occur, but may not be so obvious. Vitamin A and zinc are both necessary for the immune system to fight infections. Some people with Down syndrome may not absorb or use one or the other of these nutrients adequately. When that happens, there may be an increased number of ordinary infections (like ear or sinus infections) that may also be difficult to cure, or there might be abnormal infections (like bone infections) caused by unusual bacteria or fungi. Please see Chapter 4 for more on this subject. Some have suggested that zinc can improve growth in some people with Down syndrome, though whether an absorption problem created a deficiency in those individuals has not been shown.

Conclusion

Many gastrointestinal conditions are commonly associated with Down syndrome. These conditions may be due to anatomical, functional, or nutritional disorders, and may significantly affect the growth and development of your child if not treated. For this reason, your child's gastrointestinal system should be carefully evaluated shortly after her birth, and its functioning should be closely monitored as your child grows and develops.

Because children with Down syndrome often have a variety of special health care needs, it makes sense to use an interdisciplinary approach to assist with this monitoring process. The family doctor or pediatrician is often the best link your family has to appropriate professionals and a hospital equipped to provide the services needed. Other professionals that you may wish to consult might include a pediatric radiologist, a pediatric surgeon, a feeding team (typically made up of a physical therapist, a nutritionist or dietician, and perhaps a speech therapist), and a social worker (to guide your family to a variety of support services). Together, the problems of the GI tract can be managed and treated.

References

Abalan, F., et al. "A Study of Digestive Absorption in Four Cases of Down Syndrome, Down Syndrome Malnutrition, Malabsorption and Alzheimer's Disease." *Medical Hypotheses,* Vol. 31, 1990, 35–38.

Anneren, G. and Gebre-Medhin, M. "Trace Elements and Transport Proteins in Serum of Children with Down Syndrome and of Healthy Siblings Living in the Same Environment." *Human Nutrition: Clinical Nutrition,* Vol. 41C, 1987, 291–299.

Black, C. and Sherman, J. "The Association of Low Imperforate Anus and Down Syndrome." *Journal of Pediatric Surgery,* Vol. 24, No. 1, 1989, 92–94.

Carr, J. *Young Children with Down Syndrome,* (London: Butterworth and Co., 1975).

Dias, J. and Walker-Smith, J. "Down Syndrome and Celiac Disease." *Pediatric Gastroenterology and Nutrition,* Vol. 10, No. 1, 1990, 41–43.

Hillemeier, A.C., et al. "Esophageal and Gastric Motor Abnormalities in Gastroesophageal Reflux During Infancy." *Gastroenterology,* Vol. 84, 1983, 741–46.

Hillemeier, A.C., et al. "Esophogeal Dysfunction in Down Syndrome." *Journal of Pediatric Gastroenterology and Nutrition,* Vol. 1, 1982, 101–104.

Napolitano, G., et al. "Growth Delay in Down Syndrome and Zinc Sulphate Supplementation." *American Journal of Medical Genetics* (Supplement), Vol. 7, 1990, 63–65.

Opitz, J. and Gilbert-Barness, E. "Reflections on the Pathogenesis of Down Syndrome." *American Journal of Medical Genetics* (Supplement), Vol. 7, 1990, 38–51.

Potts, S. and Garstin, W. "Neonatal Duodenal Obstruction with Emphasis on Cases with Down's Syndrome." *Ulster Medical Journal,* Vol. 55, No. 2, 1986, 147–50.

Pueschel, Siegfried. *A Parent's Guide to Down Syndrome,* (Baltimore: Paul H. Brookes, 1990).

Simila, S. and Kokkonen, J. "Coexistance of Celiac Disease and Down Syndrome." *American Journal of Mental Retardation,* Vol. 95, No. 1, 1990, 120–122.

10 Orthopedic Issues Affecting Children with Down Syndrome
S. Michael Lawhon, M.D.

Introduction

The structure of our bodies resembles that of buildings. Where buildings have girders and beams, we have bones. Where buildings have trusses and cables, we have ligaments and tendons. Where buildings have external walls, we have muscles and skin. But that is where the similarities end. The major difference between buildings and people is that buildings are static and people are dynamic. Buildings are designed to stay in one place; we are built to move.

Bones are the structures upon which everything inside our bodies hang. They hold our bodies together. The bones of the skeleton provide support. Tissues that connect bones to other bones are called *ligaments*. Connective tissues that attaches muscle to bones are called *tendons*. Problems with the bones, ligaments, tendons, or muscles are called *musculoskeletal disorders*. The area of medicine dealing with these disorders both medically and surgically is called *orthopedics*. Orthopedists are physicians specially trained in the medical and surgical treatment of musculoskeletal problems.

The most common musculoskeletal disorders that affect children with Down syndrome involve the neck, spine, hips, legs, and knees. These include:

- *atlant-oaxial subluxation*—instability of the bones of the neck;
- *genu valgus*— "knock knees";

- *hip instability;*
- *metatarsus primus varus*—inturning of the foot;
- *patellofemoral instability*—instability of the knee cap;
- *pes planus*—flat feet;
- *scoliosis*—curvature of the spine; and
- frequent joint dislocation.

There are three major characteristics of the muscles and bones of children with Down syndrome that contribute musculoskeletal problems. People with Down Syndrome appear to have differences in their bones and in the structure of their connective tissue. In addition, their muscle tone can be low. Tone is best described as tension, such as the tension in a support cable or wire. If the cable is not taught enough, it sags. When this happens to a tendon in the human body, it is described as loose. Muscles provide tension to the tendons. If the muscle is not constricted or tense enough because of abnormalities in the nervous system, it is called low in tone or *hypotonic.*

People with Down syndrome may develop symptoms of any of the conditions listed above as a child, adolescent, or adult. If your child develops one of these conditions, you may want to consult an orthopedic surgeon. Pediatric orthopedists will usually have the most experience and expertise in treating children with Down syndrome. They can usually be found at major children's hospitals in the United States. If you need a list of orthopedists who have a special expertise in children with Down syndrome, contact the National Down Syndrome Congress or a down syndrome clinic.

Joint Dislocation

Joints are where two or more bones meet. Joints are usually cushioned with special soft tissue, called *cartilage,* to ease movement. Our bodies are made up of many joints, some which move very little, such as the bones of the skull; and some which move a great deal, such as the hips, knees, and ankles. Because of their tendency to have loose ligaments and hypotonia, the joints of children with Down syndrome are often not held as firmly in place as the joints of other children. Consequently, they are more prone to dislocated joints. When this occurs, the joints come out of their soft tissue setting—they may separate. This can result in loss of motion, pain, and early degeneration of the joint.

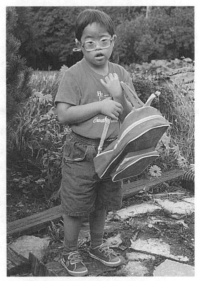

Among children with Down syndrome, the most commonly dislocated joints are the thumb, elbow, hip, and knee. A joint may become dislocated by injury, resulting in early degeneration of the joint. Joint degeneration means that the cartilage cushioning the joint breaks down. Without the cartilage cushion, bone rubs against bone, causing pain and further damage. Although joint dislocations can cause a great deal of pain, joint degeneration is usually not painful in its early stages and may not result in any major problems for your child. If the a joint degenerates significantly, however, nerves can become painfully pinched, joints can become very unstable, and basic movements like walking can become impossible.

Sometimes joints can become very unstable, and repeatedly dislocate. This may subject the joint to undue stresses; pain usually follows. Repeated dislocation may also lead to early degenerative changes to the surfaces of the bones of the joint. Degeneration may result in joint swelling and pain, particularly as your child becomes an adult. Joint degeneration is often not noticed in childhood because it occurs gradually, and can take a long time before bone begins to rub against bone.

Sometimes surgery can help reduce the amount of joint instability in early degenerative changes. However, in most cases, conditioning of the muscles to help improve muscle bulk and strength may lead to decreased instability of the joint without surgery. Also, modifying your child's activities can help prevent continued dislocation. Choosing activities that do not place unusual stresses on potentially dislocateable joint surfaces can help. Your orthopedist can help you find activities that do not strain your child's joints.

Children with Down syndrome may also have more congenital (present at birth) dislocations, particularly of the hip. They may also have more dislocations that result from minor injuries. Dislocations that are present at birth, such as congenital dislocated hip, are treated with splints and braces (*orthoses*) in order to encourage normal development of the hip joint. This treatment may last from 6 to 10 weeks to 3 to 6 months.

Dislocations caused by minor injury (such as dislocating a thumb catching a ball) may require treatment by manipulation either by a parent or physician in order to return the joint to its proper position. Sometimes, with more serious dislocations, such as shoulder dislocations, a muscle relaxant may be needed to allow repositioning the joint. Most minor dislocations, however, correct themselves spontaneously. If your child's dislocation does not correct itself, seek medical attention promptly. In transporting your child to the doctor, use a splint for comfort to keep the limb from moving. If you have any questions or concerns about any dislocation, call your child's doctor *before* you make any effort to try the place the joint back into place.

Atlanto-axial Instability

About 9 to 20 percent of people with Down syndrome have a weakness or instability of the upper two bones (*vertebrae*) of the spinal column in the neck. This condition, known as *atlantoaxial instability*, can result in potentially serious complications. It is believed to be caused by the lax ligaments common in people with Down syndrome.

Atlantoaxial instability, if present, is a serious medical concern. It can cause *subluxation* (slippage). That is, the first *cervical* (neck) vertebra (called *C1*) slips onto the second (called *C2*). Spinal cord damage may occur. Because the spinal cord contains nerves that control the movements and functions of the entire body, damage to the spinal cord could cause paralysis or even death.

The most common symptoms of atlantoaxial instability are neck pain, *torticollis* (tilting and twisting of the neck), and decreased ability to walk. The sudden appearance of symptoms may also be a signal of some other neurologic disease or of inner ear problems. That is why immediate medical attention is important. Other symptoms of atlantoaxial instability may include changes in bowel or bladder function, incontinence, changes in gait, fatigue when walking, increased clumsiness, decreased coordination, increased muscle tone in ankles or other extremities, or increased reflexes such as when you tap on your child's knee. Other symptoms may include limited neck movement, sudden preference for sitting, weakness of legs or any extremities, weakness which may come and go or become progressively worse, a worsening sense of balance, more difficulty than usual in developing motor skills, and loss of abilities such running and playing peer group activities.

Diagnosis of Atlanto-axial Instability

Because atlantoaxial instability can be present without symptoms, all children with Down syndrome should be screened for this condition. If your child has any of the symptoms of neck instability, he should be immediately examined by his doctor and referred to an orthopedist or neurosurgical physician who is experienced in evaluating this type of problem. If your child shows no symptoms, he should still be examined before enrollment in any educational or day care program that includes sports or athletic activities—usually between the ages of four and six. As Chapter 16 explains, your child should also be evaluated for cervical instability before receiving general anesthesia for a surgical procedure. Whenever your child with Down syndrome undergoes surgery, his doctors should assume that he has atlanto-axial instability, even if he has not been diagnosed with it.

A variety of physicians, including your primary care physician, orthopedist, neurologist, or neurosurgeon, can examine your child for atlantoaxial instability. It is important that the physician who examines your child be knowledgeable about this condition and familiar with the appropriate consultations and tests needed. Not all physicians are familiar with the symptoms and physical findings of atlanto-axial instability, so you may have to ask.

Your child's evaluation will consist of two parts: 1) a neurological exam to look for increased tone, muscle weakness, abnormal reflexes, and other neurological symptoms; and 2) x-ray studies. X-ray examination should consist of x-rays of the front and back of the neck, in both flexed (bent) and extended positions (*anterior-posterior and flexion-extension lateral x-rays*), as well as special views of the cervical spine. These special x-ray views of children with Down syndrome are called *odontoid* views of the cervical spine. X-rays can be taken by private radiologists, hospital radiology departments, or orthopedic clinics.

Other types of x-ray studies, including *cine radiology, tomography, computerized tomography* (CT) *scans,* and m*agnetic resonance imaging* (MRI) scans are also used on occasion. Cine radiography is a motion picture film using x-ray.

Tomography is a special computerized film of the neck. Magnetic resonance imaging is a new technique for imaging bony and soft tissue that does not use x-rays. These can provide additional information about the dimensions of the bones and spinal cord that is especially important if your child will be receiving surgery.

In diagnosing your child, the physician will carefully examine your child's x-ray films for evidence of slippage (subluxation) and bone abnormalities. If your child has normal x-rays and no symptoms, he usually will not need further screening. However, some studies indicate that cervical instability can develop in a person who has had a normal x-ray in the past. More research needs to be done, however, to establish definitively whether this condition is present at birth or develops during the growing years. We also need to learn when cervical instability first becomes evident, and whether the level of instability remains constant throughout life. For this reason, you should be aware of the symptoms of cervical instability listed above. If your child develops any of these symptoms at any time, he should be evaluated by a physician, and the exam should include appropriate x-rays.

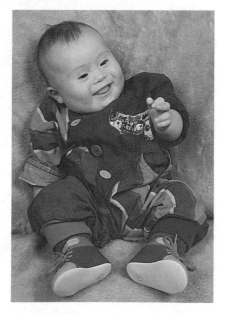

If x-rays reveal that your child does have atlanto-axial instability, his condition will be categorized according to his degree of subluxation and clinical symptoms (see Table 1). The word "interval" in Table 1 refers to the distance measured between the two vertebra. The greater the distance, or interval, the greater the po-

Table 1: Distribution by Atlas-odontoid Interval and Clinical Symptoms

Group	Interval	Clinical Presentation
1	Less than 4.5	No instability
2	Less than 6.5	Mild instability without symptoms
3	Less than 6.5	Mild instability with symptoms
4	Greater than 6.5	Gross instability without symptoms
5	Greater than 6.5	Gross instability with symptoms

tential for instability. The degree of instability is categorized by groups, with no instability being normal (Group 1). Groups 2 and 3 are mildly unstable and groups 4 and 5 are grossly unstable. Obviously, the higher the group number the greater potential for damage to the spinal cord.

Treatment of Atlanto-axial Instability

If your child has atlanto-axial instability, follow-up and treatment will depend on the diagnostic group to which he assigned. (see Table 2).

Table 2: Treatment for Atlanto-axial Instability— According to Group

Group Treatment

1. Continue screening on a regular basis

2. Limit activities which flex and hyperextend the neck; follow-up screening every three years

3. Surgical stabilization

4. Continue close observation; CAT scan to ascertain spinal cord space; consider surgery if amount of slippage or atlantoaxial space reaches 8 millimeters

5. Surgical stabilization

For children with little or no cervical instability and no symptoms (Groups 1 and 2), no treatment is needed. Screening, however, should continue on a regular basis. Usually it is sufficient to have additional x-rays done every three years. Obviously, children who are in Groups 2 through 5 may need x-rays more frequently depending on their particular condition. In addition, children in Group 2 should limit activities that might overextend the neck. Activities to avoid are listed below. Approximately fifteen percent of children with Down syndrome have cervical instability without any symptoms (Group 2) and may remain so throughout life. They are, however, considered "at risk," and thus some of their physical activities may need to be curtailed. There are no studies showing how often children with Down syndrome should be retested, but you cannot assume that the condition will not occur sometime in the future, even if your child's cervical spine is normal now. Children with normal cervical spines should be tested at between 8 and 10 years of age, and every 10 years thereafter.

If your child is in group 3, 4, or 5, he may require surgical stabilization. He will first need additional evaluations. These will include preoperative neurological testing and detailed evaluations of the cervical spine by either computerized tomography scan or MRI. It is very important to document by both x-ray and clinical exam all findings so that after surgery your child can be monitored appropriately. In this way, doctors can determine whether your child's condition is stable, improving, or deteriorating.

If you and your child's doctor decide to proceed with surgery, the first and second vertebra (C-1 and C-2) will be fused (joined) with bone grafts and, in some cases, metal wire. The bones usually come from another part of the body; most commonly the hip. After surgery, your child will need to wear a halo (a brace attached to the head to keep it stable) for a significant period of time depending on how quickly the bone grafts fuse and on how extensive the bone grafting was. Your child's spinal cord should be closely monitored following surgery to make sure that his condition is stabilizing and improving. In a few cases, the fusion does not take and may need to be repeated. In addition, there needs to be monitoring for any surgical complications such as infection. Your child's cognitive abilities will have a significant bearing on his ability to follow after-surgery care recommendations. If your child will not tolerate a halo for a period of time, he may not be an optimum candidate for surgery.

Restricting Your Child's Activities

As mentioned earlier, all children with Down syndrome should be evaluated for atlanto-axial instability before they take part in any activity that may put stress on the neck or result in an injury to the neck. Children who have symptoms or x-ray evidence of cervical instability should not take part in these "high risk" activities.

The Special Olympics Committee has put together a list of activities they consider to be "high risk." These activities are:

- butterfly stroke in swimming
- diving
- gymnastics
- high jump in track and field
- soccer
- trampoline
- tumbling
- warm-up exercises that place pressure on the head and neck muscles

Even after surgical stabilization it may not be a good idea for a child with atlanto-axial instability to take part in these activities, although the possibility of a problem is markedly reduced. Special Olympics's policy is not identical to that of the American Academy of Pediatrics Committee on Sports Medicine when it comes to recommendations on sports activities for children with Down syndrome. Special Olympics recommendations are more specific: They prohibit people with Down syndrome from participating or competing in a number of different sport activities and exercises that could place pressure on the head and neck. There is no definitive data supporting the restrictiveness of these recommendations.

There may be other activities that your child's school will not allow your child to participate in if he has atlanto-axial instability. Each school establishes its own policy; many require a medical evaluation or a signed waiver before participation. Remember, though, when physicians sign medical release forms, they are concurring that they have found no symptoms of spinal cord damage and no x-ray evidence of instability during that particular examination. This does not mean, however, that cervical instability will not develop later.

Other Disorders of the Cervical Spine

In addition to atlanto-axial instability, several other disorders of the musculoskeletal system may affect the cervical spine. Among the most common in people with Down syndrome is degenerative disk disease (*arthritis* and *spondylosis*). With degenerative disk disease of the spine, the distance between the two vertebrae, in which a cushion of cartilage sits, may narrow. As the cartilage breaks down, extra bone may be formed in the body's attempt to reinforce the area. This extra bone formation may impinge upon the nerves or cause narrowing of the spinal canal. This is called spondylosis. About 8% of people with Down syndrome will have other congenital bony defects of the cervical spine that may accelerate the beginning of degenerative disease of the spine. Degenerative disc disease is found in half of all adults with Down syndrome, which is considerably more frequent than among other people.

Scoliosis

Scoliosis is a lateral (from side to side, as opposed to front to back) curvature of the spine. People with Down syndrome have a higher incidence of scoliosis than other people. Scoliosis occurs in about 50 percent of all people with Down syndrome, and usually affects the *thoracolumbar* (the chest and mid-back) area of the spine. Most often, this curvature does not worsen. The usual result of scoliosis in children with Down syndrome is only slightly misaligned ribs with little if any effect. Close monitoring is still necessary for children whose spinal curvature is less than 20 degrees.

If the curvature of the spine becomes more severe, it can lead to spinal imbalance and significant deformity, resulting in difficulties in breathing, other cardiac and pulmonary problems, pain, and significant limitations in walking. Left uncorrected, scoliosis can cause irreversible cardiac and pulmonary problems and even death.

Early diagnosis of scoliosis greatly influences the type and effect of treatment. Your child's sex and your family's medical history is of great importance; scoliosis is more common in females and tends to run in families. Physical symptoms that suggest scoliosis are asymmetry of the back, a difference in leg length, or a changing gait. Treatment decisions are usually made following multiple evaluations by orthopedics, physical therapists, and in some cases cardiac and pulmonary specialists. Decisions are based on history, x-ray, physical examination, and the degree of curvature. Other medical problems, such as cardiac and pulmonary disease and psychological and social concerns, should also be taken into account.

Scoliosis is usually treated with a brace or cast or by surgery. Treatment choices depend on the age of your child, his or her sex, and the degree of spinal curvature. Using a brace for a child with a moderate curve of 20–40 degrees whose muscles are still maturing is common. Orthopedists try to treat scoliosis before children have stopped growing. The age at which the skeleton stops growing is variable but is usually about 14½ years in females and about two years later in males. Skeletal maturity is determined by x-ray which demonstrate fusion of the growth centers of the skeleton. The brace is usually made out of a synthetic material and is called a body jacket. The objective of the body jacket is to prevent the curve from worsening.

Surgery to correct scoliosis is usually recommended for children with spinal curvature of more than 55 degrees or a spinal curvature of more than 45 degrees which is worsening. This type of surgery usually entails inserting one or more rods to brace the spine coupled with fusing some of the vertebrae to gain stability. After this surgery your child will be in a cast for a length of time depending on the procedure performed and degree of spinal grafting needed.

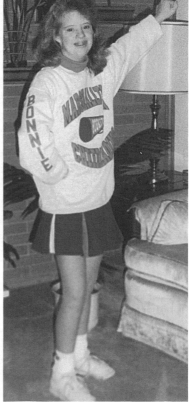

Hip Conditions

Many hip conditions can result in pain, dislocation, or limitation of movement. Hip problems are more common in individuals with Down syndrome because of joint laxity. The overall incidence of hip conditions in people with Down syndrome is not known. One study reported a rate of 11 percent.

In children with Down syndrome, the most common hip problems are: 1) *Congenital hip dislocation* (hip dislocation present at birth); 2) *acetabular dysplasia* (underdevelopment of the hip socket); and 3) otherwise normal hips that tend to dislocate.

Acetabular dysplasia is the lack of formation of the hip socket. If that socket does not completely develop, dislocation and pain often occur. Also, this problem can hinder the flow of blood to the head of the femur. In infants less than one year of age, the cause of hip instability is most likely due to congenital dislocated hips. Congenital dislocated hips are treated with a harness or brace. The harness or brace positions the hip properly to allow the hip socket to form normally. It stabilizes the ball and socket joint while the soft tissue capsule tightens. The length of time for the brace depends on the degree of dislocation and when the problem was identified. Usually, the earlier the identification the less time the harness needs to be worn. Similar bracing is the early treatment of choice in older children unless there is a significant hip joint deformity such as acetabular dysplasia.

If bracing does not correct the problem of the hip joint deformity, then surgery may be needed. The type of surgery depends on the severity of the deformity and the specific type of deformity. During the surgery, doctors try to cover the head of the femur in order to allow the hip joint to develop normally and reduce pain. Surgery to correct hip instability in children with normal hips is often delayed depending on the type and degree of instability.

As children with Down syndrome grow into adolescence and adulthood, their orthopedic problems change. To understand these problems, you need to know a little about the structure and development of the long bones of the body, such as the femur (thigh bone). The body's long bones have three parts. The *diaphysis* is the middle part or shaft of the bone. On each side of the diaphysis is the *metaphysis,* a small section of spongy bone. One each end is the *epiphysis,* which contains both spongy bone and cartilage. There is a plate, called the growth plate, between the epiphysis and the metaphysis. New bone grows in this plate and causes the bone to lengthen at both ends.

After childhood, the problems people with Down syndrome can have include *slipped femoral epiphysis, avascular necrosis of the femur head,* and *degenerative arthritis.* Both slipped femoral epiphysis and avascular necrosis affect the femur (thigh). In slipped femoral epiphysis, the bone slips along the growth plate. This can cause abnormal growth or can stop growth of the bone. With avascular necrosis, there is a lack of development of the femoral head (epiphysis), usually due usually due to restricted blood supply to bone. Without a head, the bone cannot fit properly into the hip socket. This results in early degeneration of the hip, pain, and possible dislocation. Degenerative arthritis may include degeneration of either the head of the femur or of the hip socket (*acetabulum*).

The pain associated with these conditions may be treated with nonsteroid anti-inflammatory medications such as Motrin. However, these medications may produce side effects such as GI upset or bleeding. Because many people with Down syndrome have gastrointestinal disorders, you and your physician should be cautious if you are considering treating your child's pain with anti-inflammatory medications.

If joint changes continue to get worse, as they often do, total hip replacement may be an option. In this surgical procedure, doctors cut off the head of the femur and replace it with a prosthesis; the extent of the replacement depends on the extent of the degeneration. Many young adults with Down syndrome have had successful total hip replacement. Avascular necrosis is generally treated by surgical insertion of a hip screw in an effort to stabilize the hip joint.

Knee Disorders

People with Down syndrome often have musculoskeletal disorders involving the knee, including instability, dislocation, and partial dislocation. One study has suggested that as many as 36 percent of people with Down syndrome may have significant knee problems. Knee cap or *patella* instability accounts for the majority of problematic knees. This instability is caused primarily by severe ligament laxity and lower leg misalignment (when the legs of the bone turn in or out, causing crooked legs or legs of different length). Treatment is determined by the degree of instability or pain.

Knock knees (*genu valgus*) is another knee problem more common among people with Down syndrome. In knock knees, the knees turn in toward each other so much that they knock together during walking. People with genu valgus that is severe may have significant pain and gait problems.

In general, treatment for knee cap disorders includes physical therapy and short term nonsteroid anti-inflammatory medications. Elastic knee sleeves are frequently prescribed and are especially helpful for children with dislocateable knee caps. This type of treatment can lead to better functioning and also enable your child to return to gym class and sports activities.

Surgery to improve knee cap alignment must be carefully planned and should include postoperative therapy. Without planning and close follow up, the condition may recur. Realignment procedures have not been very successful. Following surgery for realignment, dislocations or other symptoms such as pain frequently continue due to generalized joint laxity.

Foot and Ankle Problems

Children with Down syndrome frequently have minor deformities of the ankles and feet. These include:

- *pronation* (a condition in which the structure of the forefoot causes walking on the inside of the arch);

- *flat feet* (which can be congenital or can occur when the arch collapses) occurs in about eighty percent of all people with Down syndrome ;
- widened forefoot; and
- weak ankles associated with ligament laxity.

Often, children with these deformities do not have any symptoms. About half of the time, however, foot and ankle problems affect the ability to walk and, therefore, require treatment. Many children with foot problems develop corns, callouses, or blisters, and walk with a limp. Fungal infections commonly described as athlete's foot, viral infections of the skin, and contact dermatitis (a mild local irritation) are also common.

Many of these complications result from constrictive footwear. Consequently, shoe modifications can help decrease the degree of skin irritation. Instead of getting into expensive modifications, however, many parents find that a good quality, well fitted, tennis shoe with a shoe insert provides support with few skin problems. *Orthoses* (orthopedic shoe inserts) for tennis shoes and other shoes are really just plastic inserts that fit into the shoe. They can improve function and provide support and better weight balance. Remember, however, that orthoses only work when they are worn. When they are taken out of the shoe, the problems are still present. Training in proper nail and skin hygiene is also very important to maintain good foot health.

Surgery is sometimes needed to correct foot deformities that are severe enough to prevent wearing shoes or do not respond to other treatments. However, surgery is usually reserved for those individuals with very severe foot deformities that result in pain and alter or prevent walking.

Summary

People with Down syndrome frequently have musculoskeletal disorders that affect the neck, spine, pelvis, legs, ankles, and feet. Many of these disorders can be painful and make movement difficult. In addition, instability of the cervical spine is a special concern because it may lead to compression of the spinal cord and paralysis.

Fortunately, there are effective treatments that can improve these conditions or prevent them from worsening. Finding a caring orthopedic surgeon who is knowledgeable about the musculoskeletal disorders of people with Down syndrome is the first step in ensuring that your child receives the care he needs.

References

Diamond, L.S., et al. "Orthopaedic Disorders in Patients with Down Syndrome." *Orthopedic Clinics of North America,* Vol. 12, 1981, 57–71.

Lawhon, S. M., et al. "Orthopaedic Aspects of Down Syndrome."

Contemporary Orthopaedics, Vol 20, No. 4, 1990, 395–403.

Livingstone, B. & Hirst, P. "Orthopaedic Disorders in School Children with Down Syndrome with Special Reference to the Incidence of Joint Laxity." *Clinical Orthopedics,* Vol 207, 1986, 74–76.

Paulson, G.W. "Failure of Ambulation in Down Syndrome: A Clinical Survey." *Clinical Pediatrics,* Vol. 10, 1971, 265–267.

Pueschel, S.M., et al. "Atlantoaxial Instability in Down Syndrome: Roentgenographic, Neurologic, and Somatosensory Evoked Potential Studies." *Journal of Pediatrics,* Vol. 110, 1987, 515–521.

Pueschel, S.M., et al. "Symptomatic Atlantoaxial-axial Subluxation in Persons with Down Syndrome." *Journal of Pediatric Orthopedics,* Vol. 4, 1984, 682–688.

Pueschel, S.M., et al. "Atlantoaxial Instability in Children with Down Syndrome." *Pediatric Radiology,* Vol. 10, 1981, 129–132.

Pueschel, S.M., et al. "A Longitudinal Study of Atlantoaxial-Dens Relationship in Asymptomatic Individuals with Down Syndrome." *Pediatrics,* 1992, 1194–1197.

11 | Children with Down Syndrome and Leukemia

Pedro de Alarcon, M.D.

Children with Down syndrome are about twenty times more likely than other children to develop leukemia, a cancer of the blood system. Although this only amounts to about one in one thousand children with Down syndrome, this is little consolation if your child happens to be among that number. Fortunately, leukemia is more survivable now than ever before, with cure rates around 70 to 80 percent. With aggressive and early treatment, more children than ever before are being cured of leukemia and going on to live normal, healthy lives.

If your child is diagnosed with leukemia, her treatment will likely last several years and go through several phases. Her Down syndrome will affect her treatment. This chapter explains what leukemia is, how it is diagnosed, and how it is treated in children with Down syndrome. The goal: to make you a knowledgeable consumer of the medical services your child will need during this time.

What is Leukemia?

Leukemia is a type of cancer. A cancer is a tumor (a mass or lump of tissue) made up of cells from the body that are growing "out of control." In cancer, the normal processes that guide and control growth and development fail, and the cells multiply rapidly. These cells then interfere with how "normal" cells work. In leukemia, the cancer cells are abnormal blood cells.

Table 1: Characteristics of children with ALL at the time of diagnosis.

Characteristics, signs, and symptoms	Percent of children with these characteristics
Lethargy/malaise	37%
Fever/infection	32%
Pain in joints/extremities	23%
Bleeding	18%
Loss of appetite	10%
Abdominal pain	7%
Symptoms of leukemia in brain	2%
Physical findings	
Pallor	27%
Enlarged liver/spleen	27%
Bruising	18%
Swollen glands	9%

Adapted from Sallan and Weinstein in *Hematology of Infancy and Childhood* (W.B. Saunders Company, 1987).

There are many kinds of blood cells, including red and white blood cells. Most blood cells begin their formation and development in the bone marrow (the spongy material in the middle of the hip, arms, legs, and other bones). When leukemia occurs, some blood cells grow abnormally. Although there are several different types of leukemia, they all share many features. The exact variety of leukemia, however, depends on the type of blood cells that become cancerous and when in the blood cell development process they begin to grow out of control. Leukemia cells can be found in almost all types of blood cells and in blood all over the body. In most cases, leukemia cells grow faster than normal cells, and, consequently, may crowd out the normal cells. Because leukemia cells are not as developed as normal cells, they do not function as well in fighting infection. If left untreated, leukemia can destroy both the blood's ability to fight infection and its ability to deliver oxygen to the body.

Leukemias are classified in several ways. First, they are categorized as being either *acute* or *chronic* leukemias. Acute leukemias progress very quickly and, before there was effective treatment, tended to cause death in a very short period of time (a few months). Chronic leukemias progress more slowly and, before there was effective treatment, typically caused death in years rather than months.

All leukemias produce similar symptoms. These symptoms may appear suddenly or may come on slowly. They may be serious, like a life-threatening systemic (affecting the entire body) infection or hemorrhage, or there may be no symptoms at all. Most commonly, parents consult a doctor when their child has been tired and hasn't felt well for two to six weeks. The child may run a fever, look pale, bruise easily, or have obvious hemorrhages, like nosebleeds. Her stomach may look swollen because of a large liver or a large spleen. Some children complain of joint or bone pains. A few children have swollen glands. There may also be signs in the blood that laboratory tests can detect. Table 1 shows some of the changes that may be detected by laboratory tests.

The Diagnosis of Leukemia

If your child is suspected of having leukemia, she will be referred to a *pediatric oncologist*, a physician who has special knowledge of childhood cancers. Diagnosis and treatment by a qualified physician is critical to your child's survival; avoid "alternative" therapists who may promise cures through herbs, spinal adjustments, or diet.

Formal diagnostic tests for leukemia require examination of the bone marrow—the soft tissue inside the bones where most blood cells are made. The marrow is usually taken from the back of the hip or *pelvic* bone. The doctor first numbs the area with local anesthesia so that your child will not feel the needle. Then a needle is pushed into the bone and, using a syringe, bone marrow is drawn out, much like a blood test. In a

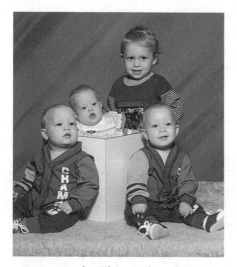

person without leukemia, this procedure is not very painful and is very quick. It only hurts for about one second (or not at all) when the marrow is being drawn out. Unfortunately, in a child with leukemia, the bone marrow is full of leukemia cells. When this occurs, there is less fluid in the marrow space, and it takes longer to get an adequate sample. This makes the process more difficult, time-consuming, and painful.

The specimens removed from the bone marrow are examined in the pathology lab. They are first carefully prepared to allow viewing under a microscope. Using special stains that mark only certain kinds of cells or certain parts of cells, the pathologist (a physician who specializes in using laboratory techniques to diagnose diseases) works with the oncologist to decide which kind of leukemia is present. Bone marrow samples are also used after diagnosis to help determine the success of treatment by making sure that all the leukemia cells are gone.

Another test used in the diagnosis of leukemia is called a *spinal tap* or *lumbar puncture (LP)*. To do this test, a very thin needle is inserted between the lower vertebrae (the bones that make up the backbone) to sample some of the fluid that surrounds the spinal cord and brain. At the lower part of the back where this test is done, the spinal cord has ended and split into thinner nerves. A needle can safely be placed here with very small risk of damaging any nerves.

Although a spinal tap is much less painful than a bone marrow test, your child might be very frightened by all that happens. The test requires your child to be still in a position very bent at the waist until the needle has been removed. Your doctor may use a local anesthetic to numb the skin before inserting the long spinal needle. Sometimes sedation is used to help calm the patient, especially if she is very frightened.

The spinal fluid that is removed is sent to the pathology lab for testing. A microscope is used to look for leukemia cells. This information helps determine how far the leukemia has spread. Spinal taps are also used during and after treatment to make sure the leukemia cells do not return.

To reduce the discomfort, some doctors give sedation to make your child sleepy, in addition to local anesthesia. If sedation is going to be used, the doctors should have the appropriate facilities to watch your child carefully. This will involve carefully monitoring her rate of breathing, heart rate, blood pressure, and the amount of oxygen in the blood while she is sedated. These precautions are very important because too much sedation can cause a child to stop breathing. Sedated children should be watched until fully awake again.

Types of Leukemia

Two types of leukemia are especially common in childhood. These are *acute lymphoblastic leukemia* (ALL) and *acute myeloid* or *myeloblastic leukemia* (AML). Among children with Down syndrome, ALL is more common in older children (over one year of age), and AML is more common in younger children (under one year of age). Young children with Down syndrome may also develop a condition called *transient myeloproliferative disorder* or *transient leukemia,* which mimics AML, producing similar symptoms, but is not really a leukemia at all. Determining which type of cancer your child has is very important, because the treatment for each is different.

Acute Lymphoblastic Leukemia (ALL)

Acute lymphoblastic leukemia is so-named because it is characterized by the rapid growth of lymphocytes in the blood. Lymphocytes are one of the types of white blood cells that fight infection. ALL is the most common form of cancer seen in children. Approximately 2000 children are diagnosed with ALL in the U.S.A. each year. In most children with ALL, the disease usually appears between ages 2 and 6.

Until the early 1960s, ALL was always fatal. With today's intensive treatment methods, however, about seventy percent of children with ALL can now be cured. Although some studies have indicated a slightly lower cure rate for children with Down syndrome, other studies have shown that the cure rate is just as high in children with Down syndrome, as long as they receive intensive treatment.

Treating ALL. The treatment of ALL begins soon after diagnosis. The first step is to get your child both physically and mentally ready for treatment. To prepare psychologically, it is important that your child and family understand the diagnosis and the treatment. You may want to talk to other families about what to expect by making contact with one of the groups described in the section on Family Support Groups and Services. You should also feel free to ask your doctor questions and to gather information from any member of your child's treatment team.

To help prepare your child psychologically for treatment, there are several things you can do. First, prepare yourself so that your level of stress is controlled and you do not frighten your child. To do this, learn as much as you can about the treatment your child will receive. Second, talk to your child about what will be happening. Describe who she will encounter, where she will go, and what will happen. Third, take your child to the hospital to show her the oncology department. It reduces fear to have a visual image of the place before your visit. Last, introduce your child to children with leukemia.

To prepare your child physically for treatment, doctors will take several steps to help her eliminate waste products from her blood. This is because treatment is designed to kill fast growing cells such as leukemia cells; however, it is not possible to kill only leukemia cells. Consequently, both leukemia and normal cells will be killed, creating a large amount of waste. Therefore, good hydration—lots of fluids—is important. It is also important for your child to begin taking a medicine called *allopurinol*. This helps clear away a waste product called *uric acid*. Doctors will also try to bring your child's blood chemistry and blood cell counts to as close to normal as possible. If your child is very low on red blood cells (the cells that carry oxygen from the lungs to the rest of the body), she may therefore receive a transfusion of red blood cells. If she is bruising and bleeding and has a low platelet count (the cells that stop bleeding), she may receive a transfusion of platelets.

The actual treatment for ALL usually consists primarily of chemotherapy. In chemotherapy, your child will be given medicines that act as poisons to fast-growing cells such as leukemia cells. There are a wide variety of medicines used, depending on the type of leukemia and the stage of the treatment. For example, your child may receive medicine orally, intravenously, or by injection into the spinal canal or into muscle. As explained below, bone marrow transplants are also occasionally used in treatment. How your child's chemotherapy is conducted may vary depending on the medical center where she is being treated. In general, however, treatment lasts $2\frac{1}{2}$ to 3 years and consists of these phases:

- induction;
- central nervous system (CNS) therapy (treating leukemia in the brain);
- intensification; and
- maintenance (see Figure 1).

Induction therapy is started as soon as possible after diagnosis. It generally takes place with your child in the hospital, but as treatment progresses it may be given on an outpatient basis. Intensification therapy is also started in the hospital, but, like induction therapy, may become outpatient therapy.

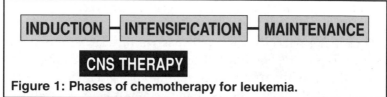

Figure 1: Phases of chemotherapy for leukemia.

Maintenance therapy, which continues for the longest time, is usually an outpatient treatment. Some parents ask why treatment is spaced out over phases. This is because it is too toxic to give all the drugs used to treat leukemia at once.

Induction therapy is the beginning of treatment. Its goal is to kill most of the leukemia cells. It lasts four weeks and uses a combination of three or four drugs. Most induction treatments include prednisone, vincristine, and L-asparaginase. Other drugs such as adriamycin or dounamycin may be added, depending on the intensity of the treatment. They too kill leukemia cells, but they act at different points of the cell growth cycle. At the end of induction treatment, the bone marrow test is repeated to see whether a *remission* has been achieved. A remission is a disappearance of all signs and symptoms of leukemia. It does not necessarily mean that your child is cured, but rather that the leukemia cannot be detected. About 98 percent of children with ALL achieve a remission at some point in their treatment.

Most cancer treatment centers now include an intensification phase following induction treatment. The goal of this phase is to kill the leukemia cells that remain after the induction phase. The drugs used during this phase will be different from those used during induction. Some of the drugs used are methotrexate, 6–mercaptopurine (6MP), adriamycin, dounamycin, cytosine arabinoside, and cyclophosphamide.

Central nervous system (CNS) therapy is given during both the induction and intensification phases if leukemia is present in the brain or if there is a risk it will spread to the brain (depending on how early the leukemia is caught). It may consist only of chemotherapy, or may combine chemotherapy and radiation therapy. The chemotherapy is given directly into the fluid that bathes the brain or into the spinal fluid. To do this, a lumbar puncture or spinal tap test is done. A sample of the fluid is taken to look for leukemic cells. Chemotherapy with one, two, or three drugs is then given through the same needle. The drugs used are methotrexate, cytosine arabinoside, and hydrocortisone.

Some children will also receive radiation therapy to the brain if their risk of CNS leukemia is high. Radiation therapy to the spine may also be used if leukemia in the central nervous system is present at diagnosis or appears during treatment. Radiation therapy consists of small, focused doses of x-rays to the brain which kill the leukemia cells and also damage other cells in the central nervous system.

Maintenance therapy begins at the end of these three phases of therapy. By this point, most of the cancer cells have been killed by one or another of the treatments, but there may still be a few leukemia cells alive. A different group of medicines is used to help your child's body "finish off" the remaining cancer. In maintenance therapy, there are more choices in the drugs to be used, and there are usually fewer side effects. As a result, this therapy is not as physically taxing on children as induction or intensification therapies. Oral medications are usually used, but sometimes drugs are given by injection and intravenously. In general, maintenance therapy lasts a long time, usually for months. In some centers, a second round of intensive therapy (*re-intensification*) may be given a few months later and then maintenance treatment is restarted. Continuing treatment for more than three years is not useful. On the contrary, it tends to increase the side effects of therapy.

Effects of Treatment on Children with Down Syndrome.
Children with Down syndrome are especially prone to complications of leukemia therapy. These include:

- infection—chemotherapy kills normal white blood cells as it kills leukemia cells, leaving the body less able to fight off infection;
- high blood sugar from L-asparaginase treatment—high blood sugar can lead to diabetes and dehydration which can then delay chemotherapy;
- *mucositis,* or an irritation of the lining of the bowel and mouth, resulting in ulcers. This irritation is generally caused by methotrexate, which is the backbone of maintenance therapy (and is sometimes used in intensification therapy). The drug causes particular problems for children with Down syndrome because they do not metabolize and excrete the drug as well as other children do. Unfortunately, it is a very effective drug against ALL and is one of the most important drugs used for treatment. If treatment will include high doses of this medicine, it is important that you be aware that extra precautions are needed, and that the dose of this medicine must be controlled carefully. Folate—a salt derivative of folic acid (part of the B vitamin complex)—can be given to help revive nonleukemia cells after methotrexate treatment.

At the end of treatment, most children with ALL will be cured. More specifically, about 60 to 70 percent of children with Down syndrome will be cured, provided their treatment includes an intensification phase. This success rate is one of the landmarks in the fight against cancer; only thirty years ago *all* children with this disease died.

Doctors are still not certain why some children with leukemia are cured and others are not, but we have learned that there are certain characteristics present at the time of diagnosis that affect chances for recovery. We call these *prognostic signs* or *indicators*. We know that if a child gets ALL at birth or during the first year of life, the prognosis is worse. If she gets ALL when she is more than ten years old, her prognosis is also worse. Another important prognostic sign is the total white blood cell count; if it is very high—over 50,000—the prognosis is worse. Some other prognostic signs: Girls tend to do better than boys, as do children who do not have obvious leukemia in their spinal fluid. As the intensity of chemotherapy has increased, many of the prognostic signs have become less reliable. Doctors use them now to select patients to get less intensive chemotherapy (if their prognostic signs are good) or more intensive therapy (if their prognostic signs are bad).

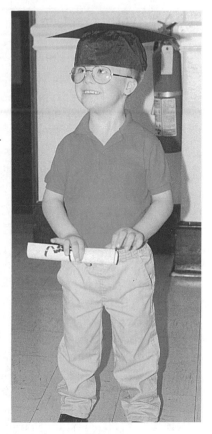

Acute Myeloid Leukemia (AML)

Acute myeloid leukemia (AML)—also known as acute non-lymphocytic leukemia (ANLL)—is the second most common form of leukemia in children. Myeloid cells in the blood, the granulocytes and monocytes, are another type of white blood cells (like the lymphoid cells) and are part of the body's immune system. They perform several jobs in helping to fight infections. In the past, it was believed that this leukemia was the most common among children with Down syndrome, but studies have since shown that ALL is more common. Children

Table 2: Types of acute myeloid leukemia (AML).	
Type	**Description**
M1	Myeloid granulocytic *(immature)* leukemia
M2	Myeloid granulocytic *(with some maturation)* leukemia
M3	Acute promyelocytic leukemia
M4	Acute myelomonocytic leukemia
M5	Acute monocytic or monoblastic leukemia
M6	Acute erythroid *(red blood cell)* leukemia
M7	Acute megakaryocytic *(platelet)* leukemia

with Down syndrome generally develop AML at a younger age than other children do. Most children with Down syndrome and AML are less than four years old, and many develop symptoms in the newborn period or the first year of life.

There are seven different types of AML, called M1 through M7 (see Table 2). The different names refer to the different phases of cell development when cancer begins and to the type of cell that would have resulted if development had continued normally. Names ending in *-cyte,* such as monocyte or granulocyte, refer to the fully mature cell of a certain type. When *-blast* is used (such as monoblast), the cells are very early in their development. The different types of AML are:

- M1—acute myeloblastic leukemia, with very immature cells (myeloblasts) that would have become granulocytes if they had developed normally;
- M2—acute myeloblastic leukemia, like M1, but with some slightly more mature cells mixed in with the immature cells;
- M3—*acute promyelocytic leukemia* (APL). Promyelocytes are also destined to become granulocytes, and are more mature than myeloblasts;
- M4—a mixture of granulocytes and monocytes (a monocyte is another type of developing white blood

cell). This type of leukemia is also known as acute *myelomonocytic leukemia* (AMMoL);

- M5—*acute monoblastic or monocytic leukemia* (AMoL);
- M6—*acute erythroid,* or red cell, leukemia, that affects the red blood cells;
- M7—*acute megakaryocytic leukemia* (AMKL) (*megakaryocytes* are the cells in the bone marrow that make platelets—the cells that stop bleeding; think of this leukemia as platelet leukemia).

All versions of AML are lumped together under the same diagnosis because children with these leukemias have about the same symptoms and prognosis and are treated with the same kinds of therapy. In addition, the symptoms of AML closely resemble those of ALL. It is only by doing special tests on the bone marrow that ALL can be distinguished from AML, and the specific type of AML identified.

Treatment of AML in children who do *not* have Down syndrome is less successful than it is with ALL. Although the cure rate for ALL increased in the 1960s and 1970s, it stayed the same for AML. During this time, only 15 to 20 percent of the children with AML could be cured. The lack of success at achieving remission was the same for children with Down syndrome and children without Down syndrome. As a result, the therapy for AML in children was intensified and the rates of remission have improved. Two major forms of intensive therapy evolved for AML, bone marrow transplantation (BMT) and intensive chemotherapy. With these forms of therapy, long-term survival and cure rates are around 45 to 50 percent of children with AML.

Recent studies have shown that children with AML and Down syndrome have a higher survival rate than other children. The survival rate overall is better than 80 percent for children with Down syndrome and AML, compared to only 45 percent in other children with AML. Clearly the children with Down syndrome are responding better to therapy than chil-

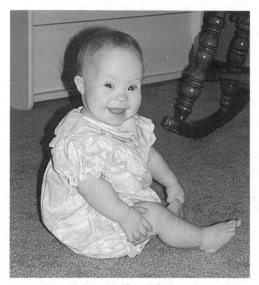

dren without Down syndrome. Research is attempting to understand why.

Treating AML. The first task in treating AML is to confirm the diagnosis. AML can appear to be another condition, *transient myeloproliferative disorder,* also called transient leukemia, which is discussed below. The symptoms are quite similar. The two conditions, however, are treated very differently. So, it is important to first make sure your child has AML and not transient leukemia. Once a diagnosis of AML is confirmed, treatment should be started immediately.

Intensive therapy is very important to treating AML. As with ALL, induction therapy is not enough. Most chemotherapy is given for one to two weeks every month in the hospital as part of a treatment plan that continues for one to two years. The treatments are often associated with serious complications, especially infection. This is because the drugs used are stronger than those used in treating ALL in order to kill the myeloid cells which are more resistant to treatment.

The treatment for AML is changing rapidly as more is learned, but it is clear that intensive therapy is needed. With intensive therapy, children with AML and Down syndrome have an 80 percent chance of good response. Still, some questions persist. For example, 15 percent of children with AML develop leukemia in their brain, yet we do not know what effect CNS therapy has on curing AML. We also do not know if maintenance therapy is necessary for AML. Further research will help improve the treatment of AML.

There are other treatments for AML, such as bone marrow transplants (BMT). Although BMT is a reasonable treatment option for children with AML, chemotherapy has been so effective that the relative merits of the two different therapies must be carefully weighed. BMT is discussed below.

Transient Myeloproliferative Disorder

A blood disorder called *transient myeloproliferative disorder,* or transient leukemia, is found almost exclusively in children with Down syndrome. Most children with transient leukemia get better spontaneously; transient leukemia does not require treatment. Some children with Down syndrome who have transient leukemia, however, develop AML later on. One study found that about 20 percent of children with transient leukemia developed another leukemia later in life. Another study found that 50 percent of the children with leukemia and Down syndrome had transient leukemia before developing AML. Consequently, it is important that children with transient leukemia be carefully monitored for the development of AML later.

As mentioned above, transient leukemia looks like AML. Because AML requires very intensive chemotherapy, it is vital to distinguish between AML and transient leukemia. This is not easy. It is still not possible to separate these conditions except by observing how they progress in a patient. There are some aspects of the symptoms and some kinds of laboratory tests that may help. These are, however, only suggestive. They cannot identify all children with these conditions. If a child with AML-like symptoms is older than one, she is more likely to have AML and not transient leukemia. Conversely, if the child is a newborn, transient leukemia is more likely. There are a variety of other characteristics that can indicate whether your child has AML or transient leukemia. No test or symptom, however, is absolute. Consequently, a period of observation and treatment of just symptoms is necessary for all infants with leukemia and Down syndrome, unless there are life-threatening complications that require the start of therapy right away.

Bone Marrow Transplants

Bone marrow transplants (BMTs) are used to treat some leukemias. BMT has been successful in curing a variety of leukemias, including AML, ALL, and chronic myeloid leukemia (a type of leukemia that is no more common in children with Down syndrome than in other people). Between AML and ALL, BMT has different success rates. BMT has a success rate of curing AML of about 60 to 70 percent. It is not used in treating ALL unless all other therapies have failed. However, in spite of the seriousness of the procedure and the risk of complications, BMT is the treatment of choice when ALL recurs while a patient is receiving chemotherapy or shortly after. In some patients with ALL and very poor prognostic signs (discussed above) who have achieved remission, BMT may be considered as the initial form of therapy instead of chemotherapy. For AML, if a matched sibling donor is available, BMT may be the therapy of choice. After chemotherapy, if AML comes back and a second remission can be obtained, BMT is the therapy of choice.

Bone marrow transplants take several forms, depending on who is the donor. A BMT can be autologous, allogeneic, or syngeneic. In an *autologous* BMT, your child receives her own treated bone marrow. In a *syngeneic* BMT, the marrow donor is an identical twin of the recipient. All other BMTs are *allogeneic*; that is, they come from a matched sibling, a parent, a relative, or an unrelated person.

BMTs can be matched or mismatched. In a matched BMT, the donor and the recipient have the same genes; autologous and syngeneic BMTs are matched. Almost all allogeneic BMTs are mismatched; that is, there are slight differences in genes that influence acceptance or rejection of the transplant. This means that even though the bone marrow of an unrelated donor can be a very close match, it is still a mismatched transplant. Mismatched BMT is generally not as effective as matched BMT.

The major concerns about treating a child who has leukemia with a bone marrow transplant are: 1) rejection of the transplanted bone marrow; 2) graft versus host disease (GVHD); 3) infection; 4) pneumonia; and 5) recurrence of the leukemia. Rejection of the bone marrow occurs when the body does not accept the new bone marrow. To have a successful BMT, the recipient's bone marrow must be killed. The immune system needs to be suppressed (using chemotherapy and radiation) so that the new bone marrow will be accepted. Thanks to chemotherapy and radiation therapy, rejection of bone marrow is not common except when the match is very poor.

Graft versus host disease (GVHD) is the opposite of the body's rejection of the transplanted bone marrow. In GVHD, the transplanted bone marrow rejects the body and begins to attack it. The organs most commonly affected by GVHD are the skin, the liver, and the bowel. However, other organs, particularly the lungs, can be affected. The greater the mismatch, the more likely and the more serious GVHD is. It is one of the causes of serious complications, and even death, following a BMT.

Patients who receive a bone marrow transplant have a high risk of serious infection, due to the drugs needed to suppress the immune system and from chemotherapy, radiation therapy, and GVHD. The risk is greatest just after the BMT, but it lasts for a long time. Pneumonia can be a very serious complication of BMT. Finally, leukemia can recur after a BMT, and represents a large portion of the failures of BMT in the treatment of leukemia.

A successful BMT requires careful balancing. Many of the complications of BMT are interrelated. Sometimes what is done to improve *engraftment*—the acceptance of the new bone marrow—may increase the risk of GVHD or infection. Efforts to decrease the frequency and severity of GVHD may increase the chances of rejecting the bone marrow, of infection, or of recurrence of leukemia. All of these risks need to be considered as each child's BMT is planned.

BMT is well tolerated by children with Down syndrome, but some side effects, such as GVHD or growth failure, may be more serious. All of these factors need to be considered while making the decision to undergo BMT.

BMTs are usually done in centers that specialize in this procedure where there are oncologists who specialize in BMTs. BMTs are very difficult and complicated procedures that generally include three parts. First, all of the bone marrow of the patient must be killed. This requires very heavy chemical doses and can be very unpleasant. Next, bone marrow from the donor is harvested and prepared for transplant. Last, the donor's bone marrow is injected into the recipient's blood intravenously. The most difficult part of a BMT is killing the recipient's bone marrow. The actual transplant is quite simple and does not require anesthesia.

Cancer Treatment Centers

It is very important that a child with leukemia be treated by a *pediatric oncologist*, a physician who has special knowledge of childhood cancers. Treatment should be carried out at a center that has experience in this area. Once the diagnosis is confirmed and the therapy started, some of the treatments may be given by other specialists, such as a pediatric cancer specialist not working at a center, or a pediatrician. In each case, however, the specialist will be under the supervision of the pediatric oncologist. For children with Down syndrome and leukemia, this is even more important because of the special concerns.

There are many centers that provide cancer treatment. Some are connected with universities or hospitals, and some are freestanding centers, such as Saint Jude's Children's Research Center in Memphis, Tennessee and Sloan Kettering Memorial Hospital in New York City. Your child's oncologist should be able to discuss the choices with you.

Family Support Groups and Services

Childhood leukemia causes tremendous fear, worry, and stress. Fortunately, there are groups that can provide the emotional support needed during this time. Most treatment centers have two types of parent organizations that support children and families affected by leukemia. Candlelighters is a national association with local chapters in most centers treating children with cancer and in the communities surrounding the centers. They provide literature and support groups for both families and children.

Centers will also have social workers, psychologists, and psychiatrists on their staff. A social worker can provide both emotional support and assistance with economic and social issues that arise when a child has a serious, long-term illness. Families can also tap the services of the center's staff psychologist or psychiatrist.

Leukemia Research

Children with Down syndrome have approximately twenty times the risk of developing childhood leukemia compared to other children. Scientists are researching why this is. Is there a connection between the extra chromosomal material present in children with Down syndrome and leukemia? Scientists suspect that trisomy 21 plays a role in increasing the risk of leukemia, but there is no clear evidence yet.

The science of molecular biology has given scientists the ability to isolate the genes that cause specific conditions, and to identify the genes responsible for specific characteristics. Everyone has genes in their cells, called *proto-oncogenes,* which can make some kinds of cancer more likely under some circumstances. Researchers have discovered that some of these are located in the same area of chromosome 21 that controls Down syndrome characteristics. Scientists have found that putting excess copies of one of these genes into normal cells can cause normal cells to grow out of control. This does not mean that scientists have discovered the gene that makes children with Down syndrome more prone to leukemia, but it does suggest a link that should be closely investigated.

Summary

Children with Down syndrome frequently have abnormalities in their blood and immune systems. In particular, they have a twenty-fold increased risk of leukemia during some part of their childhood. They are, however, no more likely than other children to develop other forms of cancer.

Early in life, children with Down syndrome may develop transient myeloproliferative disorder, or transient leukemia, a condition that is similar to leukemia but that goes away by itself. Although most children with this disorder recover, twenty percent of them eventually develop leukemia.

Recent developments in genetics have identified an area of chromosome 21 that determines the physical characteristics of Down syndrome. This area also contains a type of gene called a proto-oncogene. The study of these proto-oncogenes and that section of the chromosome 21 may soon help us to understand why children with Down syndrome have an increased risk of leukemia and other blood conditions.

ALL is the most common leukemia of childhood and is the most common leukemia in older children with Down syndrome. Tremendous progress has been made in the treatment of this disease, and today seventy percent of children with ALL have a prolonged remission and may be cured. Children with Down syndrome and ALL need to be treated with intensive therapy. With this intensive therapy the response to treatment is as good as for other children but the side effects are greater. In particular, children with Down syndrome have problems with one of the drugs used in chemotherapy, methotrexate, and special attention must be paid when this drug is used.

AML is the most common leukemia in infants with Down syndrome. AML needs to be distinguished from transient leukemia. Children with Down syndrome have a predisposition to develop a particular type of AML called M7 or megakaryocytic leukemia. Progress in the treatment of AML in children has been slow, but the use of intensive therapy or bone marrow transplants during the past five years has improved survival rates. Children with Down syndrome tolerate chemotherapy for AML as well as other children, and they respond very well to treatment. While about 45 percent of children with AML who don't have Down syndrome have a prolonged remission and may be cured, 80 percent of children with Down syndrome can have a prolonged remission and hopefully a cure of their leukemias. Bone marrow transplantation (BMT) is another way of treating AML. It is the treatment of choice when the leukemia recurs after chemotherapy.

A child with Down syndrome diagnosed with leukemia should receive treatment at a medical center that specializes in the treatment of children with cancer. These centers provide not only medical care, but also the emotional and psychological support needed by the child and the family during the treatment process. In addition, by sharing information these specialized medical centers play a major role in developing increasingly effective therapies for the treatment of children with cancer.

References

Arenson, E.B. & Forde, M.D. "Bone Marrow Transplantation for Acute Leukemia and Down Syndrome: Report of a Successful Case and Results of a National Survey." *Journal of Pediatrics*, Vol. 114, 1989, 69–72.

Miller, R.W. "Neoplasia and Down's Syndrome." *Annals of the New York Academy of Science,* Vol. 171, 1970, 637–643.

Ragab, A.H., et al., "Clinical Characteristics and Treatment Outcome of Children with Acute Lymphocytic Leukemia and Down's Syndrome." *Cancer,* Vol. 67, 1991), 1057–1063.

Rowley, J.D. "Down Syndrome and Acute Leukaemia: Increased Risk May Be Due to Trisomy 21." *Lancet,* 1981, 1020–1022.

Sallan, S.E. and Weinstein, H.J. "Childhood Acute Leukemia," in Nathan and Oski, *Hematology of Infancy and Childhood*, 3rd edition (New York: WB Saunders Company, 1987), 1028–1055.

Zipursky A., et al., "Canadian Down Syndrome Leukemia Registry. Myelodysplasia (MDS) and Acute Megakaryoblastic Leukemia (AMKL) in Down Syndrome." Department of Pediatrics, The Hospital for Sick Children and the Department of Pathology, University of Toronto, Toronto, Ontario, Canada. *Proceedings of ASPHO*, Vol. 1, 1992, 24–26.

Zipursky, A., et al., "Megakaryoblastic Leukemia in Children: A Review of Oncology and Immunology in Down Syndrome." *Progress in Clinical Biology Research,* Vol. 246, 1987, 33–56.

12 | Dental Concerns of Children with Down Syndrome

Arthur J. Nowak, DMD

Introduction

The mouth has many functions. It is the primary entry point for nutrition that allows us to develop and grow in our early years, and for maintenance and energy in our adult years. We use the mouth to produce sounds associated with pleasure and unhappiness, and for the speech we use to communicate with others. Facial expressions, produced by various movements of the lips and muscles, assist us in our social interactions with others. All of these functions require a mouth free of disease, a mouth that functions without pain or discomfort, and a mouth that is clean of debris and free of odor.

Children with Down syndrome often have unique differences in their mouths and teeth. These include smaller jaws with possibly increased tongue size, and delayed tooth eruption. In addition, there are several dental problems that are more common in children with Down syndrome than in other children, including gum disease and enamel abnormalities. This chapter explains the differences and problems that affect children with Down syndrome, and explains their treatment.

Appropriate and early oral hygiene and care are essential for children with Down syndrome. The differences they can have make them more vulnerable than other children to dental disease. Preventative care, therefore, is very important. Poor oral and dental health can harm your child's development and education. Dental cavities and abscesses can be very painful, may be very distracting for your child, and may cause school absence. This chapter reviews the best methods for dental care for your child, and explains how to find good dental care.

Obtaining good dental care that is tailored to your child's specific needs can be challenging. Often, there is a lack of health care providers trained to recognize people who have a higher risk for dental disease. This can lead to missing the early signs of problems. A crevice in a tooth that traps food can lead to a cavity; if not dealt with appropriately, the cavity may enlarge and develop into an abscess. For optimal preventive care, it is important that children who are at risk of problems get early dental care. Children with Down syndrome as a group probably are at increased risk of infection and inflammation, and may not be able to manage their personal dental care as well as other children can.

Parents sometimes do not seek early dental care for their child with Down syndrome. This may be because their efforts to cope with a multitude of other medical, social, financial, and emotional issues may crowd out concerns about dental care. Concern about teeth can too easily be left to the future. In addition, oral health can be assigned a low priority by physicians and insurance companies.

Another barrier to effective oral health care may the behavior of your child in the dentist's office. Your child's age, cognitive ability, and level of anxiety, along with inexperienced dentists and staff, can make good dental care nearly impossible. Too often parents are told to return when their child is older or can "behave" in the office. This results in delays not only in the start of professional dental care, but also in teaching parents the daily dental care they need to provide for their child at home.

Oral and Dental Development

To understand the differences in the teeth of children with Down syndrome, it helps to understand oral and dental development in general.

Oral Development

Children with Down syndrome grow more slowly than do other children, and this slower growth affects the growth of the face and head. Several facial features are linked to Down syndrome. Often, the jaws and palate are smaller, and frequently the lower jaw comes too far forward, contributing to poor alignment of the jaws. The size, surface, and position of the tongue may also be different. Controversy continues about the relative size of the tongue. Some doctors believe that the tongue is larger than normal; while others believe that the tongue is normal in size but that the oral cavity (the inside of the mouth) is smaller, forcing the tongue out of the mouth. The tongue is often more furrowed, creating crevices that retain food and plaque. Retained food may foster bacteria growth and contribute to bad breath, but probably does not have any other health effects.

Children with Down syndrome may also have dry mouths *(xerostomia)*. Although some studies show reduced saliva flow, the dryness is most likely due to an open mouth and mouth breathing. In addition, the lips of children with Down syndrome may be badly fissured and dry, leading to splitting, bleeding, inflammation, and discomfort. These conditions are so common that they are almost expected in people with Down syndrome. Treating dry and inflamed lips is discussed in Chapter 7. Children with Down syndrome also have a higher incidence of clefting of the soft palate, which can affect swallowing and the sound of speech. Usually there is no special treatment for the clefting, although in the worst cases surgery may be necessary.

Dental Development

Both the primary ("baby") and permanent teeth begin to develop before your child is born, and complete their development as he grows. Studies of tooth development in unborn babies have shown that the primary teeth begin to form at about 6 weeks, while permanent teeth begin to form at about 12 weeks after conception. Studies have not been done specifically for babies with Down syndrome, so it is not known if this is any different for them.

In most children, teeth usually emerge in a predictable sequence. The lower front teeth erupt first, and are followed by the upper front teeth; later the teeth toward the back of the mouth appear. The ages when these events happen are extremely variable. The first tooth appears anywhere from 4–6 months of age out to 28–30 months. In children with Down syndrome, the range is also wide but a bit delayed, ranging from 12–18 months out to 30–48 months for first tooth eruptions.

Once tooth eruption starts, children with Down syndrome have no unusual teething problems, although the sequence of emergence is often different from other children. For instance, your child's upper teeth may show up first, then some teeth toward the back, followed at last by the lower teeth. In addition, there is also a higher prevalence of congenitally (congenital means that a condition is present at birth) missing primary or permanent teeth, misshapen teeth that may have extra points or cusps, or teeth that are much smaller than normal.

Irregularities of the enamel surface of teeth are also quite common, appearing as discolored pits of varying sizes. Not only can these teeth be unattractive, they can also retain food and plaque that cause tooth breakdown.

With the delayed eruption of teeth there can also be a delay in the loss of the primary teeth. If the primary teeth do not fall out, they can block the space where the permanent teeth go. This can cause the permanent teeth to erupt in the wrong position and result in crooked teeth. Sometimes baby teeth actually wear away to nothing instead of being pushed out by the erupting permanent teeth; at other times they may need to be removed to make room. No tooth should be removed until it is certain that there will be a permanent replacement.

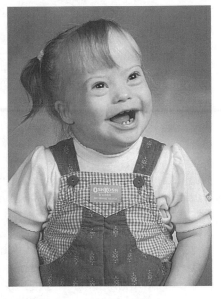

Dental Disease

The two most common diseases that affect teeth and surrounding tissues are cavities, whose medical name is *caries,* and *periodontal,* or gum, disease. Both diseases can affect children with Down syndrome.

Many studies have found that children with Down syndrome actually have fewer caries but more gum disease than do other people. The experience of dentists seems to verify this finding, although cavities and gum disease can vary from person to person.

It is difficult to determine the reason for the lower incidence of cavities in children with Down syndrome. Dentists are not sure whether the low incidence of caries is due to the late eruption of teeth, differences in the immune system, diet, daily oral hygiene, frequency of missing teeth, mouth breathing, or differences in saliva or salivary flow.

The need for good oral health care increases with age. Doctors are learning that people with Down syndrome between the ages of 20 and 48 have significantly more dental disease than do younger people with Down syndrome. As a generation of children with Down syndrome who have received good dental care grows, the incidence of dental disease may decline. That is why good dental care and hygiene now is so important.

Early Intervention

As with most diseases, early intervention can interrupt the process of dental disease and prevent it from causing more serious injury. Because children with Down syndrome have a higher risk of oral and facial disorders, they should see a dentist shortly after their first teeth appear. If no teeth have erupted, the first visit should be at or before one year of age.

Some general practice dentists are more comfortable than others with patients who have special needs. A specialist in dentistry called a *pediatric dentist* has additional training and experience with children who have special needs, and can provide more comprehensive, ongoing, state-of-the-art dental care. The office staff of a pediatric dentist will likely be knowledgeable about and comfortable with children who have special needs. All of this can contribute to a positive dental experience for you and your child.

Your child's first dental appointment has four major goals:

1. To review the special oral-facial and dental characteristics of your child;
2. To discuss the process that leads to cavities and gum disease;
3. To examine your child; and
4. To talk with you about beginning a comprehensive preventive care program that you can follow.

You will learn how to clean your child's teeth and gums. If no treatment is required, a schedule of future visits will be arranged. More about dental visits is discussed below.

Dental Care

Good dental care involves many elements, including toothbrushing, anti-cavity treatments, diet, sealants, mouthwashes and rinses, and dental visits. This section reviews all the parts of good dental care.

Toothbrushing

The major cause of dental disease is a film of bacteria and debris that forms on teeth. It is called *dental plaque* and is made up of a complex network of bacteria and food. Acid that is produced in the plaque by the bacteria as they digest food softens enamel and irritates the tissue surrounding the teeth. As the enamel softens, the tooth erodes, causing a "cavity" to form. The irritation of the gums is the periodontal disease mentioned before. Good oral health requires the regular removal of plaque and bacteria; this disrupts the production of acid.

Brushing and flossing remove plaque. Both activities require manual dexterity and an understanding of the shape and position of teeth. Most children master these activities as they age and develop good coordination of the muscles of their hands, arms, and mouth, while learning daily routines from their family. Children with Down syndrome may be delayed in gaining these skills for several reasons. Coordinated control of the arms, fingers, and hands often is slower to appear, at least partly due to low muscle tone. Communication problems may get in the way if your child does not completely understand what is expected. The expectations we place may also be problems; the difficulty of the task may be beyond your child's abilities when you are ready to turn the responsibility over to him. You may need to physically do the brushing and flossing for your child beyond the age when a child without Down syndrome could manage the task alone.

Toothbrushing should start with the appearance of the first teeth. You can easily clean the teeth as part of your child's going-to-bed routine. Visibility and accessibility are important. Try having your child lie down; this gives you a good view into his mouth. You can use one hand to open your child's lips for better visibility. A wet toothbrush gently applied to the surfaces of the new teeth can quickly and safely get the job done. As your child grows, additional effort and time will be needed to clean all the teeth.

As your child grows and is more able to cooperate with the brushing and flossing, using a mirror can be helpful. If you both sit or stand in front of a large mirror during the brushing, your child can keep an eye on what is happening, and attempt to mimic what he sees. One way to do this is to brush your child's teeth completely first, then hand him the brush while you clean your own teeth. Then your child has the chance to watch you and try to match your actions visually, while remembering how it felt when you did the brushing.

Toothbrushes are available in a number of sizes, shapes, and colors. Manual toothbrushes are most commonly used, but recently motorized brushes have begun to be popular again. There are many styles on the market, with new ones coming out regularly. Whatever device you select, appropriate handle size, head shape, and bristle softness are important. The handle size depends on who is doing the brushing; if your child is to use it, it should be easy to hold and keep in motion during brushing. The head shape and size need to match well with your child's mouth and teeth. Soft bristles are always recommended for safe care of the teeth and gums. Your dentist should be able to recommend toothbrushes.

Brushing should be performed systematically so that all surfaces of the teeth are cleaned. Plaque sticks tightly to the enamel crevices and in the area close to the gumline. The bristles must be directed into these areas, using a vibrating, circular motion.

As new teeth erupt and move closer together, it will be more difficult to clean between the teeth. Passing dental floss through the spaces removes the plaque and cleans the tissues between the teeth. Most children do not have the manual dexterity to floss, so you need to do this for them until they master the skill. Once again, it may take longer for a child with Down syndrome to become independent in flossing. Many methods are available and your dentist and his or her staff can teach you the best method for your child. Thorough brushing and flossing should be performed at least once a day, preferably before bedtime. Ideally, your child can be instructed to brush after each meal, to remove food and debris.

Toothbrushes need to be cleaned after each brushing and allowed to dry thoroughly between uses. Leaving the brush wet creates a risk of bacteria or mold growth. The simplest way to clean a toothbrush is to rinse with cold water and shake well to remove most of the water. Generally most brushes need to be replaced about every three to six months depending on the frequency of their use. Children and adults should never share brushes, no matter how well they are cleaned or sterilized between uses.

Anti-Cavity Treatments

Oral health depends on eliminating the causes of cavities and gum disease. One common technique is to use chemicals that modify tooth surfaces and make them disease resistant. These substances are as effective for people with Down syndrome as for anyone else. The best known and best researched dental preventive agent is the mineral *fluoride*. Years of research and thousands of reports have confirmed that using fluoride reduces or even eliminates dental caries. Whether applied to the surface of the tooth directly by a dental hygienist or dentist, by the use of a fluoride toothpaste, or by drinking fluoride in water, it hardens previously softened enamel and slows or even stops the development of cavities.

Fluoride is available to your child in a number of forms. In infancy, it should be added to his diet depending on the feeding method you select. Breast milk contains very little fluoride, making the use of a liquid supplement important. Most powdered infant formulas also contain very little fluoride (although soy products may have higher amounts). The water used to mix with the powder may have either added or natural levels of the substance. Most communities test their water sources for fluoride as well as other things, so you should be able to sort out how much you are giving your baby if you mix up the formula yourself. If you use bottled water, this may be more difficult. Some bottlers will list the contents if you ask, but that information is not always available. If you use formulas that are concentrated or ready-to-use, it may be difficult to discover how much fluoride is present.

For children who have moved beyond formula or breast-feeding, if the drinking water contains optimal fluoride, no supplements are required. If not, oral supplements can be prescribed by your physician or dentist. When your child begins toothbrushing, a small amount of fluoridated toothpaste can be used daily. Depending on your child's overall risk of dental disease, additional fluoride (in the form of a daily and semi-annual topical applications) may also be a good idea. For instance, a child with low fluoride intake who eats a diet with lots of sweets, is at higher risk of cavities, and more likely to benefit from the treatment.

Fluoride treatment is not completely free of risk. It should be carefully monitored by you and your child's dentist. If the fluoride concentration in the drinking water is unknown, a water sample should be analyzed. If fluoride levels are too low, a supplement can be prescribed according to your child's age and risk factors. Too much fluoride, especially during the critical time when the permanent teeth are developing enamel (when a child is around 2 to 4 years of age), can cause the enamel to be pitted and discolored. This is called *fluorosis*. Finally, fluoride use is not limited to children. Fluoride should be used throughout life; adults also benefit from daily fluoride use to prevent caries.

Diet

As explained above, plaque is a major cause of dental disease. To survive in your child's mouth, the bacteria in plaque require nutrients. These nutrients can come from a variety of sources, including the foods we eat. Although the majority of foods pass through the mouth quickly, some collect in and around the teeth. The bacteria in plaque digest this food to produce the energy they need to survive. This digestion produces acid. If this process continues day after day without interruption, tooth enamel will be softened and eventually break away to form a cavity.

The same process that produces the acid that causes tooth decay, irritates the gum tissues around the teeth as well. If this is allowed to continue, the gum tissue becomes infected and plaque builds up along the roots of the teeth. Eventually the bone surrounding the teeth weakens, and in time the tooth will loosen as its bony foundation is lost.

In addition to daily plaque removal through brushing and flossing, limiting the nutritional sources of plaque is an important preventive strategy. Unfortunately many parents and most children have difficulty in sticking with a diet that promotes oral health. Poor diet is encouraged by advertisements for foods that are high in carbohydrates. Carbohydrates, especially sugars, are easily digested by the bacteria in plaque to produce acid. The longer the bacteria are exposed to the carbohydrates, the more acid is produced. So carbohydrates that stay near the teeth longer are worse than foods that quickly leave the mouth. Sticky, gooey foods and candies are likely to coat the teeth and remain close to bacteria, while hard candies or sweet liquids dissolve rapidly.

You need to begin early to teach your child good eating habits. For example, you should discourage the use of nighttime and nap-time bottles after your child's teeth appear or after your child's first birthday. Repeatedly drenching teeth with sweetened liquids causes a breakdown of the enamel, especially on the upper front teeth. The crowns of the teeth can

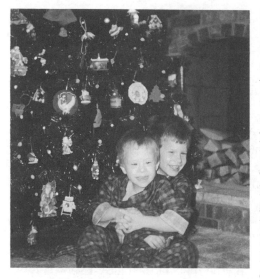

crumble to the gumline, necessitating removal. Most physicians encourage weaning by the time children are able to drink from a cup. Beyond this age, a bottle often serves more as a convenience for parents than as a good source of nutrition for your child. For a child with Down syndrome, drinking from a cup may come a bit later.

Offer your child a well-balanced assortment of foods. Portions should be age appropriate. It may be hard, but try not to bribe or coerce your child into eating the foods you offer. New foods should be introduced as your child's tastes mature. Children should not raid the pantry and refrigerator. Desserts, including carbonated beverages and candies, should be regulated. Good eating habits should be learned early in life, because your child will soon be off to school where food choices will be made without your guidance. Chapter 17 discusses diet and nutrition for children with Down syndrome in detail.

Sealants

The biting surfaces of teeth are at high risk for cavities because they contain little irregularities, like tiny crevices, that may hold the food and plaque on the tooth. If plaque is allowed to remain, the acid it produces will quickly soften the enamel and a cavity will develop.

In recent years, a plastic coating has been developed that can protect the surfaces of teeth. This product, called *sealant,* can be applied to the teeth by a dentist or by another dental specialist with minimal discomfort. Numerous studies report excellent results with the use of sealants. To be effective, the sealant must be used on a tooth that has come in far enough so the tooth surface can be kept dry during application. The tooth surface is first cleaned and etched with a mild acid. The sealant is put in place and then hardened.

Sealants do not protect the smooth sides of a tooth. They can be used on both primary and permanent molars, but usually it is the permanent teeth that are sealed because the crevices and fissures on the biting surfaces are much deeper than on the primary teeth.

Mouthwashes and Mouth Rinses

Because brushing and flossing are difficult, there has been hope that alternative methods for reducing plaque around the teeth would be developed. One possibility is using mouthwashes or rinses that either kill the plaque-causing bacteria or interfere with their growth. The goal is for these antimicrobial solutions to be both effective and safe.

For years antimicrobial solutions have been available in Europe, but they have only recently been made available to United States consumers. One solution that has been extensively studied and has consistently reduced plaque and gum disease, called Peridex™, contains the chemical chlorhexidrine. When this solution is used twice a day as a rinse, plaque shows an average of 50 percent reduction. Unfortunately this rinse requires a prescription.

Over-the-counter products that are available without prescription have been widely advertised and promoted for many years. They contain a variety of antimicrobial agents, including sanguinarine, stannous fluoride, quaternary ammonium compounds, and hydrogen peroxide. These include Cepacol™, Listerine™, and Gel-Kam™, among others. All of these products are effective to some degree, depending on their use. More recently, "prebrushing" mouth rinses have also become available as over-the-counter products. One of these is Plax™. Unfortunately, studies have shown no benefit from these products. Although they probably do no harm, without clear benefit they may just be adding more to your daily routine, and are not usually recommended by dentists or physicians.

Dental Visits

Dentists traditionally schedule patients for six-month visits for a dental examination and teeth cleaning. However, there is little evidence to support the need for six-month examinations. Instead, you and your dentist should schedule return visits on the basis of your child's risk of developing dental disease. These factors include:

- Your child's history of past dental disease;
- Your child's access to fluorides, whether systemic (taken internally) or topical (applied to the surface of the tooth);
- The level of daily oral hygiene that can be provided by or for your child, including the thorough removal of plaque;
- Your child's diet and eating patterns;
- The quality of the your child's tooth enamel;
- The alignment of your child's teeth; and
- Your child's ability to understand the importance of good oral health.

The schedule for your child's return visits should be customized to reflect his risk factors. There may be times when more frequent observation and treatment is necessary. At other times, visits may be less frequent.

X-rays, also called radiographs, are used to look for problems with teeth and the bones of the jaw that might be hidden inside the tooth, or below the gums. Like dental visits a schedule tailored to your child's needs should be established. Dental radiographs should not be taken on a routine basis, but rather based on your child's risk of oral disease. Periodic radiographs to check for cavities between the teeth are important, especially in children who have high caries rates. For children with no caries or very low caries rates (like many children with Down syndrome), radiographs may be scheduled every two to three years. Taking radiographs to detect other oral or dental problems will depend on your child's oral health status. The amount of radiation exposure in dental X-rays is very low when modern equipment is used, and even lower than the exposure from medical X-rays.

In some cases radiographs will be impossible because of your child's age or inability to cooperate. To get a successful X-ray of your child's teeth, he needs to sit still for a few seconds while holding a piece of cardboard between his teeth. This may be painful or frightening, and your child may resist cooperating. Sometimes a child may need to be sedated to obtain the necessary films. You may be able to help prepare your child for the experience by talking about what will happen so there are fewer surprises.

Choosing and Working with a Dentist

It is important to begin dental care when your child is very young, and to develop and maintain a relationship with a dentist who is knowledgeable and comfortable with your child. An office staff who too are comfortable with children with special needs is very helpful. If is usually possible to find a dentist who has had experience treating children with Down syndrome. In fact, many family practitioners are able to work with children with special dental needs. Ask other parents and inquire at your local Down syndrome parent group, local branch of The ARC, or at the nearest developmental clinic. In addition, the organizations listed at the end of this chapter can assist you in finding a dentist with experience in treating children with Down syndrome.

It is important to provide your child's dentist with a comprehensive medical, social, developmental, and dietary history, including information about your child's primary physician and any specialists involved in his health care. Your dentist may want to discuss your child's medical history with these other professionals so that he or she has a complete picture of your child and his health. It could be important to know if your child has any medical conditions like heart disease or drug allergies that could affect his dental treatment. Penicillin is frequently used with teeth cleaning and filling if your child has heart disease; if he has an allergy to penicillin there would need to be another choice made.

Like other children, your child may well dislike visiting his dentist. It may require more work to obtain his cooperation. Methods to examine frightened or uncooperative children vary. If your child is an infant under three years of age, your dentist may use the "knee to knee" position. The parent and dentist sit knee to knee, and create a cradle to support your child. This position stabilizes your child's movements, while providing excellent visibility and accessibility to the mouth. It also allows you to follow along as the dentist carries out the examination.

If your child's experiences with dentists have not been too traumatic, you may find that there are fewer problems with cooperation as time goes by. You may be able to help defuse fears by encouraging your child to play out roles with dolls or drawings. Letting your child play at "being the dentist" with your own teeth and a flashlight could, for instance, let your child walk through the process and become less worried about the unknown.

As your child grows, the dental chair will be more convenient. Some dentists request that parents be present to assist with the exam, while others may prefer to have parents remain in the reception room. Either approach can be appropriate; it all depends on the style of management preferred by your dentist. If you are uncomfortable with the style suggested by your dentist, then you should discuss it openly at the first opportunity. Techniques that work very well for one child may not work for another. If you feel that your dentist's approach is not the best for your child, you need to talk about it.

If your child is resistant or combative, your dentist may ask you to help. A hand or arm placed on an anxious child can provide a calming effect. Sometimes more restraint is necessary, either by someone holding your child firmly, or through the use of devices such as straps. Obviously, the use of these techniques should come after trying other options, and only be used when really needed. You may need to discuss with your dentist whether the procedure can be postponed, and attempt to prepare your child for the next time by behavior modification techniques. If this isn't effective, or if the procedure just can't wait, your dentist may suggest a medication to calm your child. If more extensive treatment is necessary, your dentist may suggest a general anesthetic, given in an out-patient surgical center or the hospital, depending on the community resources and your child's health.

Treatment techniques for all of the dental conditions mentioned here are the same as those used with any child. To restore a tooth destroyed by decay, your dentist may recommend using stainless steel crowns. If primary teeth need to be removed, space needed for the permanent teeth should be maintained with an appliance that holds the space open until the permanent tooth has emerged. If teeth are affected with discolorations, by fluorosis or after the use of certain medications such as tetracycline, or have irregular enamel, tooth color plastics can be applied to re-contour the teeth and create an attractive smile. If permanent teeth are missing, a false tooth, or prosthesis, can be fabricated from a variety of materials. Whether it is a "fixed" or a "removable" prosthesis would depend upon your child's ability to manipulate and care for it.

Because gingival (gum) disease is common in children with Down syndrome, it is important to regularly examine and clean the teeth and the tissue around the teeth. The crevice between the teeth and gums where the collar of the gum meets the tooth must be frequently cleaned in order to ensure gingival health. In cases of gingival disease, surgery may be necessary to make it easier to keep the area free of plaque and debris. This kind of surgery would be performed by your dentist or a periodontist, and might include recontouring the skin to cover the tooth base. Sometimes the removal of diseased bone is necessary. Comprehensive mouth care after the surgery is even more important, because careful cleaning is essential to a successful outcome.

People with special health care needs often benefit greatly from more frequent professional observation and care. This is often true for children with Down syndrome. Your child may need this additional care, even though some insurance plans only allow two follow-up visits per calendar year. Private health insurance sometimes provides coverage for routine dental care, but often require a preauthorization when hospitalization and general anesthesia are necessary, and do not always guarantee payment. More importantly, you should be very careful when purchasing insurance to be sure coverage is available to children with special health care needs. Some companies exclude children with Down syndrome.

If your child has a heart condition or has had heart surgery, your child's dentist and physician need to work together. Because heart disease and heart surgery can cause disruptions in the blood flow in the heart, there is an increased risk of cardiac infection if bacteria is introduced into the bloodstream. Mouths normally harbor quite a lot of bacteria that can enter the bloodstream if the inside of the mouth, especially the gums, are cut or begin to bleed. This can often happen during dental exams, teeth cleanings, cavity repair, and oral surgery. Most physicians prescribe antibiotics to be taken before and after dental treatment for children with Down syndrome who have heart conditions or who have had heart surgery. This can prevent infection. Most physicians can provide you with SBE (*subacute bacterial endocarditis*) prophylaxis cards, notices that alert other health providers to your child's heart condition requiring antibiotic treatment before invasive dental procedures. Your child's need for prophylaxis may change with time, or after surgery, if the risk of infection diminishes. Your dentist should talk with your child's physician about the need for antibiotics, and also review the drug of choice, dosage, and method of administration. Heart conditions and their effect on dental care are also discussed in Chapter 3.

Orthodontics

This dental specialty involves the analysis of the fit of teeth and jaws, and correcting problems by aligning crooked teeth, changing the shape of the jaws, or some combination. Children with Down syndrome may have a variety of dental, facial, and mouth malformations. Like other children they can have crooked teeth, but they may also be more likely to have other conditions that require repair or treatment. These conditions include:

- constricted maxilla (a narrow upper jaw);
- delayed eruption (teeth that come in late);
- delayed exfoliation (baby teeth that are lost late);
- hypotonic (having little muscle tone) lips;
- large or small tongue (also with low tone);
- missing teeth;
- mouth breathing (which may result from other jaw and mouth abnormalities, or may be due to sinus or nasal problems; the drying of tissues that results can interfere with good hygiene.)
- open bite (upper and lower teeth that don't touch in the front when the mouth is closed);

- posterior crossbite (teeth that don't come together properly at the back of the mouth);
- prognathic mandible (lower jaw that extends out past the upper jaw);
- reduced palatal height (the upper palate inside the mouth is flat, rather than domed); and
- small teeth.

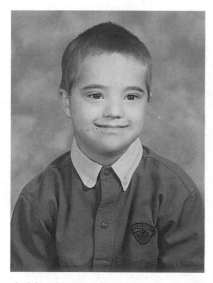

These malformations can result in altered function, different appearance, and difficulty in providing good oral health care.

Treatment through orthodontic care depends on many criteria, but your child's manual dexterity and ability to understand instructions are important because they affect his ability to comply with the treatment. In evaluating treatment options, consider the modifications of your child's diet (inability to eat favorite or common foods because of the presence of the braces), numerous appointments, and financial responsibilities. Long-term treatment for as long as 2–5 years is usually necessary, due to the growth patterns and low tone of facial and oral muscles found with children with Down syndrome. This long-term treatment can impose long-term stress on parents and children, through changes in diet and the demands of frequent cleaning and other care. You should closely consult your child's dentist and an orthodontist.

Summary

Your child's oral health contributes to his overall health. Poor oral and dental health can harm your child's development and learning. Children with Down syndrome often have unique mouth or teeth characteristics. This is why early and continuous dental care and monitoring is important.

Early intervention, before disease begins, followed by regularly scheduled examinations, allows your child's dental team to closely monitor and work with your child to repair and even to prevent problems. Working as a team—a team that includes you, the parent—they can achieve their goal: a child who enjoys a mouth that is healthy, functional, and attractive.

Resources

Many organizations exist to help you meet the dental and oral health care needs of your child. There are three organizations you can contact to get the names of dentists (both in the U.S. and internationally) who have experience in treating children with special health care needs. These organizations are:

American Academy of Pediatric Dentistry
Suite 700, 211 E. Chicago
    312/337–2169

Academy of Dentistry for the Handicapped
211 E. Chicago Avenue
Chicago, IL 60611
    800/544–2174

National Foundation of Dentistry for the Handicapped
Suite 1420, 1600 Stout Street
Denver, CO 80202
303/573–0264

Schools of dentistry usually have special clinics that offer services to children with special needs. Children's hospitals or university teaching hospitals are also good sources of dental care.

Financial assistance for dental care for your child with Down syndrome may be available in your state. This kind of financial assistance varies from state to state, and even from community to community. Some states have excellent programs to support parents while others have very little if any support. Your state's department of human services may be able to provide you with information about financial assistance programs for dental care. Your local public health nurse may also be helpful, as well as your local school's special education staff.

References

Barnett, M., et al. "The Prevalence of Periodontitis and Dental Caries in a Down's Syndrome Population." *Journal of Periodontology,* Vol. 57, 1986, 288–293.

Borea, G., et al. "The Oral Cavity in Downs Syndrome." *Journal of Pedodontics,* Vol. 14, 1990, 139–140.

Entwistle, B. and Casamassimo, P. "Assessing Dental Health Problems of Children with Developmental Disabilities." *Journal of Developmental and Behavioral Pediatrics,* Vol. 2, 1981, 115–121.

Ettinger, R., et al. "Toothbrush Modifications and the Assessment of Hand Function in Children with Hand Disabilities." *Journal of Dentistry for the Handicapped Patient,* Vol. 5, 1980, 7–12.

Fischer-Brandies, H. "Cephalometric Comparison between Children With and Without Down's Syndrome." *European Journal of Orthodontics,* Vol. 10, 1988, 255–263.

Fischer-Brandies, H., et al. "Craniofacial Development in Patients with Down's Syndrome from Birth to Fourteen Years of Age." *European Journal of Orthodontics,* Vol. 8, 1986, 35–42.

Fox, L. "Preventive Dentistry for the Handicapped Child." *Pediatric Clinics of North America,* Vol. 20, 1973, 245–257.

Grossman, E., et al. "A Clinical Comparison of Antimicrobial Mouth Rinses." *The Journal of Periodontology,* Vol. 60, 1898, 435–440.

Modeer, T., et al. "Periodontal Disease in Children with Down's Syndrome." *Scandinavian Journal of Dental Research,* Vol. 98, 1990, 228–234.

Nowak, A.J. "The Special Patient: Challenges of the 80s." *Special Care in Dentistry,* Vol. 2, 1982, 175

Nowak, A.J. "Dental Disease in Handicapped Persons." *Special Care in Dentistry,* Vol. 5, 1984, 66.

13 | Medical Issues Related to Sexuality and Reproduction
Thomas E. Elkins, M.D.

Introduction

Gynecologic care—health care that deals with a woman's reproductive tract and with the issues of reproduction and sexuality—is perhaps one of the least emphasized areas of health care for teenaged girls and women with Down syndrome. For example, a recent study showed that this is the one area of health care that is still relatively unavailable to persons with mental retardation in some states in this country. But gynecologic care is just as important for women with Down syndrome as it is for other women. Like all women, women with Down syndrome may have menstrual irregularities that require treatment, and have a chance of developing cervical, breast, or other cancers. In addition, they often require *more* counseling and guidance than usual about menstrual hygiene, reproductive issues, and appropriate sexual behavior.

While your daughter is a teenager, it is largely up to you to ensure that she receives the gynecologic care she needs. This can seem like a daunting prospect, but with the support of a good gynecologist, you can teach your daughter to take responsibility for her own care. Most women with Down syndrome are quite capable of good menstrual hygiene and of looking after their own reproductive health.

The First Gynecologic Exam

Most women have an initial pelvic examination, Pap smear, and breast examination by age eighteen. It goes without saying that adolescents with Down syndrome should have the same health care. The American College of Obstetrics and Gynecologists, a national group of physicians that sets standards to certify obstetricians and gynecologists, recommends that all women have a pelvic exam by age eighteen, regardless of symptoms or menstrual function. Generally, the start of menses before age ten, or beyond age eighteen, would merit a visit to the gynecologist. If your daughter develops problems of any type related to her menses, such as hygiene problems, irregular or heavy bleeding, pain or dysmenorrhea, premenstrual behavior problems, seizures during menses, or cessation of menses, you should seek medical care.

Finding a gynecologist with knowledge and experience in treating women with Down syndrome can be challenging, but the situation is improving. First, there are some specialized gynecology programs for women with disabilities. These are usually connected to university centers and are often associated with pediatric and adolescent gynecology specialists. Some private gynecologists may also have an interest in providing care for women with disabilities. Usually, these physicians can be identified through your local Down syndrome parent organization or through your local branch of The ARC (formerly called the Association for Retarded Citizens). More specialized programs are being developed. The North American Society for Pediatric and Adolescent Gynecology has made care for women with disabilities a national concern, and has developed training programs aimed at improving availability of appropriate services. Contact that organization to help find local members who can be resources to meet your needs.

To prepare your daughter for her first pelvic exam, be sure to request pre-examination counseling and education; these services are not automatically offered. Nurses or social workers on staff may spend a significant amount of time with you and your daughter discussing the exam, using life-like dolls, pictures, or slide presentations. Ask the gynecologist about using newer techniques that can make the pelvic exam much more relaxed than in the past. For example, it is possible to use Q-tip Pap smears that avoid placement of vaginal speculums, and to assess uterine and ovarian size painlessly through transabdominal pelvic ultrasonography (using high frequency sound waves). Even with these ad-

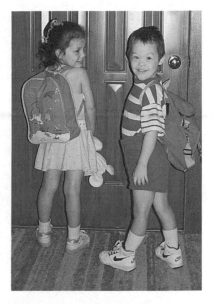

aptations, it is possible that your daughter may be so anxious that all she is able to do at the first visit is put on a gown. Often repeat visits are required to accomplish a pelvic examination. For young women who find the pelvic exam very difficult, relaxing medications such as oral ketamine and midazolam may be suggested. As with any use of sedatives, there are some side effects which may limit their use to people who need them most.

After your daughter's first pelvic exam and Pap smear, the gynecologists will let you know when the next Pap smear should be done. A woman with no symptoms of unusual bleeding or discharge, who is not sexually active, and who has had a prior "normal" Pap smear does not necessarily need a yearly Pap smear, although the recommendations may vary depending upon the circumstances and the experience of your child's physician.

Menstrual Hygiene

Most young women with Down syndrome have a regular, monthly cycle. The regular menstrual cycle begins after initial irregular bleeding episodes that usually follow the start of growth of both armpit and pubic hair. The average age of "menarche," or the age when menses begins, has been falling steadily in America over the past 25 years. It is now about 10.5 to 11.2 years of age. Young women with Down syndrome usually follow a similar pattern, with menarche ranging from 11 to 13 in some surveys. As with other physical traits, women with Down syndrome may show a wide range of characteristics, with some having delay in menarche beyond age 18 with no identifiable cause other than Down syndrome. However, the majority of young women with Down syndrome have regular ovulatory menstrual cycles.

Menstrual hygiene is often a major concern for families, but worries about menses before they begin are typically worse than warranted. Most young women with Down syndrome can manage their menstrual cycles quite successfully with proper training. Some may need medications to help control menstrual flow as a part of their hygiene training. You can learn more about teaching their daughter menstrual hygiene by talking with either your child's physician or her special education teacher. Your child's gynecologist can prescribe medications to shorten, lessen, or even eliminate menstrual flow. Newer oral contraceptive tablets that contain very low doses of estrogen and more potent levels of progestin result in minimal menstrual flow patterns that are more easily managed.

If your daughter has certain health conditions, however, she should not take oral contraceptives with estrogen. Women who have seizure disorders, limited mobility (e.g., paraplegia), diabetes, or liver disorders run the risk of developing side effects such as clotting disorders or increased seizures, headaches, or gallstones. If your child cannot take estrogen tablets, other medications may be helpful.

Progestin-only daily tablets or longer-lasting injections with medroxyprogesterone acetate (Depo-Provera) may reduce and even eliminate menstrual flow. These drugs, like all medications, may cause side effects, including fluid retention, drowsiness, lethargy, depression, headaches, acne, and occasional agitation. In almost all instances some level of estrogen or progestin medication can be found that helps and has minimal side effects. Physician guidance should be used in starting and continuing any of these medications.

In very rare instances, hysterectomy (surgical removal of the uterus) may be considered to help a woman with Down syndrome manage her menstrual hygiene. For example, a woman with heavy menses flow and severe behavior management problems may be considered for a hysterectomy. However, this is a very high-risk alternative. Surgical risks include hemorrhage (bleeding) (1 percent to 3 percent), aspiration pneumonia (inflammation of the lungs from breathing in food, vomit, or other material) (1 percent to 5 percent), deep venous thrombophlebitis with pulmonary embolus (blood clot that forms in or travels to the lungs), damage to bowel-bladder-ureter (1 percent to 2 percent), infection (5 percent), and even death. Because of the risks, this procedure should only be a last resort.

Menstrual Disorders

At some point in their lives, many women experience some kind of menstrual disorder—heavy, painful, scanty, nonexistent, or irregular menstrual flow. These types of menstrual disorders can result from a variety of causes, including certain disorders that may be associated with Down syndrome. Some of the more common causes of menstrual disorders are discussed below.

Thyroid Abnormalities. As Chapter 5 explains, Down syndrome is often associated with thyroid abnormalities, including *hyperthyroidism* (overactive thyroid) and *hypothyroidism*

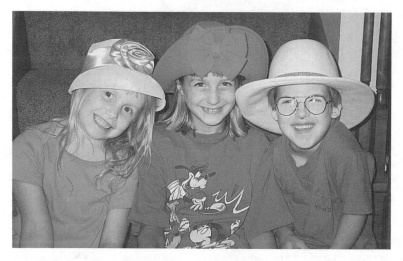

(underactive thyroid). These abnormalities may cause significant menstrual irregularities that range from excess flow to no periods at all *(amenorrhea)*. Occasionally, the first symptom of thyroid disease in women is menstrual dysfunction. *Menorrhagia* (heavy prolonged menses) often accompanies hypothyroidism, for example. Correction of thyroid dysfunction may eliminate some menstrual problems. Your child's doctor should consider a thyroid test if your child has irregular menstruation.

Some kinds of brain tumors and other central nervous system (CNS) disorders cause early menstruation (precocious puberty), and may also be associated with some causes of mental retardation like Down syndrome. In general, menses occurring before nine years of age should alert you to take your child to a gynecologist or pediatrician. Vaginal bleeding in very early childhood (before age 3 or 4) could indicate a pelvic tumor, and should require a visit to the gynecologist or pediatrician.

Poor Nutrition. Poor nutrition, which is often seen in people with mental retardation, can lead to menstrual dysfunction. Excessive weight can be associated with irregular, heavy menses, and even endometrial cancer at an earlier age. Endometrial cancer is cancer of the lining of the uterus. It usually does not occur before age 45, but has been found in extremely obese women as early as ages 15 to 17. The usual symptoms include heavy, irregular vaginal bleeding that persists over long periods of time. A gynecologist would need to help decide on and manage treatment choices if a diagnosis of endometrial cancer is made.

Extreme weight loss is less common among women with Down syndrome, but when it occurs may be associated with scanty, irregular menses, or amenorrhea. Obviously, it is simpler to prevent nutrition-related problems than to treat them. Chapter 17 offers guidance to help you ensure that your child receives optimal nutrition.

Pre-Menstrual Syndrome

Young women with Down syndrome, like most other women with mild mental retardation, often have pre-menstrual syndrome (PMS) in response to the changes in hormone levels that accompany the menstrual cycle. PMS symptoms in these young women resemble those seen in most women in America. These include headaches, irritability, bloating, weight gain, breast tenderness, depression, sadness, and fatigue, that all occur within 3 to 7 days of the onset of menses. Some women may respond to reassurance, relaxation-oriented counselling, control of their diet, or exercise. Others may require the use of mild diuretics (to relieve bloating), mild analgesics (for pain), or oral contraceptives (to modify hormonal swings) in order to control bothersome symptoms.

In women with Down syndrome who have more severe levels of mental retardation, symptoms may be especially severe. About 5 percent to 15 percent of people with Down syndrome fall into this category. It is not uncommon, for example, to see self-destructive behavior, increased seizure activity, hyperactivity, increased irritability, or angry outbursts.

This increase in symptoms appears to be related to the young woman's inability to verbalize feelings of unrest or agitation. Sensitive attempts to improve communication, particularly during times of stress, can improve behavior and help with managing the symptoms of PMS.

Oral contraceptives or similar medications can help to reduce the hormonal swings associated with PMS. For young women with severe symptoms, elimination of menstrual cycles may be the most appropriate therapy. This may be accomplished temporarily with gonadotropin-releasing hormone treatment—injections with medications that suppress activity of the pituitary gland. For longer times, cycles may be eliminated with high doses of Depo-Provera, danocrine, or continuous oral contraceptives. Occasionally, high doses of psychotropic medications such as proloxin, lithium, or thorazine may be required to control violent symptoms; these may also raise prolactin levels, leading to amenorrhea.

Reproductive Concerns

The majority of women with Down syndrome have regular menses, and are usually ovulating and capable of having children. There are not studies specifically tracking pregnancy in women with Down syndrome. One review of over thirty pregnant women with Down syndrome found that approximately fifty percent of their offspring had Down syndrome, and that one-third of the other offspring had other conditions. There is very little proof to date that males with Down syndrome are fertile, except perhaps in one or two instances that have been reported. As community involvement and socialization skills increase for both males and females with Down syndrome, however, these instances can be expected to increase.

Because women with Down syndrome tend to be short, they are likely to have small pelvic bone dimensions (this is true for all women with short stature). This makes delivery by cesarean section more likely. Also, heart defects and thyroid disease may adversely affect pregnancy and delivery, and both of these conditions are more common in people with Down syndrome.

Not surprisingly, reproductive concerns are common among young women with Down syndrome and their families. Counseling about socialization and sexuality is very important. It is especially important to discuss contemporary risks of sexually transmitted diseases, to reinforce the need for safe sex practices.

The use of contraceptives may be important in freeing young women with mild to moderate mental retardation to experience sexual relationships without unnecessary fear or risk of pregnancy. Normal fertility is maintained by levels of two hormones, estrogen and progesterone, that cycle up and down through the month. Many contraceptives work by adding higher or steadier levels of one or both of these hormones. Low estrogen oral contraceptives are often used and also have a number of positive effects besides contraception:

- menstrual flow is diminished and regulated;
- painful periods (*dysmenorrhea*) become painless;
- rates of endometrial and ovarian cancer are reduced (below the rates of women not taking oral contraceptives);
- endometriosis (a condition in which the lining of the uterus invades other tissue in the pelvis) is suppressed;
- some kinds of ovarian cysts are reduced; and
- some sexually-transmitted diseases, such as gonorrhea, are partially prevented.

As mentioned before, the risks of treatment with these contraceptives must also be considered. Sometimes they are not appropriate to use. There are newer, long-acting medications that use progestin such as Depo-Provera™ (injected into the muscle) and Norplant™ (implanted under the skin) which may also be considered. These carry the risks discussed earlier

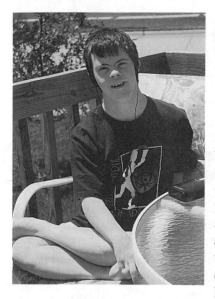

for oral contraceptives, and may increase irregular menstrual bleeding, making menstrual hygiene more difficult.

Other types of contraceptive are usually not as good choices for women with Down syndrome. Contraceptive methods that rely on a barrier—such as a diaphragm or a contraceptive sponge—require motivation and physical skills. Intrauterine devices usually increase menstrual flow and hygiene problems. They also carry a significant risk of infection, usually heralded by pelvic pain. Women with Down syndrome may be less able to identify the severity of their pain or to verbalize their symptoms clearly, so infections could become far advanced before treatment is sought.

Sterilization of people with mental retardation continues to be a controversial topic throughout the United States. In 1927, the U.S. Supreme Court authorized involuntary sterilization for people with mental retardation. This was followed in 1942 with a ruling that completely reversed the earlier view, and proclaimed reproduction an inalienable right for all people, including people with mental retardation. In 1973, federal regulations declared that federal funds could not be used to sterilize persons who were "mentally incompetent." The confusion at state levels continues, with court cases pending in a number of states. Since the 1964 case of *Stump v. Ohio,* in which a judge was rebuked for authorizing sterilization, many officials are reluctant to issue such court orders. Cases in many states follow the working of *In re Hays* or *In re*

Grady. Both of these cases urge that alternatives to sterilization be sought in every case, and that surgical sterilization be performed only as a last resort. This is consistent with an American College of Obstetricians and Gynecologists Ethics Committee statement on the issue.

Other Concerns about Sexuality

Although the use of contraceptives relieves some parental concerns related to the sexuality of young women with Down syndrome, other concerns often remain. For example, many parents are concerned about teaching their daughter appropriate sexual behavior. In fact, at a special program at the University of Michigan established to provide gynecology services for women with mental retardation, parents' concerns most frequently included inappropriate touching or other concerns about socialization.

Masturbation is a concern of parents that may not be discussed due to embarrassment. The simplest answer to this concern is information: according to surveys, this is a normal private behavior for many adults. The focus of discussion should be on privacy, so that the young woman can be socially acceptable without being made to feel "bad" or guilty.

Many parents are also worried about the possibility that their daughter might be sexually abused. Unfortunately, this concern is well founded, as perhaps 20 to 40 percent or more of people with mental retardation are sexually abused.

The best way to deal with these types of concerns is to ensure that your daughter receives effective counseling about appropriate private and public behaviors. To guard against sexual abuse, your daughter should be taught the principles of group security; silence about last names and phone numbers; avoidance of strangers; and appropriate socialization, even within families. This counselling should begin in childhood. Families and care providers are essential partners in the counseling process, which should make use of repetition, audio-visual aids, patient participation, and follow-up. Many special education programs are beginning to provide counselling. Some areas have special counselling services available, often through local universities, and most parent groups are aware of local resources.

Gynecologic care for women with mental retardation is receiving increased attention from today's gynecologists. This makes it more likely that you will be able to find appropriate and compassionate care for your daughter. In some cases, however, you may need to educate your family physician, and gynecologist as well. You will definitely take a major role in educating your daughter, as young people with Down syndrome first learn about appropriate health care and hygiene from their parents. The result of increased levels of interest and experience on the parts of patients, families, and physicians will lead to better health care for all women with Down syndrome.

Male Sexuality and Reproduction

Most discussions about the sexuality of males with Down syndrome focus on infertility. While few men with Down syndrome have been known to father children, this is not an absolute. For any particular person, all bets are off. Appropriate sexual behavior is essential to teach.

Infertility does not mean impotence. Most males with Down syndrome experience the changes of puberty on about the same timetable as anyone else. The primary sexual characteristics that develop during puberty include hormone changes, the ability to manufacture sperm, and several physical changes to the sexual organs. Secondary characteristics include pubic & facial hair, muscle changes, and a deeper voice. There may be some delay in the appearance of some of the secondary sexual characteristics, such as facial hair. By late adolescence, most young men with Down syndrome will have finished the physical changes of puberty, and will be capable of full sexual function.

Most will also experience the emotional changes of puberty and adolescence. Many teenagers with Down syndrome are well aware of the developing relationships around them, and want to have similar friendships and experiences. They may have fewer social opportunities to build friendships with young women, and may be hampered by problems with communication. Consequently, frank discussions of sexuality are at least as important for these young men as for other teenagers.

Discussions of sexuality need to include the issue of sexual abuse in addition to more typical issues. Young men with Down syndrome are seldom perpetrators of rape or other sexual abuse, but may be vulnerable to abuse themselves. An understanding of socially-appropriate sexual behavior is an important part of adolescence which is sometimes difficult to get across.

Conclusion

The increased success with which both young men and young women with Down syndrome are gaining independence in education, employment, and community living means that more and more of them will be asking for similar control over their sexual lives. As parents, you may need to help prepare your child to cope with the wide variety of decisions that are part of that independence.

References

Calderone, Mary and Johnson, Eric. *The Family Book about Sexuality* (New York: Harper and Row, 1981).

Calderone, Mary. *Talking with Your Child about Sex* (New York: Random House, 1982).

Edwards J. and Elkins T.E. *Just Between Us: A Guide to the Socialization and Sexuality Training of Persons with Mental Retarda-*

tion for Parents and Professionals (Austin, TX: Ednick- Pro-Ed Publications, 1989).

Elkins T.E. and Anderson H.F. "Sterilization of Persons with Mental Retardation: Legal and Ethical Concerns." *Journal of the Association for Persons with Severe Handicaps*, Vol. 17, No. 1, 1992, 19–26.

Ethical Concerns in Sterilization of Persons with Mental Retardation. (Washington D.C.: American College of Obstetricians and Gynecologists, Committee on Bioethics, 1988).

Haefner H.K. and Elkins T.E. "Contraceptive Management for Female Adolescents with Mental Retardation and Handicapping Disabilities." *Current Opinion in Obstetrics and Gynecology*, Vol. 3, 1991, 820–824.

Kramer, Rosalyn. *Understanding and Expressing Sexuality—Responsible Choices for Individuals with Developmental Disabilities* (Baltimore: Paul H. Brookes, 1992).

In re Grady, 85 N.J. 235; 426 A.2d. 467 (1981).

In re Hayes, 93 Wash. 228; 608 P.2d. 635, 640 (1980).

14 | Neurology of Children with Down Syndrome
Phillip Mattheis, M.D.

Introduction

Neurology is the study of the nervous system, which includes the brain, spinal cord, and all the nerves of the human body. Our nervous systems help to control most of the functions of our bodies as we adapt to the world around us. The brain is the center of the system, and is the source of thoughts, and personality, and the behaviors that others see as we go through life.

Down syndrome affects the nervous system in a number of ways. Most of the time these neurologic differences do not cause illness or problems that need medical treatment. The effects usually appear as differences in thought, speech, and learning. Muscle control, another important function of the nervous system, is also different in most children with Down syndrome, affecting the rate and timing of how they learn to use their muscles to eat, crawl, walk, and talk.

In some respects, neurologic effects are the most important, and least understood, of all of the conditions that can be different in children with Down syndrome. Most of the nonmedical problems that we know about, including communication, education, and behavior, come from the differences in the way the nervous system works.

For children with Down syndrome, these cognitive and developmental patterns have frequently been placed in the category of *mental retardation.* The definition of this designation has changed a bit over time, but has always been meant to identify people who had significantly less mental ability than the "normal" population. Generally, children are considered to have mental retardation if they score lower than 70 on IQ tests. Unfortunately, many times the tests or testers do not consider language problems or specific learning difficulties that might interfere with performance. In addition, the test results are usually assumed to be permanent, with no recognition of the possibility of growth. As a consequence, the label "mental retardation" provides little hope for the child and family and little insight for doctors and teachers.

While there is no question that the development of movement and speech and language abilities is different in children with Down syndrome, the difference is probably more in the delayed emergence of skills and slower responses than in absolute differences. For example, almost all children with Down syndrome learn to walk and talk, but they may learn these skills later than other children. Delays slow the learning process, but vary from person to person. When slowed learning is combined with the prejudices of "mental retardation," the result can be lowered expectations, which can lower your child's potential.

Cognitive differences are probably better understood as *learning disabilities* than as mental retardation. When careful attention is given to specific learning and language problems, many children with Down syndrome do "better than expected." The current generation of children in the U.S. are, as a group, receiving much more individual educational attention; as they grow and develop (with continued support) they will test the true limits of their abilities. There has long been known to be a wide range of ability in people with Down syndrome, but as expectations and educational supports are improved, we may find that most people are closer to the high end of that range.

Pediatric neurologists study the nervous system of children. Most focus their efforts on describing the causes of neurologic problems, and providing medical treatment for those conditions that can be changed. Few people with Down syndrome require the services of a neurologist for medical problems.

Developmental pediatrics is a relatively new medical specialty that focuses upon neurologic differences and disabilities that challenge a child's ability to learn and grow within the community. The work of developmental pediatricians is only partly medical, however. Realizing a person's full potential as a member of his community is the ultimate goal, and involves collaboration with a variety of other professionals, including educators, therapists, and counselors.

This chapter discusses the neurology of children with Down syndrome from the perspective of developmental pediatrics. As in other chapters, the workings of the nervous system will be described, and problems common in people with Down syndrome will be discussed. There will not be a lot of talk about therapies that address developmental delays; other books and resources will be mentioned.

What Is the Nervous System?

In many ways, the brain is like a computer, serving as the control center of the body. The spinal cord and nerves are the wiring that carry messages to and from the computer. This combination of computer and wiring is the mechanical and electronic "hardware" of the nervous system. "Software" is the set of instructions that tells the computer what to do.

Man-made computers are designed for specific tasks. The simplest computers perform just one task, like an oven thermostat that ignites the gas flame as the oven cools, and turns it off again when the oven temperature rises. It works through a simple switch that turns on or off depending upon the message from a temperature sensor in the oven. The temperature selected, or *programmed*, by the cook, controls how the computer responds to temperature readings from the sensor. The design and function of such a simple computer is all in the way the parts are wired together.

More complicated computers perform many more tasks, and consequently have more complicated designs. A computerized house heating system can vary the temperature in every room, and adjust by time of day or day of the week. There are many more switches and sensors, and more programming is needed to tell the computer what to do. Still, the design and function is in the wiring, and the job is limited to temperature control.

The machines most of us think of as computers, like the laptop device I used to type this chapter, are much more complicated than house thermostats. There are literally millions of on/off switches in the *hardware* of my little laptop, wired together in ways that make many different operations possible. This computer can run many different kinds of programs to do many different kinds of tasks, some simultaneously. The "programs" are special sets of instructions that tell the computer what to do when I give it a message, like pressing a key on the keyboard. These programs are the *software* of the system—the parts that can be changed quickly and simply without messing with the wiring.

The human nervous system is much more complicated than any man-made computer, making us capable of doing a great variety of tasks with our minds and bodies. There are many automatic adjustments like body temperature and heart rate which help our bodies to adjust to the outside world and to the demands we place on ourselves. The automatic part of the nervous system controls these functions without our thought; we can't do much to directly affect them. There really is no "software" involved, and only a small part of the brain is needed. This automatic part of the nervous system is just like the temperature control on the oven mentioned above. In humans, this part of the nervous system is the first to develop, and is usually working well at birth.

We are born with all the nerve cells we will ever have; in fact, at birth most of us have many more brain cells than we will ever use. Many of these nerve cells are not yet connected into working pathways; they are not yet "wired" into the system. Those which are hooked together may not be as well insulated as they need to be to work efficiently. During childhood, these connections and insulation develop and mature. Some of this normal development includes the death of nerve cells when they are not used. If damage to the brain occurs at a very young age while many of these "extra" cells are still alive, they may serve as "spare parts" to re-

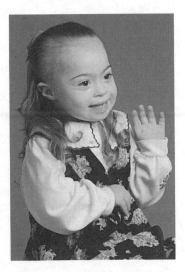

place damaged cells. Consequently, very young children can survive brain injury like strokes or infection that would kill an adult. In children with brains that are different for other reasons, such as Down syndrome, those extra cells may also help compensate for the differences. This is a subject scientists are only beginning to understand.

Most of the things we do, like talking or walking, are at least partially voluntary. We may not be aware of how we control the muscles that do these things, but we can choose when to start and stop. We learn to do these kinds of tasks as part of our development as children. The rate at which we get new skills depends upon how well the body's muscles and bones are put together, and how well the brain can coordinate them. Usually skills become more automatic with practice. Most of us do not need to pay attention to how we walk or run, or how we make words with our voices.

Other, more complicated actions like singing, or algebra, take a lot of practice and special training to get right. These learned skills are our software programs, which tell the computer what to do and how to do it. But how we are wired and how well the machinery of our bodies work, have a lot to do with what we can learn. Some people can sing beautifully from the first try, and without special training. Others of us couldn't carry a tune in a bucket, despite hours of practice with the best teachers. Running smoothly and quickly comes easily to some, while those with very loose joints or poorly organized muscles may have trouble walking steadily for more than a few feet. Thus the quality of our computer, of our wiring, and of our body's machine, all play strong roles in just how we develop and in how we learn

What each of us does with our lives is limited partly by what the software and the computer can get us to do. At least as important, however, is what is expected to be possible. At this point in time, we probably know *less* about the potential of people with Down syndrome than ever. Many previously presumed limits have been proved wrong for at least some people, and we have no good way to predict for others.

Early infant stimulation programs are helping many children with Down syndrome to develop faster and to higher levels. Many if not most children learn to read when given the opportunity. Probably the safest route is to give every child the same opportunities to learn as everyone else, with recognition of any special needs (like speech therapy) they may have.

How Does the Nervous System Do Its Job?

A mature, functioning body and nervous system works like a computer and machine. As described above, there are many operations which the computer controls automatically and without conscious effort, like breathing and heart rate. For example, if you are running and your body needs more oxygen, your brain gets chemical messages and responds by speeding up your heart and respiratory rates. When the outside temperature is too hot your body sweats; low temperatures trigger shivering and the closing of the blood vessels in your skin in order to limit heat loss.

Movement is more complicated than the automatic functions. It requires coordinated muscle actions, which are started by nerve messages. The simplest movements are called *reflex arcs,* and involve one muscle and one nerve pathway to and from the spinal cord. The reflexes checked by your doctor (such as tapping the knee with a rubber mallet) are examples of spinal reflex arcs.

Nerves in muscle tendons sense how tightly stretched the muscles are, and have been programmed to keep a certain tension even at rest. This programmed tension is the resting *tone* of the muscle, and depends upon messages from the brain, how awake and alert the person is, and how well the muscle works.

Complicated movements require the actions of several muscle groups, working with careful timing and balance of their forces to accomplish a task. For example, turning a page of this book requires muscles that work against each other across your shoulder, elbow, and wrist to direct your hand and fingers to the edge of the page. As your fingers and thumb move to grasp the page, muscles in your arm again work across the shoulder, elbow, and wrist to finish moving the page. Special parts of the brain provide motor planning to co-ordinate this timing and balancing. Messages from the brain's motor planning center are sent to the areas that control each specific part of the body and trigger signals to the individual muscles needed. As the body repeats certain actions over and over, the planning sequence is learned, and moves to another part of the brain where it is remembered. As the movement is repeated, it becomes more automatic. For example, this pattern is true for learning to play a musical instrument.

Very complicated actions, such as speech, require more steps. Speech has its own planning center in the brain and a number of special nerve pathways. *Receptive language,* or the understanding of the words of others, depends upon hearing to detect the sound of the words; the ear converts sound to nerve impulses which are then translated by the brain. The meaning is interpreted or processed in several other regions and compared and contrasted with memory and learning. The meaning that the brain assigns leads to thoughts and is called *expressive language*, which becomes the words one wants to say in response. These responses are sent to the speech planning center, which controls the signals sent to the muscles that make words. These include muscles in the mouth, tongue, and throat as well as the chest and diaphragm. Facial muscles, also controlled by the brain, make the expressions we use to help make our meaning clear. If any part of this complex network is out of sequence, or works at a different pace, speech is less successful. If parts of the system do not work well in early childhood (when most of us learn our speech and language skills), learning and communication can be impaired.

The processing of information into thought is the *cognitive function* of the brain. It is the most complicated of all nervous system functions. It depends upon the interaction of many, many nerve groups and pathways. The development of concepts and judgement requires learning about consequences of actions and reactions. This type of learning requires a system that works smoothly and consistently to deliver messages both in and out of the brain's computer. If the messages do not come in dependably, or are received, transmitted, and interpreted differently day to day, learning does not happen very effectively. Because of the differences in the brains and nerves of people with Down syndrome there are differences in how they learn.

Common Neurologic Differences in People with Down Syndrome

Anatomy

The brains of people with Down syndrome tend to be somewhat smaller than those of other people. The importance of this difference is not entirely clear, however, because brain and head measurements have not been carefully compared to the heights and weights of the same bodies. Small people have small heads and brains; and people with Down syndrome tend to be smaller than others. The shape of the brains may be a bit different from normal, with a little less distance front-to-back. This also reflects the usual shape of the skulls of people with Down syndrome.

The brain cells of people with Down syndrome may be different. In brains which have been studied under microscopes, some brain areas appear to have fewer nerve cells when compared to brains of people who did not have Down syndrome. Some nerve cells may be made slightly different, and the way messages are sent may also vary a bit. Not many studies have been done on this topic, so little is known for sure.

Aging affects the nervous system in each of us, though the changes may occur at a faster rate in people with Down syndrome. Particularly with injury, changes can occur in our brains. Some of these differences, called *plaques* and *tangles,* are seen very often in some older people's brains. This is especially true in people with Alzheimer's disease.

Plaques have been found in brains of many older people with Down syndrome, and seem to occur at younger ages. Plaques are always found in the brains of people who have Alzheimer's disease, but can also be seen in the brains of some individuals who do not have the memory and personality changes that are part of that condition. Tangles are seen in most brains of people with Alzheimer's disease, and are less likely to be found in others. Tangles do not seem to be especially common in the brains of people with Down syndrome. Alzheimer's disease is discussed further below.

Functional Differences

Muscle tone, as described above, is the amount of stretch in a resting muscle. Tone is controlled by the brain, and helps keep muscles ready to act. A muscle with low tone is like a

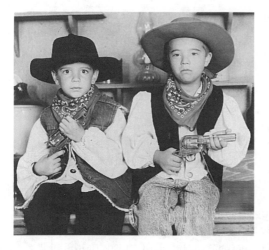

flagpole rope with a lot of slack; to move the flag you have to pull up all the slack first. The slack rope may be just as strong as one that is tighter, but takes more pulling to get the job done. One advantage of low tone is that it is "cheaper"; fewer calories are needed for more relaxed muscles. On the downside, however, muscles that burn fewer calories while at rest increase the chance of weight gain (this is discussed in detail in Chapter 17).

Most people with Down syndrome have lower tone than normal, at least as babies. There may be some differences in the way the nerves in the muscles work, but most of the lowered tone is felt to be *central,* or due to the way the brain works. Lower tone, or *hypotonia,* can have a lot of effects. Many babies with hypotonia have feeding problems, at least initially. Walking often comes later in children with lower tone. Hypotonia can affect speech in several ways, by making clear articulation difficult, and by slowing learning when muscle action is unpredictable.

In many individuals, speech problems are limited to articulation—how sounds are put together to form words. In others the trouble goes deeper. *Verbal apraxia* is the term used when the brain's speech planning center is affected, and may be more common in people with Down syndrome. Because the speech planning center does not work very well, people with verbal apraxia have greater difficulty creating the sequences of sound that make up words. Most of us discover as infants how to make a variety of sounds, and then explore different combinations. For example we learn that -*at* plus *b-,* *c-,* and *s-* produces *bat, cat,* and *sat.* As we grow older we learn meanings for the many sounds we hear, and are able to easily mimic those sounds. Verbal apraxia does not affect the understanding of meaning, but makes producing each sequence of sounds a new experience. Some people must learn to make each word as a separate process, and may need to keep practicing because they forget how to say words they don't use very often.

Other kinds of apraxia can also occur to disrupt the planning and learning of other movements. These may affect activities like walking and running, or the use of the fingers and hands. Whether these kinds of apraxia are more common in people with Down syndrome is not known.

How we think is not at all well understood in any of us, with or without Down syndrome. People with Down syndrome may exercise poorer judgement than others, but how much of this is due to learning problems, low expectations, poor role models, or direct effects on the brain is not known. Many kinds of learning disorders have been identified in children without Down syndrome, but very little is known about how often these occur in children with Down syndrome. A major problem in the use of the label "mental retardation" is the assumption that that term explains fully the problem and does not require looking any further.

Treatment of Neurologic Problems in People with Down Syndrome

The differences in muscle tone, speech and language, and thought production are present to some degree in many or most people with Down syndrome. In most cases, treatment involves recognizing the need for extra help and more time for learning. Very often, just changing expectations allows big changes in ability.

The need for specific therapies for your child with Down syndrome should be decided by his needs, not by the existence of Down syndrome. Many children with Down syndrome benefit from speech therapy, but others do not need that service. Physical therapy (PT) may be helpful for a child with loose joints and low tone who is trying to start walking, but there is not good evidence that PT is needed for every child.

Educational strategies should also recognize the particular needs of each child. There is not a "Down syndrome program" that meets the needs of all children with Down syndrome, any more than there is a "cerebral palsy program," an "autism program," or an "African-American program" to meet the needs of every child in these categories. Educational programming targeting the level of mental retardation ("educable," "trainable," "mild MR," "severe/profound MR") also tends to ignore the details that define the individual needs of real children.

Medical treatment of the neurologic differences in children with Down syndrome is usually not necessary, or helpful. A number of treatment programs have been designed by various people which attempt to change speech, or muscle tone, or learning abilities through the use of medications, vitamins, or other treatments. These may be presented as medical therapies, or as non-traditional treatments. Several of these programs are discussed in more detail in Chapter 15. None of the therapies have been proven to make any real change in the children treated. Most of these programs are expensive, or require a lot of time and trouble; some, like sicca cell therapy, can actually be dangerous. In most cases the people who have developed the programs are unwilling or unable to do studies that could prove the value they claim. Often the changes seen or claimed after the treatments can be explained by increased expectations and other resources being made available. This is not to say that there can be no treatments that will work, but that every claim should be tested to prove its value. When proponents refuse to participate in testing of their methods, suspicion is warranted.

There are some neurologic conditions that occur in children with Down syndrome that improve with appropriate medical therapy; these are discussed in the next section.

Other Neurologic Problems Which May Be More Common in People with Down Syndrome

Seizures

Seizures are abnormal changes in consciousness that are caused by changes in nerves in the brain. Often these changes are like "short circuits" in the electrical messages between nerves. There are several types of seizures.

When many nerves are involved, the result may be what is called a *grand mal seizure,* with loss of consciousness and stiffening of the muscles, followed by body shaking and then relaxation with sleepiness or confusion. This type may also be called *tonic-clonic* or *major motor* seizures. *Petit mal* or *absence* seizures also include loss of consciousness, but usually do not affect motor ability. This type occurs in children, and may look like a staring spell, or even go unnoticed.

Partial seizures usually are limited to only part of the body, and consciousness may not be affected. Probably fewer nerves are involved, sometimes in just one part of the brain. A particular type of seizure called *infantile spasms* appears in infancy, and includes a particular pattern of arm and leg movements that is very recognizable. Infantile spasms may occur in babies who do not have Down syndrome, and do not respond well to treatment in those babies. This type of seizure is more common in children with Down syndrome, but when it occurs, responds better to medicine.

The best general statement about seizures in people with Down syndrome is that they are more common than in the general population, but usually respond to treatment with *anticonvulsants* (antiseizure medicines). Control of seizure disorders almost always requires the help of a neurologist, at least to diagnose the condition, and to help to get treatment started.

The usual times for seizure disorders to appear are with brain growth and development in children, after a brain injury of any kind (at any age), and as part of aging. Seizures can be part of Alzheimer's disease, but new seizures in an older person with Down syndrome do not always mean that person is developing Alzheimer's disease. The pattern of seizures can also change with age, and require altering medicine dosage or changing anticonvulsants.

Sometimes complete control of seizures is not possible because of drug side effects or other problems. You may need to decide how many seizures are acceptable compared to sleepiness or other side effects. The degree of control may also vary because of external factors. Illnesses, fevers, changes in sleep pattern, and the use of other drugs or alcohol can all affect how well seizures are controlled.

Attention Deficit/Hyperactivity Disorder (ADHD)

Many children with Down syndrome have attention problems in school and with their families, but that fact alone does not bring with it the diagnosis of ADHD. Many children (even children who do not have Down syndrome) have learning or communication problems, and those who do tend to have trouble paying attention or are easily distracted. Often in those cases, when the learning and communication issues are addressed, the attention problems get much better. The same is true for children with Down syndrome.

There is not at this time conclusive evidence that ADHD is more common in people with Down syndrome, but as mentioned above, learning and communication problems are common. The diagnosis of ADHD in your child should be made only after careful evaluation of communication and learning abilities, as well as vision and hearing, with particular attention to the appropriateness of the education program he is receiving. When the diagnosis of ADHD is correct, children with Down syndrome usually respond to the usual treatments with stimulant medications like methylphenidate (Ritalin™) or dexedrine.

Autism

Autism is a diagnosis that includes severe communication limitations, very abnormal development of relationships with others, and odd or repetitive patterns of behavior. Autism is probably not one single condition, but is instead a common cluster (or syndrome) of symptoms, with a number of different causes. Physicians, psychologists, and others who make this diagnosis do not always agree on when it is appropriate. Some use the label very often, to include individuals within a wide range of symptoms. Others reserve the term to describe those people who have more severe symptoms, with a particular focus upon the lack of ability to form real human relationships.

Some children with Down syndrome may seem to meet the criteria for autism. As mentioned above, however, communication problems are common in children with Down syndrome, and should not be the primary reason for diagnosing autism. Similarly, compulsive or slightly odd behaviors can often occur in people with Down syndrome as well as in other children with language limitations. Many parents report that their children with Down syndrome seem obsessed with a need to close doors. Others may tend to shake strings or socks, or engage in other behaviors interpreted as *self-stimulatory.* These behaviors may be called *autistic tendencies,* but do not by themselves justify the use of the diagnosis of autism.

Most children with Down syndrome are very social, and do not demonstrate the primary autism symptom of defective relationship formation. In fact, this "socialness" is often a strategy used by children to overcome communication difficulties. Children with autism, on the other hand, tend to treat other people as objects, or as sources of gratification. Kids who seek out human company for interactive play or physical and emotional comfort are probably not autistic.

In any case, there is seldom a particular advantage to adding the diagnosis of autism to a person with Down syndrome. There is some danger, however, because many people see autism as a "hopeless" condition without much chance for change or response to treatment. Adding autism to the list may, for instance, make speech therapy less available to treat the language problems that may have prompted the diagnosis in the first place.

Behavior Problems and Psychiatric Illness

Many children and adults with Down syndrome may at times have behaviors that cause problems for them and those who know them, but there is little evidence that the behaviors are directly part of Down syndrome. Most of the time, careful analysis shows the problems to be focused around communication and expectations. In fact, sorting out the causes of misbehavior is often the easy part. Usually changing the environment, through closer attention to choices offered and improvements in communication, helps to decrease inappropriate behaviors. Because these changes require family, friends, or support staff to alter *their* style or habits, success may be hard to accomplish. Success requires making adjustments to the environment at home, school, or work, not in "fixing" the person with Down syndrome.

There is little evidence that psychiatric illness is significantly more common in people with Down syndrome. Depression can be a frequent problem, but is usually a reaction to the facts of life. People with Down syndrome are no more or less likely to be depressed by unfortunate circumstances than anyone else, but they *are* more likely to face difficult situations that can lead to depression. Times of transition bring increased risk of depression and other reactions such as aggression or regression. Changes in employment or home setting, loss of a friend or family member, or prolonged illness are challenging to any of us. Depression is a frequent response to these kinds of situations for many people, particularly if the stress is compounded by communication problems or a limited support system. Antidepressant medications may help 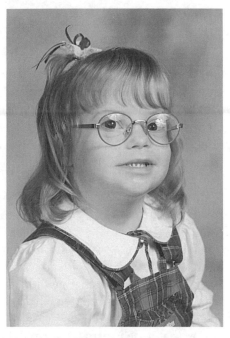 somewhat, but the best treatment for these individuals is attention to the primary problem that brought on the reaction.

Functional analysis is a type of psychologic assessment that attempts to sort out the reasons behind behaviors, and can be very useful in trying to understand aggressive or self-injurious actions. Very often the source of problem behavior is impaired communication. The behavior may be driven by a desire for escape from an uncomfortable situation or undesired task, or may be a bid for attention. Often the person does not like his choices, he does not know that he can choose, or cannot make his choice understood. Treatment consists of changing the environment to better meet that person's needs, and includes providing choice more often and paying closer attention to communication efforts.

Alzheimer's Disease

Alzheimer's disease is a condition that affects older people with and without Down syndrome. It typically changes brain function. This change is often called *dementia*. Dementia is seen as a gradual loss of memory and self-care skills, as well as changes in personality. The brain changes can be seen under microscopic exam; the plaques and especially the tangles mentioned earlier in this chapter can be seen. There are also changes seen on brain images like CT or MRI scans that may help make the diagnosis.

In most people the condition appears with age, in the late 70s or 80s. In a smaller group the problems are seen at younger ages, sometimes as early as the late 40s or early 50s. Down syndrome has come to be associated with early Alzheimer's disease, but the evidence is a bit confusing.

One type of brain change linked to Alzheimer's disease—brain plaques—is associated with abnormal differences in a gene on the 21st chromosome. In people with Down syndrome that gene is usually normal, but because of the extra 21st chromosome there may be more of that normal gene. Simply having more of the gene that can produce plaques, may not be the same as having the usual amount of an abnormal gene that produces plaques.

Studies of a large number of brains of people with Down syndrome have shown many to have the plaques and, to a smaller degree, the tangles seen in Alzheimer's disease. However, the people these brains belonged to had almost all lived in institutions for much of their lives, and little was known about their memories and abilities. When details of the lives of the people studied are known, however, the brain changes often do not correlate to changes in behavior, memory, or function. Although there are changes in the brains of people with Down syndrome, these changes do not always result from Alzheimer's disease.

One possible explanation for the confusion in diagnosing Alzheimer's disease in people with Down syndrome is that the brain changes described may occur for several reasons; when one has the condition called Alzheimer's disease, there is also dementia. In people with Down syndrome the brain changes may be a bit different, come about for very different reasons, and may not necessarily lead to dementia.

A few studies have begun to follow older people with Down syndrome as they age. One such study in New York focuses upon people living in independent or supported, non-institutional settings. The first report, after five years of visiting with these folks, has reported many fewer signs of dementia or other functional change than would be predicted if early Alzheimer's disease were common in people with Down syndrome.

Studies of people with Down syndrome who lived in institutions have reported a stronger connection between Down syndrome and Alzheimer's disease. But these studies are too narrow to draw conclusions about *all* people with Down syndrome. For example, people with Down syndrome who have been raised and live in a community (and not in an institution) cannot be compared scientifically to people whose lives were spent in institutions.

Many people with Down syndrome do have changes in ability as they get older, but there may be a number of different reasons for the changes, such as thyroid disease, worsening heart disease, depression, vision or hearing problems, or some other medical condition. There may indeed be an increase in the incidence of early Alzheimer's disease in people with Down syndrome, but the diagnosis should not be made until every other possibility has been considered. Certainly, life-changing decisions should not be made about a person with Down syndrome just because they are thought to be at higher risk of getting Alzheimer's disease. This condition is discussed further in Chapter 18.

Conclusion

Neurologic differences are common in people with Down syndrome. Most affect the way people think, speak, and act, and do not require the services of a neurologist. Cognitive ability varies tremendously from child to child. Very little is understood about the reasons for these changes. A child development assessment team, including a developmental pediatrician and various therapists, may be helpful in making school programming decisions to give your child the best possible shot at reaching his full potential.

Some neurologic conditions are more common in people with Down syndrome. Seizures happen more often, but usually respond very well to medication. The assistance of a pediatric neurologist is often necessary to manage seizures. ADHD, autism, and other conditions that include abnormal behavior are probably not more common in people Down syndrome. Children with Down syndrome respond to behavior management techniques as well as any other children. The most important facet of behavior management is to look carefully at communication and appropriateness of expectations as possible causes of problems.

References

Buckley, S. "The Development of the Child with Down Syndrome: Implications for Effective Education" in Pueschel, S.M. & Pueschel, J.K., eds. *Biomedical Concerns in Persons with Down Syndrome* (Baltimore: Paul H. Brookes Publishing Co. 1992), 29–70.

Carr, J. "Annotation: Long Term Outcome for People with Down's Syndrome." *Journal of Child Psychology and Psychiatry,* Vol. 35, No. 3, 1994, 425–439.

Devenney, D.A., et al. "Aging in Higher Functioning Adults with Down's Syndrome: An Interim Report in a Longitudinal Study." *Journal of Intellectual Disability Research,* Vol. 36, 1992, 241–50.

Florez, J. "Neurologic Abnormalities" in Pueschel, S.M. & Pueschel, J.K., eds. *Biomedical Concerns in Persons with Down Syndrome* (Baltimore: Paul H. Brookes Publishing Co. 1992), 159–173.

Kumin, Libby. *Communication Skills in Children with Down Syndrome: A Guide for Parents* (Bethesda, MD: Woodbine House, 1994).

Rogers, P.T. and Coleman, M. "The Central Nervous System" in Rogers, P.T. and Coleman, M. *Medical Care in Down Syndrome: A Preventive Medical Approach.* (New York: Marcel Decker, 1992), 201–224.

Rynders, J.E. "Supporting the Educational Development and Progress of Persons with Down Syndrome (with comments by Fredericks, H.D.)," in *Caring for Individuals with Down Syndrome and Their Families: Report of the Third Ross Roundtable in Critical Issues in Family Medicine* (Columbus, OH: Ross Products Division, Abbott Laboratories, 1995, in press).

Wisniewski, Silverman, and Wegiel. "Ageing, Alzheimer Disease and Mental Retardation." *Journal of Intellectual Disability Research,* Vol. 38, 1994, 233–239.

15 | Alternative and Unconventional Therapies in Children with Down Syndrome
Don C. Van Dyke, M.D.

Introduction

Children with Down syndrome can have significant, ongoing medical and developmental problems. Sometimes, standard medical treatment cannot solve some of these problems, such as mental retardation and recurring leukemia. The frustration that follows may lead parents to seek "alternative programs" and "unconventional therapies" in an effort to help their child.

Most medical treatments are developed over a long period of time. Scientific methods are used to study the effectiveness of a possible treatment and its side effects. Standard medical therapies are tested through a long period of clinical practice and objective studies. The results are treatments and therapies that are known to be both effective and safe.

Alternative or *unconventional* therapies do not follow standard medical practices. These therapies and treatments are often developed employing methods and standards different from those used to develop conventional treatments. They are frequently based on individual beliefs, subjective reports, or the experience of only a few individuals. Consequently, these methods may not be as thoroughly tested for effectiveness and safety before being offered to patients.

Other therapies may be controversial. Occasionally, different treatment approaches are used for the same condition.

For example, a medical problem may be treated by surgery in one country and by medicine in another. In addition, doctors may disagree over the best treatment choice for a condition, but usually the treatment outcome is the same.

Some therapies have no scientific or medical basis, but arise from superstition, unfounded claims, or simple greed. On the other hand, some alternative therapies have led to new and helpful treatments. For example, previous studies did not indicate any positive effect from therapies that use growth hormone to treat children with Down syndrome who have growth failure and short stature. However, with the recent availability of synthetic human growth hormone, there is pre-liminary evidence that treatments using growth hormone might be helpful for some children with Down syndrome. Likewise, past studies did not find giving thyroid hormone ex-tract to be beneficial. However, later studies indicated a high incidence of thyroid disease in older people with Down syn-drome. These older people did benefit from treatment of thy-roid dysfunction with hormone replacement therapy. Experiences such as these have shown that therapies must be carefully analyzed to separate the acceptable from the unac-ceptable.

Alternative therapies fall generally into four groups:

- medical
- physical
- educational
- surgical

This chapter describes some of the more commonly advo-cated therapies in each of these groups. In addition, it also provides guidelines to help you decide for yourself whether it would be in your child's best interest to try an alternative ther-apy.

Medical Therapies

Medical therapies, the term used to describe medical treatments, consist of the use of surgery and medicine to treat diseases and other conditions. Such therapies are usually prescribed and monitored by a physician or an assistant under the direction of a physician. For example, reducing blood pressure through medicine is a medical treatment. Some "alternative therapies" use medical treatment; despite the label, however, you should carefully consider any medical therapy suggested for your child. This chapter reviews the alternative medical therapies that have been and may still be suggested for children with Down syndrome.

Cell Therapy

Children with Down syndrome were first given injections of preparations containing freeze-dried animal cells in the 1960s. Proponents of cell therapy, also called *"sicca cell therapy,"* believe that injected fetal cells activate brain growth and growth of other organs. It was felt that the embryonic tissues caused revitalized cells to become the foundation for tissue regeneration. Cell therapy was frequently combined with other therapy, including education, speech therapy, and physical therapies. In addition, vitamins, minerals, and other preparations might be given. According to some proponents, cell therapy resulted an increase in I.Q.; improved motor, speech, and social abilities; and increased height, head circumference, and brain size.

Some oral and written reports have praised cell therapy. Yet research dating back as far as 1964 reports negative results. Recent studies add weight to the scientific view that cell therapy is not helpful in the treatment of Down syndrome. Even so, a small number of parents in the United States continue to try cell therapy for their children. In some cases, they travel with their child to other countries for treatment, or

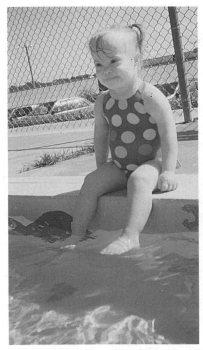

they may get freeze-dried material in the mail to be used for injection.

The New Hope Parents Association of Huntsville, Alabama, a parent support group, supports cell therapy for children with Down syndrome. They claim that no large, double-blind study (an objective study in which some patients receive the cells while others receive a placebo; neither group knows which they receive) has been done that proves cell therapy to be effective or ineffective. Although this therapy has not been tested by a double-blind trial, the existing body of published literature indicates that it has no effect on the growth or function of children with Down syndrome. In fact, some risk may accompany this therapy. A child may have an allergic reaction to the cell materials that are injected; this reaction can include anaphylactic shock, which can be fatal. Currently, there appears to be renewed interest in human fetal cell therapy (some physicians in Russia are strong advocates of it), but there is still no scientific data showing it to be effective.

Vitamin Therapy

There are many alternative therapies based on vitamin supplements. These include *orthomolecular* therapy and *megavitamin* therapy. As described by the proponents of orthomolecular therapy, individuals are given supplements of minerals and vitamins that are normally found in the human body in order to provide an "optimum molecular environment" for the developing mind. In megavitamin therapy large doses of vitamins are given in an effort to stimulate cognitive development.

Vitamin therapy had a resurgence in 1981 with the work of Dr. R.F. Harrell and others, who noted improvement in I.Q. scores in some children with mental delays, including some individuals with Down syndrome, following treatment with megavitamins and minerals. Later research that tried to replicate this study did not get the same results. Since then, the American Academy of Pediatrics has advised against the use of megavitamin therapies because of the potential risks involved. Fat soluble vitamins (such as vitamins A, D, and E) are toxic if taken in large doses over a period of time. Large doses of vitamin A can cause liver problems, nausea, vomiting, growth impairment, increased intracranial pressure, anaphylactic shock, and death. Large doses of vitamin D can result in weakness, fatigue, headache, vomiting, diarrhea, growth problems, and renal (kidney) problems. Large doses of vitamin E can lead to liver problems.

Despite the potential hazards, parents and some medical practitioners continue to attempt to treat cognitive delays in children with Down syndrome with vitamins. In one clinical review of 190 histories of individuals with Down syndrome, 19 percent had received megavitamin therapy at some time. According to the American Academy of Pediatrics, there has been no evidence establishing the effectiveness of megavitamin therapy, despite the claims. The evidence does not show that giving megavitamins to your child will improve her cognitive abilities, muscle tone, or speech.

For some children with Down syndrome who have malabsorption conditions, supplementary vitamins or minerals may, however, be appropriately prescribed. For more information on malabsorption syndromes, see Chapter 9.

Growth Hormone

In the past, human growth hormone was extracted from the pituitary glands of cadavers and given to children with Down syndrome in an attempt to increase their height. Research found, however, that this therapy was ineffective except in the rare case when a child's decreased growth was actually caused by a lack of human growth hormone. The risks of human growth hormone treatment are discussed in Chapter 5.

Currently, growth hormone therapy is once again attracting attention. The recent availability of synthetic human growth hormone now makes additional research possible. A 1991 study concluded that growth hormone made using molecular genetic techniques may produce growth in height and head circumference. Other preliminary studies indicate that synthetic human growth hormone might be effective in promoting growth if it is started at an early age.

Therapy with synthetic growth hormone is a rapidly developing area of research that may potentially benefit children with Down syndrome. However, many more studies need to be done. As Chapter 5 explains, there are concerns about an increase in the incidence of leukemia with the use of growth hormone. So, if you are considering synthetic growth hormone treatment for your child, you should understand that at present the data regarding its effectiveness are preliminary, and that there may be some risks. Check carefully before participating in any studies or therapies involving the use of human growth hormone .

Zinc/Selenium Supplements

Zinc and selenium are known as *trace elements,* or *micro-nutrients,* and are present in some diets. Zinc plays a role in the function of enzymes (it is called an enzyme *co-factor*). It is vital for white blood cell function, immunity, and metabolism. Selenium also is required for certain enzymes to work ef-

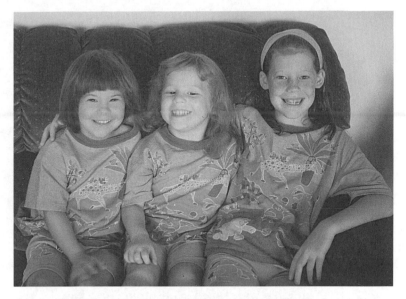

fectively. If there is not enough selenium in the body, problems can occur.

Some children with Down syndrome may have deficiencies in their immune system (discussed in detail in Chapter 4), including low T-cell levels. These deficiencies in some cases may be associated with low blood levels of zinc and selenium. Some preliminary research suggests that these trace elements may improve immune system function and growth. In such studies, zinc and selenium were given as part of a dietary supplement. The data is preliminary and no specific dosages for zinc and selenium treatment have been determined. Once again, working only with reputable studies.

Other Drug Treatments

Besides the treatments described above, many other attempts have been made to find a relationship between specific medications and an improvement in physical, mental, and social functioning in individuals with Down syndrome. Many drugs and their derivatives have been used or suggested for use in treating the symptoms of Down syndrome. Some of these compounds have included dimethyl sulfoxide (DMSO), glutamic acid and its derivatives, dihydroepiandrosterone, vitamin E, pituitary extract, 5–hydroxytryptophan, and piracetam.

Dimethyl Sulfoxide (DMSO). DMSO, a solvent, has been claimed to improve the intellectual functioning of children with Down syndrome. Studies of its use did not demonstrate any significant improvement in either cognitive function or behavior. At present, DMSO is used only to treat a specific type of bladder problem *(interstitial cystitis)*. It is toxic to the liver and bone marrow.

Piracetam. Piracetam is a new drug with a structure similar to a neurotransmitter (a chemical present in the nervous system that enables nerve impulses to travel from one nerve cell to another); it is believed by some to enhance learning and memory. This claim has stimulated interest in using the drug to treat children with Down syndrome. There have been some studies on the use of piracetam in adults with Alzheimer's disease and in children with learning disabilities and dyslexia. However, there have been no scientific studies on the use of piracetam in people with Down syndrome, and there are presently no studies into its use in people with Down syndrome. Its effectiveness and safety have not been established, and parents should be cautious.

Other Compounds. Numerous compounds have been used in an attempt to improve cognitive development, growth, and physical appearance. These compounds include glutamic acid (an amino acid that acts in nerve transmission), dihydroepiandrosterone (a steroid), vitamin E, and 5–hydroxytryptophan (a serotonin precursor or building block that functions in nerve transmission). Studies of these compounds showed that they had no significant effect in children with Down syndrome. Some, such as dihydroepiandrosterone (given in the past to children with short stature before human growth hormone was used), have not been used for many years.

Surgical Therapy

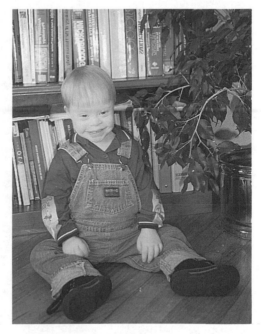

The most commonly suggested alternative surgical therapy for children with Down syndrome is *cosmetic* surgery (surgery that is not necessary for physical health). Surgery may be attempted to reduce tongue size, enlarge the nose and chin, change the appearance of the eyes, or reshape the face.

Tongue reduction surgery has been performed in an attempt either to lessen tongue protrusion or to improve articulation or speech intelligibility. Chapter 8 covers this procedure in detail; preliminary data suggest that it has no effect on articulation or speech intelligibility.

The other types of plastic surgery commonly used are intended primarily to change appearance so that Down syndrome features are less noticeable. Children with Down syndrome may have mid-facial hypoplasia (incomplete or abnormal development of the middle of the face) with a flat nasal bridge, flat chin, and sometimes mandibular (jaw) problems. Plastic surgery has not been particularly successful in altering these features. As with all plastic surgery, there are significant risks from anesthesia, scarring, and infection. The surgery is expensive and usually not covered by health insurance.

There is a wide spectrum of opinions about plastic surgery for children with Down syndrome among people with Down syndrome themselves, their parents, peers, doctors, and teachers. This will be an area of continued, long-term studies in an effort to determine whether these surgical procedures actually improve the quality of life for individuals with Down syndrome.

Physical and Communication Therapies

Most children with Down syndrome receive a variety of educational and other therapies as part of their early intervention or special education programs. Often, these therapies are essential to helping them make optimal developmental progress. You need to beware of extremes in therapy programs, however, whether it's focus is physical, occupational, education, or speech therapy. It can be frustrating and emotionally traumatic to spend a great deal of time, energy, and money only to achieve minimal results. On the other hand, you may feel strongly that exploring some new or alternative therapy is worth the risk. Whatever your choice, learn as much as you can about the therapy program before you invest in it. Some therapies that you should approach with caution include patterning and facilitated communication.

Patterning

Patterning—a program of therapy based upon frequent repetitive motion, sometimes for two to four hours daily, five days a week—has been proposed as a therapy for children with Down syndrome. In patterning your child's limbs are moved passively by a therapist in an effort to initiate primitive newborn patterns and gradually progress to more advanced movement patterns. The controversial aspect of this approach is that it requires a great investment in terms of time, people,

Table 1: Summary of alternative and controversial therapies.	
Alternative therapy	**Research shows:**
Pituitary extract	*No benefit,* to cognitive and social development
Glutamic acid	*No benefit*
Thyroid hormone	*No benefit,* except for those who have underactibve thyroid *(hypothyroid)*
5–hydroxytryptophan	*No benefit*
Dimethyl sulfoxide (DMSO)	*No benefit* to cognitive or speech development
Sicca cell/cell therapy	*No benefit* to cognitive function
Megavitamin/minerals	*No benefit* to cognitive function
Zinc/selenium	*Possible positive effect* on immune system, needs further controlled studies
Plastic surgery, facial	*Controversial;* numerous issues and many unanswered questions, research continues
Patterning	*Controversial,* no strong data to document benefits
Human growth hormone	*Strong interest,* preliminary data shows significant increase in height and head size; concern in use with children prone to leukemia

and effort. Studies show minimal short-term results and no long-term results. Proponents, however, continue to argue that these therapies have not been appropriately evaluated.

Facilitated Communication

Facilitated communication is a technique in which another person assists someone with a communication impairment to sign, write, or type a message. In facilitated communication, the facilitator holds a child's arm or hand to enable her to produce meaningful messages. In the last three years, it has aroused much interest and publicity, for it appears to improve the communication abilities of children with autism, Down syndrome, and other disabilities. It is practiced in a variety of settings, including public and private schools.

Controversy continues about the effectiveness of facilitated communication. Recent studies have shown that this technique does not work. It is, however, still widely used in schools and is still under study. It is a therapy that requires further careful evaluation.

Questions Parents Should Ask about Alternative Therapies

Making a decision about an alternative treatment or therapy can be very stressful. There are many considerations to balance. Hope and love for your child can sometimes conflict with making a rational decision. But careful weighing of the potential benefits with the potential risks is critical. If you are considering an alternative or controversial therapy, ask yourself the following questions:

1. Has your doctor or therapist provided you with written, convincing, easily understood information about research documenting the benefits of the therapy?
2. What are the possible risks of the procedure or therapy?
3. Do the benefits outweigh the risks?
4. Does your child want the therapies?
5. What kind of follow-up care is needed? How your child will be monitored? Who will monitor? How often will she be seen?
6. What are the long-term results? How are these documented?
7. What are the costs? Will insurance cover all or part of them?

Often your child's doctor will be able to answer your questions. Sometimes, your doctor may not be knowledgeable about a specific alternative therapy. If so, there are several ways to obtain more information, such as by contacting the National Down Syndrome Congress and the National Down Syndrome Society. Other parents can be a great source in your hunt for information.

Summary

As a parent you want to help your child as much as possible. In some cases, the health care profession seems to offer very little encouragement. While new research generates new hope, some yields only false promises. Alternative and unconventional treatments may go on to become accepted, conventional treatments—or they may create only controversy, confusion, and frustration (see Table I).

At present, there is no "cure" or "ultimate treatment" for children with Down syndrome. Appropriate medical care, developmental stimulation, physical therapy, and educational intervention all can play a role in helping your child develop fully. As we learn more about children with Down syndrome, these interventions will evolve to provide even greater benefits.

References

Bidder, R.T., et al. "The Effects of Multivitamins and Minerals on Children with Down Syndrome." *Developmental Medicine and Child Neurology,* Vol. 31, 1989, 532–537.

Fackelmann, K. "New Hope or False Promise?" *Scientific News,* Vol. 137, 1990, 168–170.

Golden, G.S. "What's New in Controversial Therapies?" *Update,* May 20, 1992. An abstract presented at the 12th Annual Conference on Developmental-Behavioral Disorders.

Golden, G.S. "Controversies in Therapy for Children with Down Syndrome." *Pediatrics in Review,* Vol. 6, 1989, 116–120.

Golden, G.S. "A Hard Look at Fad Therapies for Developmental Disorders." *Contemporary Pediatrics,* 1987, 47–60.

Golden, G.S. "Controversial Therapies." *Pediatric Clinics of North America,* Vol. 31, 1984, 459–469.

Pueschel, Siegfried M. *Biomedical Concerns in Persons with Down Syndrome,* (Baltimore: Paul H. Brookes, 1992), 289–300.

Sparrow, S. and Zigler, E. "Evaluation of a Patterning Treatment for Retarded Children," *Pediatrics,* Vol. 62, 1978, 137–150.

Van Dyke, D.C., et al. "Alternative and Controversial Therapies," in *Clinical Perspectives in the Management of Down Syndrome* (New York: Springer-Verlag, 1990), 208–216.

16 | Anesthesia and Surgical Concerns for Children with Down Syndrome
Frederic A. Berry, M.D.

Introduction

When children with Down syndrome require surgery, care must be taken to ensure that the surgery is safe and as painless as possible. All surgery causes some pain, but the goal must always be to minimize it. Anesthesia is critically important because it is how doctors make sure that your child's surgery will not cause him excessive pain. In addition, general anes-

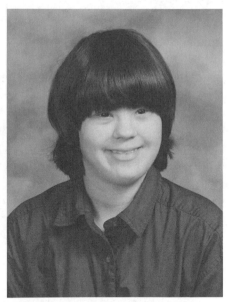

thesia reduces or eliminates psychological trauma because your child is asleep during the procedure. Anesthesia is also critical for surgery because surgery requires your child to be absolutely still. General anesthesia allows this, making delicate surgical procedures possible. This makes the surgery safer for your child.

Despite the benefits of anesthesia, care must be taken in using it with children with Down syndrome. Children with Down syndrome have a higher incidence of medical problems that require surgery, and they have more frequent problems with anesthesia. This chapter reviews the concerns with using anesthesia and explains how anesthesia should be used. In addition, the chapter explains the basic procedures used in most surgeries. This will give you a clearer picture of how anesthesia is used. If you know what to expect, the experience can be less frightening and intimidating.

Before Surgery

There are many issues that must be considered by parents and doctors before any surgery. *All* surgeries need to be carefully planned. Concern for the health, safety, and emotions of your child must come first. Every doctor should share these concerns with you.

A visit with the anesthesiologist before surgery will allow you to discuss any anesthetics your child has received in the past and whether or not there were difficulties. It is very important during this visit for you to share with the anesthesiologist any concerns and fears you have. The anesthesiologist will discuss the various risks of anesthesia. Try making a list of questions ahead of time. Sometimes, there is so much information that you can forget the questions you really wanted answered. Do not hesitate to ask for understandable explanations about the procedures that will be used.

Communication

When a child undergoes surgery, the entire family shares the anxieties of the experience. As parents, you will unquestionably feel a great deal of emotional pain when your child faces surgery. You need emotional support, as well as information. During the anxious period surrounding surgery, good communication among parents and professionals is crucial.

Good communication is not a luxury; it is a basic factor in good medical care. You need to feel free to communicate your concerns to the medical team.

The medical "team" includes all the professionals involved in the care of your child. Obviously, some people are more visible and more available to you than others. If your child is admitted as an inpatient, the people you will have most contact with are the nurses; the doctors will visit periodically (and often unpredictably) throughout the day. If the surgery is done as an outpatient procedure, the surgeon and the person providing the anesthesia may by your primary contacts.

The medical team also has a responsibility to communicate realistically with you about their concerns. If communication is not good, frustration and anger can develop, even when medical care is effective and appropriate. These emotions may be felt by you or by the members of the medical team, and can jeopardize the success of treatment.

Studies show that effective communication is crucial to any patient's satisfaction with medical care. However, the very nature of modern medical care can lead to frustration with the enormous amount of paperwork, repetition, delay, and wasted time. Sometimes a parent mistakes frustration with "the system" for frustration with medical care.

Sometimes improving communication is as simple as deciding on a regular schedule for you and the physicians to meet each day during hospitalization; other times it may take more of an effort by the doctor to understand your questions. If you write down your questions ahead of time, it is easier to get them answered. Not only do you remember to ask, but sometimes just the process of writing things down may help you to understand what it is you really want to know.

When unhappiness or frustration occur, it is important for you and the medical team to freely communicate with each other. This clears the air and makes it easier to provide the best medical care possible for your child.

Medical Conditions and Anesthesia

Children with Down syndrome have a high incidence of conditions that require surgery. About half of all children with Down syndrome have congenital heart disease, and this frequently requires surgical intervention. Newborns with Down syndrome have a high incidence of intestinal obstruction. Leukemia is more frequent in young children who have Down syndrome, and this may require bone marrow transplantation. Sleep apnea, caused by many factors, can lead to upper airway obstruction. These and other conditions are discussed throughout this book.

The good news is that many congenital heart defects can now be repaired. Most children will have *curative* surgery, which cures the condition. A few children have heart defects so severe that only *palliative* surgery can be performed. This is surgery which results in an improvement of the condition, but is not a cure. Heart conditions and their treatment are discussed in detail in Chapter 3. However, the effects of heart conditions and heart surgery affect the use of anesthetics in the future.

Even when surgery has "repaired" a heart defect, your child's heart may never be completely "normal" (this is discussed in Chapter 3). Children with congenital heart disease may be subject to a type of infection of the heart called *subacute bacterial endocarditis*. This infection can result from certain types of operations that cause bacteria to get into the blood stream. These surgeries include any surgery on the nose, throat, teeth, kidneys, bladder, and intestinal system. For this reason, these children may require antibiotics during certain surgeries.

Children at risk for endocarditis need to take antibiotics to ward off infection from surgery, and this has an effect on anesthesia. Opinions differ as to exactly when the antibiotics need to be given. Unfortunately for children, the guidelines of the American Heart Association suggest giving antibiotics 30 to 60 minutes before anesthesia begins. Some doctors and anesthesiologists take these guidelines as rules, rather than suggestions. This timing, however, may conflict with the goal of keeping pain and discomfort to a minimum. The only way that antibiotics can be given 30 to 60 minutes before surgery is intravenously or by an intramuscular (into the muscle) injection. Both of these techniques are painful. Studies have shown that antibiotics are just as effective when given orally two hours before surgery or intravenously shortly after the anesthesia begins. With these methods your child feels no pain. If your child is having outpatient surgery (surgery that does not require staying in the hospital) and will return home the same day, you will need to give him antibiotics for 2 or 3 days after the surgery. If your child is hospitalized for the surgery, the hospital staff handles giving the antibiotics.

Risk Factors

Every surgical procedure, no matter how minor or routine, carries with it at least some risk. Low risk surgeries include placement of ear tubes or oral surgery to repair dental problems. High risk procedures include most heart repairs as well as repair of spinal injury due to neck instability. There are both risks of the surgery itself and risks from the anesthesia.

The risks of surgery and anesthesia arise from two factors. The first is whether or not your child has any underlying medical conditions. For example, a child with Down syndrome may have a congenital heart defect; this underlying condition creates certain risks. In addition, a child's condition, such as poor nutrition that results from feeding problems, may delay healing and increase the chance of infection following surgery. The other risk factor is the surgical procedure itself. A child with a congenital heart defect who is having a tonsillectomy faces, first, the increased risks of anesthesia in a child with a congenital heart defect; and, second, the risks associated with the tonsillectomy.

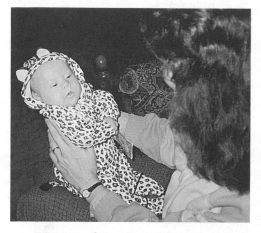

In addition to the risks all children have from anesthesia, children with Down syndrome may have special anesthetic concerns that can complicate the surgical procedure and add to the risk of surgery. These concerns are discussed below.

Timing of Surgery. When surgery occurs has a big effect on risks. Surgeries are described as either *elective* or *emergency*. Emergency surgery is surgery that must be done immediately to treat a condition that presents a serious threat to health. An appendectomy to remove an infected appendix or the repair of a badly broken bone are both considered emergencies surgeries. Surgery that can be safely done at a future date is called elective surgery. For example, placement of ear tubes is considered elective surgery; it can be scheduled around everyone's convenience. However, elective does not mean unnecessary; some life-saving surgeries can be delayed until children are old enough or big enough. For example, the timing of surgery to repair heart defects can often be planned for when your child is best able to handle it.

The repair of many but not all congenital heart defects and most other surgeries for children with Down syndrome are planned, and are thus considered elective surgeries. The advantage of this is that parents have time to find information about the risks and benefits of the anesthetic and the surgery. You have time to prepare yourselves and your child for the surgery.

By definition, *emergency* surgery cannot be anticipated or postponed. You do not have time to develop the same level of comfort that you can with elective surgery. Most of the common reasons for emergency surgery—accidents that cause broken bones, appendicitis, and the like—are no different for a child with Down syndrome than for any other child. But children with Down syndrome are more prone to some conditions leading to emergency surgery that are less common. Children with heart disorders sometimes get worse quickly and need emergency surgery, and children with unstable necks are at higher risk of sudden injury that might require an operation.

Emergency surgery is also more common for newborns and very young children with Down syndrome compared to other children, and this can present some special problems. For example, emergency surgery to correct an intestinal blockage may be needed for a newborn infant with Down syndrome. Surgeries like these can be especially wrenching emotionally because they occur at the same time parents make their first adjustment to the news that their baby has Down syndrome. The addition of the acute anxieties of surgery can be overwhelming.

Today hospital staff are usually much more familiar with the needs of families facing surgery for a very young child, and can provide valuable support. Children with Down syndrome receive the same health and surgical care as any other child, and their parents can receive the same support as other parents. And there are things you, as parent, can do to make the surgery less stressful for your child.

Just like other children, children with Down syndrome may need emergency surgery due to any of the more common problems of childhood, such as appendicitis or a broken leg. In these circumstances, you do not have the time to develop the same degree of comfort with the upcoming surgery as you would with elective surgery. Your child's pain or discomfort may make it very difficult for him to understand exactly what is happening. Your frustration with your inability to prepare your child for surgery may add to your own distress.

Even during emergencies, it is important for you to explain to your child, in a simple and truthful way, what can be expected. Comfort your child by explaining that you will be there when he goes to sleep and when he wakes up. Tell your child that there will be medicine available so that the surgery won't hurt. One of the major fears children have is a fear of injections, or "shots." In studies, this is the number one fear expressed by most children. Health care workers have made a concentrated effort to reduce the number of injections that are given to children. Medications can usually be given by mouth (orally) or through a child's IV (intravenous) line. If your child asks about shots, it is difficult to give an answer unless you know exactly what the medical team plans for your child. Sometimes the best answer is "I don't know, but I do know they won't give you any shots unless you really need them to get well."

Common Anesthetic Risks. Children with Down syndrome are usually small at birth, and during infancy and childhood grow more slowly than other children. The high incidence of congenital heart disease may be partly responsible for this, but even children with Down syndrome who are free of congenital heart disease have slower growth. Small size can affect surgical and anesthetic procedures.

During some surgeries a plastic tube is placed into your child's trachea (the air passage that goes from the mouth to the lungs). It is called an *endotracheal tube.* Your child gets oxygen and anesthetics through the endotracheal tube. These tubes are important for surgery, but extra care must be taken in their use with children with Down syndrome.

One of the results of a child's smaller size is that the usual formulas for determining the size of his endotracheal tube, which are based on age, can't be used. Smaller tubes than your child's age may indicate must be used. In addition, children with Down syndrome often have *congenital subglottic stenosis*, a narrowing of the area of the trachea just below the vocal cords. This narrowing can make it difficult to insert the endotracheal tube. If the area becomes irritated and swollen due to the tube, your child may not be able to breath easily. Many children develop noisy breathing called *stridor*. Stridor occurs more frequently in infants and children with Down syndrome than in other children. Anesthesiologists should be aware of this risk and plan for using a smaller tube than usual.

Atlanto-Axial Instability. As discussed in Chapter 10, *atlanto-axial instability* refers to instability of the spine (vertebrae) where the head joins the neck. This instability allows the two vertebrae to slip too far forward and backward, called *subluxation*. The result is that the bony edges of the vertebrae can press on the spinal cord, which can cause temporary or permanent damage.

Your child's surgical team, including the anesthesiologist should know if your child has atlanto-axial instability. Even though about 10 percent of people with Down syndrome have abnormal neck x-rays that suggest atlanto-axial instability, only 1 to 2 percent show any symptoms. Anesthesiologists are concerned about the potential for neck instability because of the way anesthetics are given, as well as how your child's head is positioned during and after surgery.

Children with Down syndrome who have a potential for instability have increased risk during anesthesia for two reasons. First, the placement of an endotracheal tube requires tilting the head back to extend the neck. Muscle relaxants are often used to make it easier to insert the tube. In addition, inserting the tube may require opening your child's mouth very wide which also extends the neck. Every member of the surgical team needs to be aware of the potential for cervical spinal cord damage from extending the neck during surgery.

The second period of risk for children with a potential for spinal cord damage is during the period of awakening. When children awake from anesthesia, they may be confused and frightened, and can sometimes struggle and thrash about.

Even though the risk of spinal cord damage during anesthesia is extremely small, your child's anesthesiologist needs to be aware of the possibility and plan to avoid it. Lastly, after surgery, your child should be examined for any signs of spinal cord damage that might have occurred during surgery.

Anesthesia During Surgery

Preparation for Anesthesia and Surgery

It is helpful to talk with your child about the upcoming anesthesia and surgery. Let your child ask questions; listen carefully and answer thoughtfully and honestly. You are the best judge of your child's ability to understand, and of when to begin talking about an upcoming surgery. It is a good idea to coordinate this with your family doctor, anesthesiologist, and surgeon, so that both the timing and the information are appropriate.

A visit to the hospital before surgery can be helpful by taking away some of the mystery; fear of the unknown is a large part of the anxiety for anyone who needs an operation. Several children's books have been written about hospitalization; one good book from Children's Television Workshop is called *Grover Visits the Hospital*. It answers common questions many children have about doctors, hospitals, and operations. Reading a book with your child can be a nonthreatening way to bring up the topic, and can help you to uncover any particular questions or secret fears your child may have. If a family member or friend has been in the hospital or has had surgery, perhaps your child could benefit from talking to him or her. You should be careful, however; not everyone has good experiences in the hospital; your child does not need to hear someone else's horror stories.

Pre-Medication and the Induction of Anesthesia

Prior to the beginning of surgery, your child will be admitted to the hospital. Sometimes this occurs on the day before the scheduled operation if your child is ill or if there are tests that need to be done first. Other times the admission happens just before the time of surgery. Many operations are now done as "outpatient procedures"; this means that your child is expected to go home the same day of the operation, after recovery. The choice depends upon the surgery planned and your child's medical condition.

The exact sequence of events before the start of surgery also varies from child to child. Usually an intravenous (IV) line is placed in a vein. Your child may be asleep when this is done, but sometimes that might not be possible. IVs are small plastic tubes that are placed in larger veins to allow doctors to give your child fluids and medicines during and after the surgery. These tubes or *catheters* are placed using small needles which guide the tube into the vein. When the catheter is in place, the needle is removed and the IV is taped to keep it from falling out. Some children have veins that are very hard to find; others have veins that are fragile and break easily. Children with Down syndrome are more likely to have both problems. Most of the time IVs are put in the hand or arm, but your doctor may choose to use a vein in a foot or even the scalp if necessary. In addition to IV lines, your child may have wires attached that monitor his breathing, heart rate, and blood pressure during the surgery.

There are two times during the anesthetic process when there is a potential for emotional trauma for both you and your child. The first is when you are first separated from each other. The second is when the anesthetic is begun. These transitions need to be and can be handled so as to minimize emotional trauma. You should make it clear to your child's surgical team that you want them to help make this time as easy as possible.

There are several ways to ease the initial separation before surgery, and to make the start of anesthesia (called *induction*) more peaceful. The longer you can remain with your child before surgery, the better. However, some medical centers are not designed to allow you to remain with your child in the area near the operating room. Always ask to stay with your child as long as possible, but cooperate with the hospital staff's directions.

In order to make it easier for your child to be away from you, he may be given "pre-medication." These consist of sedating medicines like Valium that will help your child relax, reduce anxiety, and blur his memories of the event. Unfortunately, pre-medications may not taste very good, and some children will not readily take them. Similar medicines can be given as a suppository in your child's bottom, but that is not a popular method for children over age four. If getting the pre-medication into your child causes a lot of commotion it may not be worth the trouble because the purpose of pre-medication is to make the operation go more smoothly for your child.

A second, sometimes difficult time comes when anesthesia is started. This is when you may be required to leave your child. Medical centers typically use one of three approaches, again depending upon their facilities. In some medical centers, your child, with or without pre-medication, will be taken into the operating room where the anesthetic is begun. Usually parents are not allowed in the operating room with their child. However, in some hospitals, you will be allowed to come into the operating room for the induction of anesthesia. To do this, you must wear a surgical cap, gown, and mask. The third approach is a separate room to start the anesthesia where you can be with your child. No cap, gown, or mask are needed.

With children younger than 7 or 8 years, anesthesia is usually begun by breathing a gaseous anesthetic through a mask. For older children, anesthesia begins when sedatives such as pentothal or propofol are given to the child through the IV line. A technique frequently used for children younger than 5 or 6 years who do not cooperate in breathing an anesthetic gas from a mask is to use a drug called Brevital. This is a rectal suppository that can be given with the parents' help. With Brevital, your child will usually fall asleep within 5 to 7 minutes. This allows a quiet separation and a peaceful beginning of the anesthetic.

For infants younger than a year, parents are usually not permitted to be present. For older, more cooperative infants and children, however, parents may be allowed to be present for the induction of anesthesia if facilities allow. Not every medical center and not every anesthesiologist is experienced with allowing parents to be present for the induction of anesthesia. It is difficult for a child to *not* be frightened by anesthetic procedures. When allowed, your presence can be reassuring. With a little extra time and effort a peaceful separation and anesthesia induction can be accomplished.

When a drug such as pentothal or propofol is given intravenously, sleep is induced within 30 to 60 seconds and there is usually no excitement or struggling. When anesthesia is begun by breathing through a mask, it takes several minutes for the child to become anesthetized. During this period, there may be some crying and struggling as the child loses consciousness. Some children may get agitated for a short period of time. In addition, in some children, anesthesia makes them feel as if they are falling just before they completely lose consciousness. They often put their hands and legs out as if to catch themselves. You need to understand these behaviors ahead of time so that you will not be alarmed and can ease your child's fears. As soon as your child loses consciousness, a nurse or other staff will guide you to a waiting room while the anesthesiologist takes your child into the operating room.

Certain situations may complicate the induction of anesthesia, and they cannot be predicted or completely prevented. One problem is if your child has a narrow or obstructed air-

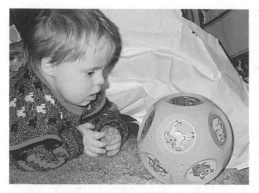

way. If there is concern about your child's airway, the anesthesiologist may ask you to leave. The reason is that the anesthesiologist needs to be free to focus entirely on your child. A well-trained medical team can very efficiently open airways with suction, with placement or re-placement of a breathing tube, and with medicines. If one or more of the team is distracted by you, however, the teamwork may suffer. It is in your child's best interest if you leave immediately if you are requested to do so.

You may feel that you are not emotionally suited to be present for the beginning of the anesthetic. If you feel your presence would make a difficult situation worse for your child, you should not feel pressured to stay. Indeed, it would be a mistake. The primary reason for you to be there is to provide emotional support to your child—but it is difficult to be supportive if you yourself are upset.

Another source of stress to parents during surgery is the time you spend waiting for your child's surgery to be completed. This time can often be longer than you have been told to expect. Sometimes the actual surgery may be delayed for simple reasons, such as trouble with an IV line or problems with equipment. Similarly, procedures following surgery (*post-operative* routines) may keep your child in the operating room for some time after surgery has been completed. In many hospitals, parents are informed of these delays; asking staff to extend this courtesy to you can help you avoid needless worry.

It may be helpful to know that even routine surgery can *seem* to take forever. It isn't uncommon to find yourself remembering every unlikely risk or complication of surgery that you have ever heard anyone mention. You may also find that being in a hospital waiting room calls up memories of past illnesses and injuries that may add to your level of anxiety.

Many parents report that time passes more quickly if you have others to share the wait with you. Ask anyone that can help you—family, friends, professional—to come to the hospital, and ask anyone who would add to your stress to wait at home. Your local family support group may be able to give you the names of experienced families who can help you prepare for your child's surgery as well as provide moral support on the day of the operation.

After Surgery

As the surgeons are finishing up their work by cleaning up the surgery site and dressing the wounds, the anesthesia team will begin to wake your child. The anesthesia medicines are cut back or stopped. If a machine has been breathing for your child, the tube is removed from the airway, and your child is allowed to breathe on his own. At this point, the action usually moves to the recovery room next to the operating suite. Here your child will be closely watched until he is "stable."

If the surgery was done as an outpatient procedure, your child will remain in the recovery room until he is fully awake and his doctor is satisfied that he is stable enough to go home. Vital signs (heart rate, breathing rate, and blood pressure) must be completely normal. Bleeding must be stopped, and dressings must be securely in place. Pain must be under good control with medicines that can be given at home.

If the plan was for inpatient recovery, or if there were complications requiring further treatment, your child will be moved to a hospital unit where the nursing team can monitor his progress. Vital signs are followed, and again, pain and bleeding must be under good control. Fluids are usually given by IV until the patient is clearly able to tolerate drinking. This may take several days after some surgeries.

Sometimes the recovery is expected to be complicated and require very close observation; in those cases your child is moved to the intensive care unit directly from the operating room. If your child has open heart surgery, it is likely that he will be taken to the intensive care unit with many tubes and monitors still attached, where the nursing team will be very busy with the details of his recovery for several days. You should ask your child's surgeon where your child will go after surgery and what to expect when you visit him there.

Post-Operative Pain Relief

The use of medicine to relieve pain from surgery has changed a lot during the past ten years. In the past, children did not receive the same pain relief after an operation as adults did. Because of the awareness that children suffer from surgical pain just like adults, better anesthesia techniques as well as other pain relief techniques are now increasingly used with children.

Doctors may use a variety of medicines to control the pain from surgery. There are two major forms of anesthetics: 1) local or regional and 2) general. Anesthesia during the operation uses several kinds, especially *anesthetics,* which cause numbing or loss of all sensation. General anesthetics work on the entire body, while regional and local anesthetics are used for smaller parts of the body where the surgeon works.

There are a variety of methods to provide post-operative pain relief. One of these is to use regional anesthesia called an *epidural*. With an epidural, anesthetic is injected at the base of the spine (this is just like what many mothers receive during delivery). *Analgesics* control pain without the loss of consciousness or numbing. Very often *anti-inflammatory* medicines like Tylenol™ or Motrin™ are used to help with the pain of swelling and with injury that affects muscles and bones after the cutting and bruising of surgery. *Narcotics* such as morphine and fentanyl are a special class of medicines that change the way the brain receives pain messages. These drugs are particularly useful for severe pain immediately after surgery, when there are post-operative procedures like traction, or when tubes or drains are left in the body that can cause continuing pain. Usually the need for narcotics decreases over several days and the anti-inflammatory medicines are strong enough to deal with the pain that remains.

Technology has provided new and more effective ways to provide post-operative pain relief in some cases. For a child who is old enough to understand, PCA—*patient controlled analgesia*—can be used. This technique involves the use of a pump that provides a pre-set dose of pain medicine through your child's IV line. When your child feels discomfort, he can press a button and a small dose of narcotic is automatically injected into the IV line. The dispenser does not allow a patient to give himself too much medication. If your child cannot use the PCA system, you or a nurse can evaluate the level of his pain and press the button.

Research shows that effective pain relief improves surgical results and shortens hospital stays. Each of the techniques for relieving pain are very safe, greatly increase comfort after surgery, and present few risks. Do not hesitate to ask your child's doctors to help your child with pain relief at every stage of his time in the hospital.

Post-Operative Anesthesia Concerns

A major concern after surgery for children with Down syndrome is the potential for post-operative complications, particularly those that involve the respiratory system because respiratory complications occur more often in children with Down syndrome. Often after surgery, secretions collect in the airway. Usually, patients cough to clear these secretions, although it can be painful. However, people who have low muscle tone, such as children with Down syndrome, can have additional difficulty in coughing up fluid. The result is that children with Down syndrome may need to breathe through an endotracheal tube for longer than is usual. Most anesthesiologists will choose to leave the endotracheal tube in place for several hours or perhaps overnight if there is any sign of a problem. Your child will be carefully watched, either in the recovery room or the intensive care unit for normal awakening and vital signs.

Some children develop respiratory difficulty after the endotracheal tube is removed. Sometimes the upper airways become chronically swollen and irritated by the endotracheal tube, making it hard to breathe normally after the tube is removed. These children require very close observation, and sometimes need to have the endotracheal tube re-inserted. When that occurs, the endotracheal tube may remain in place for several hours or perhaps even several days. A tracheotomy may need to be performed. During a tracheotomy, a small opening is made through the trachea (which is located at the base of the voice box or *larynx*), and a breathing tube is inserted. This allows your child to breath while his swollen airways heal. After healing, the opening is allowed to grow shut. A tracheotomy is rarely necessary, but you should realize it might be needed if your child has severe airway problems.

Children with Down syndrome also have an increased occurrence of *obstructive sleep apnea*, a condition in which breathing may briefly stop during sleep. Sleep apnea is discussed in detail in Chapter 8. Apnea may be caused by the underdevelopment of the face and the jaw bone. The result is that the tongue, tonsils, and adenoids do not fit normally in the oral cavity, and can obstruct breathing. In addition, a small flat nose can make breathing through it more difficult. The bottom line for your child's medical team is that his breathing will need close monitoring.

Children with Down syndrome also have more frequent infections of the respiratory system, such as colds, ear infections, tonsillitis, and pneumonia (discussed in Chapter 8).

These infections can increase the respiratory complications of anesthesia and surgery. Infection and secretions hinder the work of the respiratory system during and after anesthesia and surgery. For this reason, doctors usually request that children be free of infection for a period of 4 to 6 weeks before surgery. However, many children with Down syndrome never have a period this long between infections, and at times surgery needs to be performed either immediately after or even during a respiratory infection. Physicians and parents must carefully weigh the risks and benefits of surgery against the risks and benefits of delay or cancellation.

Many children with Down syndrome also have less muscle strength compared to other children as a result of *hypotonia*, or low muscle tone. Muscle strength is very important for coughing, breathing, and—to use an anesthesiologist's term— for "maintaining the airway" (keeping the airway clear of mucus, secretions, and blood, and ensuring irritation has not caused swelling) Anesthesiologists carefully assess your child's ability to breath through his nose and mouth and his ability to remove secretions by coughing. Lower muscle tone makes it harder for the muscles of the throat and tongue to cough, and to maintain a normal airway when there are increased secretions due to anesthetics. And, when the muscles of the chest and the diaphragm are weak, your child's ability to cough and breathe is reduced.

Pulmonary Hypertension

Breathing problems can sometimes cause a condition called *pulmonary hypertension,* or increased blood pressure within the lungs. Breathing problems reduce the level of oxygen in the blood stream—if you cannot breath well, less oxygen gets into the lungs and, consequently, the blood. This can cause the blood pressure within the lungs to rise for several reasons (for example, the heart responds to the body's lack of oxygen by pumping more blood to the lungs), resulting in pulmonary hypertension. Pulmonary hypertension increases the stress on the heart muscle because the heart has to pump harder against the higher pressure in the lungs in order to deliver blood there. Children with Down syndrome have an increased occurrence of pulmonary hypertension; they may have a physiological predisposition for it. Children with pulmonary hypertension caused by airway obstruction may require a tracheotomy in order to maintain normal levels of oxygen in the blood stream, reduce blood pressure within the lungs, and decrease stress on the heart. This should be reviewed carefully with your child's medical team. During and after surgery, your child's blood pressure should be measured so that pulmonary hypertension can be diagnosed and treated promptly. Depending on the surgery (for example, heart surgery) monitors that directly measure pulmonary blood pressure may be used.

Atropine and Children with Down Syndrome

Many years ago, it was felt that children with Down syndrome were especially sensitive to the effects of atropine, an important drug used during surgery to help maintain a healthy heart rate. Atropine reduces sweating and increases the heart rate. The result in some children was an apparent increase in body temperature, and children with Down syndrome were thought to be particualrly sensitive to this problem. However, several recent studies have demonstrated that children with Down syndrome are neither more nor less sensitive to atropine and similar drugs, such as glycopyrrolate, than are other children.

Non-Surgical Medical Procedures

Anesthetics are needed for some diagnostic as well as therapeutic (treatment) procedures. Diagnostic procedures that may require the use of an anesthetic include CT (computerized tomography) and MRI (magnetic resonance imagery) scans. These procedures require your child to remain perfectly still. The therapeutic procedures include spinal taps and minor surgery such as stitching lacerations.

In non-surgical procedures, the anesthesia process begins with the anesthesiologist evaluating your child's general medical condition. With children with Down syndrome, there is often a medical record with reports by the various specialists who have been involved in his care. The anesthesiologist will look for drug allergies, heart conditions, pulmonary problems, and a family history of problems with tolerating anesthesia.

If your child has congenital heart disease, for example, a cardiologist has usually evaluated him. Children with congenital heart disease may need surgery for a non-cardiac condition such as sleep apnea (discussed in Chapter 8). In this situation your child's anesthesiologist should get a report from the cardiologist to determine if his heart disease is stable—that is, not changing or getting worse. If your child's heart condition is stable, then elective surgery can be planned. If he has been scheduled for elective surgery, but his heart condition worsens, it is very important to re-evaluate him. And, if his heart disease is not stable, any type of elective surgery should be delayed until the heart condition can be further evaluated.

Choosing a Hospital for Your Child's Surgery

Choosing a hospital for your child's surgery can be difficult. There are often several choices. Should your child's surgery be done in a community hospital, a teaching center, or a specialty care hospital with a pediatric unit?

Start by talking with your child's primary care physician. Find out from him or her what medical care is available in your location. If the anesthesiologists and surgical staff of a community hospital have experience in treating children with

Down syndrome, then that hospital may be a good choice. If the surgery is major, your child may need to be referred to a teaching hospital or a tertiary care hospital with specially-trained staff and more advanced technology. These decisions may be made by your insurance company or your health maintenance organization (HMO).

Summary

Tremendous progress has been made in the last decade to improve the surgical treatment of many of the conditions children with Down syndrome can have. Surgical procedures have been improved, including anesthesia. Although the anesthesia risks discussed in this chapter cannot be eliminated entirely, they can be managed through preparation and planning. You child's medical team can work with you to ensure that any surgery your child requires goes smoothly and is as free from pain and fear as possible.

Surgery does not affect just your child; it affects your whole family. All members of the health care team, parents and professionals alike, need to recognize this fact and to support each other through these anxious times. In preparing for surgery, do not be shy about asking questions, and don't be shy about asking for explanations that you can understand. Be assertive in making sure you feel comfortable with the treatment your child is receiving. The medical team is there to help you and your child. Surgery is a team effort among families and professionals. You as a parent are part of the team.

References

Beilin B., et al. "Anaesthetic Considerations in Facial Reconstruction for Down's Syndrome." *Journal of the Royal Society of Medicine,* Vol. 81, 1988, 23–26.

Berry, F.A. *Anesthetic Management of Difficult and Routine Pediatric Patients,* (second edition) (New York: Churchill Livingston, 1990), 426–428.

Kobel, M., et al. "Anaesthetic Considerations in Down's Syndrome: Experience with 100 Patients and a Review of the Literature." *Canadian Anaesthetic Society Journal,* Vol. 29, 1982, 593–598.

Moore R.A., et al. "Atlantoaxial Subluxation with Symptomatic Spinal Cord Compression in a Child with Down's Syndrome." *Anesthetic Analgesia,* Vol 66, 1987, 89–90.

Sherry, K.M. "Post-Extubation Stridor in Down's Syndrome." *British Journal of Anaesthesia,* Vol. 55, 1983, 53–55.

Williams, J.P., et. al "Atlanto-Axial Subluxation and Trisomy-21: Another Perioperative Complication." *Anesthesiology,* Vol. 67, 1987, 253–254.

17 | Nutrition and Children With Down Syndrome
Peggy L. Pipes, R.D., M.P.H.

Introduction

Diet and nutrition for children with Down syndrome are often sources of great concern for parents. All parents want their children to eat a healthy diet, to grow, and to have fit bodies. Because of some of the differences in children with Down syndrome, however, these goals can be harder to achieve. Although no nutrition concerns have been identified that are common to all people with Down syndrome, some questions are asked often, including:

- When will my child be ready to eat more than pureed foods?
- Is it inevitable that my child will become overweight?
- How can I help my child learn better feeding behavior?
- Will vitamin or nutritional supplements help my child?

In addition to these concerns, some children with Down syndrome have medical problems, such as constipation, which diet changes can help. Also, the slower growth rate of infants and young children with Down syndrome sometimes raises concern that they may not eat enough to support normal growth.

There is nothing inherent in Down syndrome that causes children to eat or reject certain foods. Food preferences and food choice are most often cultural, familial, and behavioral. Children with Down syndrome living in America have the same type of food preferences as many other American children. In trying to get your child with Down syndrome to eat a

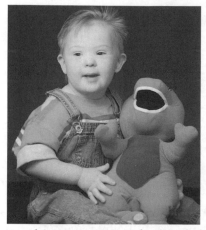

balanced, healthy diet, I have one piece of advice: Ignore the Down syndrome.

For a variety of health reasons, many children with Down syndrome do require special nutritional counseling and guidance. In addition, problems can often be prevented by monitoring physical growth and energy intake, identifying appropriate feeding strategies, and teaching appropriate feeding behaviors.

Nutritionists, or dietitians, are the health professionals who have training and experience in evaluating nutritional needs and problems. When seeking nutritional advice, be certain that the nutritionist is registered with the American Dietetic Association, and has been licensed or certified by the state. This will help assure that the information you receive is reliable and accurate. Any person (including someone selling a "nutritional" product or supplement) can call him- or herself a nutritionist.

Nutritionists have the expertise to look at all the social, economic, emotional, and medical factors that contribute to the what, why, how, and when of eating. They then can work with you to design a dietary pattern for a healthy lifestyle for your child.

This chapter reviews the nutritional needs of children with Down syndrome and discusses some of the dietary problems they may encounter.

Nutritional Needs of Children with Down Syndrome

Children with Down syndrome require the same nutrients as all other children. They eat the same foods, and need the same type of healthy diet. As with other children, proteins, fats, carbohydrates, vitamins, and minerals are all necessary for health and growth. Because the growth of children with Down syndrome can be different, however, parents often are concerned about diet. This section explains the basic nutritional needs children with Down syndrome have and discusses their effect upon growth.

Feeding as a Developmental Process

As your child grows, her ability to handle foods changes with the maturing of her eating and swallowing skills. Food supports the developmental process as your child moves from liquid to semi-solid food to table food. As the texture of the foods increases, your child's ability to chew and swallow also changes to adapt. Many of the same muscles and movements used in eating are also used in the development of speech. That is why an increase in sound production often happens at the same time as your child's ability to handle more complex foods increases.

It is important for children with Down syndrome to have appropriate kinds of foods offered when they are developmentally ready. This means that changes in foods offered should not be based upon your child's age in months or years, but upon her chewing and swallowing abilities. Table 1 lists some of the developmental landmarks that indicate when children are ready to progress in feeding.

Semi-solid foods should be offered when your child is able to handle the additional texture and swallow without choking. Usually this is begun by mixing a small amount of dried cereal with your baby's milk or formula, and feeding several spoons with one of the feedings. As your baby shows she can handle

Table 1: Developmental stages of readiness in feeding.

Developmental landmarks	Change indicated	Examples of appropriate foods
Tongue laterally transfers food in the mouth Voluntary and independent movements of the tongue and lips Sitting posture can be sustained Beginning of chewing movements *(up and down movements of the jaw)*	Introduction of soft, mashed table food	Tuna fish; mashed potatoes; well-cooked mashed vegetables; ground meats in gravy and sauces; soft diced fruit such as bananas, peaches, pears; liverwurst, flavored yogurt
Reaches for and grasps objects with scissor grasp Brings hand to mouth	Finger-feeding *(large pieces of food)*	Oven-dried toast, teething biscuits, cheese sticks *(food should be soluble in the mouth to prevent choking)*
Voluntary release *(refined digital grasp)* Rotary chewing pattern	Finger-feeding *(small pieces of food)* Introduction of more textured food from family menu	Bits of cottage cheese, dry cereal, peas Well-cooked chopped meats and casseroles, cooked vegetables and canned fruit *(not mashed)*, toast, potatoes, macaroni, spaghetti, peeled ripe fruit
Places lips at rim of the cup Understand relationship of container and contained	Introduction of cup Beginning self-feeding *(messiness should be expected)*	Food that when scooped will adhere to the spoon, such as applesauce, cooked cereal, mashed potatoes, cottage cheese
Increased rotary movement of the jaw Ulnar deviation of wrist develops Walks alone	More skilled at cup and spoon feeding May seek food and get food independently	Chopped fibrous meats such as roast and steak Raw vegetables and fruit *(introduce gradually)* Food of high nutrient value should be available
Names food, expresses preferences; prefers unmixed foods Goes on food jags Appetite appears to decrease		Balanced food intake should be offered *(child should be permitted to develop food preferences without parents being concerned that they will last forever)*

From: Pipes, P.L. and Trahms, C.M. *Nutrition in Infancy and Childhood* (St. Louis; Mosby Year-Book, 1993).

the new food, you can offer more with each feeding, and then include the new food at more of the feedings as well. It is usually best to only add one new food at a time. If your baby has problems with a particular food, it may be difficult to identify which is the source if several are added at once.

When you have added several cereals to your child's diet, you can begin to add other similar-textured foods, such as fruits and vegetables. These may be commercially available foods, or strained or ground foods you have prepared yourself. Sometimes using home-prepared versions of your family's typical diet can help your new baby "grow into" that diet and may help avoid food dislike problems.

When you offer a solid food for the first time, try cutting it into small pieces that your child can easily move from one side of her mouth to the other as she begins to learn to use the muscles of her mouth to handle foods. Placing the food between the back teeth can help with these movements. Foods

that are
moist, such
as ham-
burger in
gravy, tuna
fish, or spa-
ghetti sauce,
are more eas-
ily accepted
than drier,
harder
foods, such
as steaks and
roasts.
Young chil-
dren often
do not de-

Table 2: Suggested finger foods for young children.
► Oven dried toast
► Zweibach toast
► Arrowroot biscuits
► Graham crackers without honey
► Cheerios, Kix or Toasted Oat Rings
► Banana slices *(cut in quarters)*
► Soft, cut-up fruit *(skin or peel removed)*
► Canned fruit, avoid grapes
► Soft apple slices *(skin removed)*
► Canned or well-cooked vegetables *(green beans, broccoli, carrots)*
► Cheese sticks, hard cheese only *(cheddar, Monterey Jack, Swiss)*
► Large curd cottage cheese
► Fish sticks *(no bones)*
► Small pieces of tender meats *(small meatballs, pork, or chicken)*
► Scrambled egg yolk *(after child is one year old, use the whole egg)*

velop very effective chewing until they have been eating solids
for some time; it is important to give them pieces small
enough to swallow without much chewing.

Vegetables should be well cooked. Soft, raw fruits, such as
bananas and ripe pears, are often better accepted than those
canned in syrup, which may be too slippery. Finger foods are
often more desirable than spooned foods because your child
can eat them without help. Appropriate finger foods are
shown in Table 2.

Physical Growth

Children with Down syndrome often grow more slowly
than other children. This growth difference begins before
birth and continues until between 3 and 5 years of age. By the
age of 5 years, the average height of children with Down syndrome is noticeably less than the average height of children
without Down syndrome. By the beginning of adolescence,
children with Down syndrome are typically 1 to 2 inches

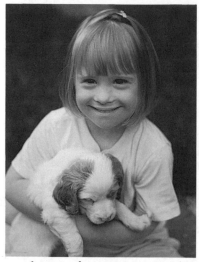

shorter than other children the same age. Conditions like heart disease or hypothyroidism can affect growth if they are present. Rarely, children with Down syndrome may have a deficiency of growth hormone, but there is no evidence that this cause is any more common among children with Down syndrome than in other children. Currently, researchers have not pinpointed why children Down syndrome often grow more slowly than other children.

Today, growth charts developed specifically for children with Down syndrome are available and in widespread use. Heights and weights plotted over time on these growth charts show how your child with Down syndrome is growing and gaining weight compared to other children the same age who also have Down syndrome. As with any child, the velocity of growth, or how fast your child is growing, is more important than her actual place on the chart.

To effectively monitor your child's weight gain in relation to height, the growth charts used to follow typical children can be also consulted to take advantage of the special weight-to-height curve plotted there which is not included on the Down syndrome charts. The chart shows how heavy your child is for her height compared to the general population. For example, if your child's weight-to height ratio is 90 percent, it means she is heavier for her height than 90% of the population. See Figures 1–3.

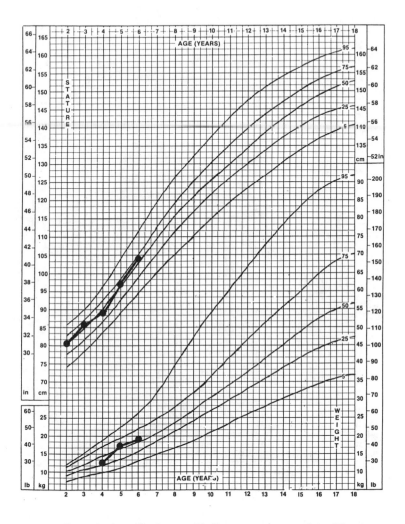

Figure 1: Growth chart for boys with Down syndrome, 2 to 18 years of age.

Energy Requirements

Children with Down syndrome generally require fewer calories than other children the same age. Slower growth rates can often mean smaller bodies. Thus, even though there may not be a medical reason for the slower growth rate, there

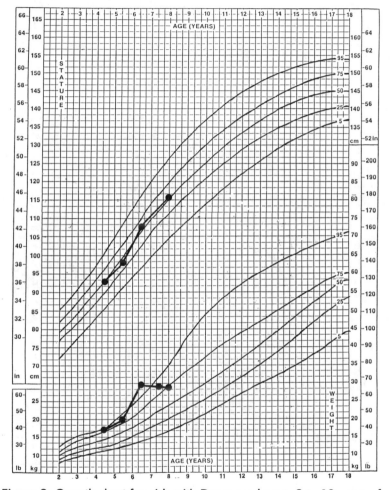

Figure 2: Growth chart for girls with Down syndrome, 2 to 18 years of age.

can be medical consequences to your child if she becomes overweight.

The body uses the energy food provides through metabolism, a complex process that occurs in every cell. During metabolism, the cell converts fuel (food) to energy (calories). Every person has their own unique rate at which metabolism occurs, but it is true for everyone that more energy is used—or metabolized—during physical activity than at rest. The basal metabolic rate, the amount of calories used by a person when they are at rest, has been shown to be measurably lower in some people with Down syndrome than in others. Their so-called "cost of living" is lower; they burn less energy than other people, and, consequently, may need less fuel (food) to meet their body's energy demand.

Another important factor in determining your child's energy requirements is how many calories she expends during activity. Low muscle tone (hypotonia) and lower levels of activity may mean that she uses up less energy than other children. This means that your child with Down syndrome needs fewer calories than another child involved in the same kind of activities and lifestyle.

The best way to assess whether your child's diet has the right energy supply is to regularly chart her height and weight on a growth chart. The ratio of weight to height plotted on the growth curve shows how her body is using calories to grow. If her rate of weight gain is much less than her rate of linear growth (height), then she should be eating more calories. However, if your child is gaining weight much faster than she is gaining in height, then her calorie intake needs to be reduced. For children with growth problems, following the progress of this ratio over time can be very helpful in seeing if diet adjustments are having any effect.

Children with Down syndrome are not genetically programmed to achieve a predetermined body shape. There is nothing in Down syndrome that forces people with the condition to be obese or to have a wide body shape. If your child is overweight, most of the time it is because more calories are taken in as food than are burned in growth or activity.

Another useful technique used by nutritionists to follow growth rates is measuring your child's body fat. The least expensive, most readily available technique to do this is by measuring skin folds, using metal calipers. When done regularly by a nutritionist, physician or trained staff person, and when combined with weight and height measurements, skin folds help to assess the effects of diet and activity changes in children with Down syndrome. It shows the amount of your child's weight that is made up of fat tissue.

Treatment for the Overweight Child

It is much easier to prevent obesity than to cure it. By monitoring growth, excessive weight gain can be identified early. Reducing fat intake, monitoring portion sizes, and increasing appropriate physical activity, are usually sufficient to reduce the rate of weight gain and prevent obesity. However if the ratio of weight to height (described above) is at or above the 90th percentile, some kind of treatment to correct obesity may become necessary.

Obesity is a serious health problem; it can cause high blood pressure, diabetes, heart problems, and joint problems. Although it is possible to limit excessive weight gain, weight reduction in any child is an extreme measure. Unless the obesity is causing medical problems, weight reduction will probably not be necessary, because your child's growth will help to correct things. If weight can be kept from increasing, as height increases, your child will "grow out" of the weight problem.

To reduce the rate of weight gain, it is important to reduce fat in the diet. Fried foods, butter and margarine, sauces and gravies, and high-fat snack foods like chips and cookies should be limited or eliminated. Table 3 shows the caloric content of some typical snack foods. Low-fat or skim milk should also replace whole milk. Desserts and sweets should be a small part of the diet. Portion sizes should be controlled.

As high-calorie foods are reduced in the diet, they should be replaced by less "energy dense," lower calorie foods like fruits and vegetables. The goal is not just to reduce fat and sweets in the diet, but to meet a balance of energy needs and other necessary nutrients.

Table 3: Approximate energy value of common snack foods offered young children.

Food	Portion Size	kcal
Cheese cubes	1/4 oz.	25
Hard-boiled egg	l/2 medium	36
Frankfurter, 5" x 3/4"	1	133
Pretzel, 3" x 1/2"	1	20
Potato chips	10	114
Popcorn with oil and salt	1 cup	41
Bread stick, 4 1/2"	1	38
Saltines	1	12
Graham cracker	2 squares	55
Animal cracker	1	11
Brownie, 3"x 1"x 7/8"	1	97
Chocolate cupcake	1	51
Vanilla wafer	1	18
Yogurt, plain	1/4 cup	40
Homogenized milk	3 oz	60
Chocolate milk	3 oz	80
Cauliflower buds	2 small	2
Green pepper strips	2	2
Cucumber slices	3 large	2
Cherry tomato	each	3
Raw turnip slices	2	5
Dill pickle, large	1/3	5
Apple wedges	1/4 medium apple	20
Banana	1/2 small	40
Orange wedges	1/4 medium orange	18
Orange juice	3 oz	35
Grape juice	3 oz	60
Lemonade	3 oz	40

From Adams, C.F., "Nutritive Value of American Foods in Common Units," in *Agriculture Handbook No. 456* (Washington, D.C.: U.S. Department of Agriculture, 1975,); reprinted in Pipes, P.L. and Trahms, C.T., *Nutrition in Infancy and Childhood*, fifth edition (St. Louis: Mosby Year-Book, Inc., 1993).

By mid-childhood, many children with or without Down syndrome have developed strong food preferences which can be difficult to change. While there are a few children with Down syndrome who have problems with chewing or swallowing that make some foods difficult to eat, there is nothing about Down syndrome that makes your child taste things differently or react differently to foods. Often food preferences reflect the choices made by others in the family, and are supported by the kinds of food available in the home. Chang-

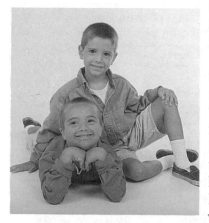

ing the diet of one person in a family often means change for everyone else.

Successful weight control almost always requires a real, lifelong change in the "diet" of the individual or family; repeated cycles of the latest fad "diet" followed by a return to the same old bad habits almost never works. Do not expect your child with Down syndrome to change her eating habits while the rest of your family continues to eat as before. Few people have such strong determination that they can cheerfully watch their family eat foods forbidden to them.

Food Preferences and Nutrition

Healthy children may occasionally refuse to eat enough good food to support normal growth, for a variety of reasons. There may be a need to exert independence, or a desire for control over parents. Most preschoolers go through periods when their appetites are finicky and unpredictable, when they "don't like milk," or refuse to eat fruits and vegetables. Short periods of such behavior probably have no effect on growth, but if those refusals last for months, your child may not be getting enough of certain nutrients like vitamins and minerals.

If your child refuses to drink milk or is one of the few who truly cannot digest it well, other sources of calcium will need to be found. Calcium is needed for the growth of bones and teeth. Our bones get most of their calcium when we are children, adolescents, and young adults; it is hard to add calcium to bones when one has reached adulthood. Without enough calcium in the bones as an adult, *osteoporosis* (weak bones that have too little calcium and break easily) is much more likely. Calcium is available in milk and milk products such as cheese and yogurt, and (in smaller amounts) in

---

Table 4: Calcium equivalents.

1 cup whole milk =	1 cup skim milk* 1 cup 1% or 2% milk 1 cup buttermilk 1 cup (8 oz) yogurt	= 300 mg calcium *(approx)*
3/4 cup milk =	1 oz cheddar, jack, or Swiss cheese	
2/3 cup milk =	1 oz mozzarella or American cheese 2 oz canned sardines *(with bones)*	
1/2 cup milk =	2 oz canned salmon *(with bones)* 1/2 cup custard or milk pudding 1/2 cup cooked greens *(mustard, collards, kale)*	
1/4 cup milk =	1/2 cup cottage cheese 1/2 cup ice cream 3/4 cup dried beans, cooked or canned	

*Some low-fat or skim milks and some low-fat yogurts have additional nonfat dry milk (NFDM) solids added. Some labels will read "fortified." These products will contain more calcium than indicated here.

From: Lucas, B.," Normal Nutrition from Infancy through Adolescence," in Queen, P.M. and Lang, C.E., editors, *Handbook of Pediatric Nutrition* (Gaithersburg, MD: 1993).

---

a variety of other foods, including vegetables (broccoli, spinach, collard and beet greens), nuts and seeds (almonds, sunflower seeds), seafood (oysters, canned salmon), and other foods like molasses and legumes (navy beans, soybeans, tofu). Table 4 shows the calcium content of certain foods compared to milk.

Vegetables are sources of many nutrients, but are also frequent focuses of food dislikes. Most vegetable refusals will be short-lived if they aren't rewarded, or given too much attention. During times when your child refuses vegetables, continue to offer very small portions (1 teaspoon). If you ignore the refusals, but praise your child when the food is tasted, there is less chance that her behavior will turn into a power struggle (which makes things much harder to correct).

Another important nutrient is iron. This mineral is used to build blood cells and muscles, and is important to the growth of brain and nerve cells. Low iron is the most com-

Table 5: Some common sources of non-heme iron.

Item and portion	mg. iron
Cereal and grain products	
Infant cereal, 4 tablespoons, dry	6.8
Cooked cereals	
Malt-o-Meal, 1/2 cup	1.3
Ralston, oatmeal, Cream of Wheat, enriched rice, 1/2 cup	.7
Ready-to-eat cereals	
Total, Product 19, 1/2 cup	9.0
Wheat Chex, 1/2 cup	7.0
Raisin Bran, 1/2 cup	4.0
Bran Flakes, 40%, 1/2 cup	2.8
Corn Flakes, 1/2 cup	.3
Other sources	
Wheat germ, 1 tablespoon	.5
Enriched bread, whole wheat bread, 1 slice	.6-.8
Flour, enriched, 1 cup	3.2
Flour, unenriched, 1 cup	0.9
Cooked beans, peas, legumes, 1/2 cup	1.3-3.0
Cooked greens *(spinach, beets, mustard)*, 1/2 cup	1.5-2.0
Green peas, frozen, 1/2 cup	1.3
Dried fruit, about 1/4 cup	1.0-1.5
Nuts, most kinds, 2 tablespoons	1.0

mon nutritional deficiency in North American children, largely because of the changes in the "typical American diet" which have occurred.

Iron is found in many foods, and in two forms; both kinds are needed by the body. Red meats (primarily pork and beef) contain one kind, called *heme iron,* which is very easy for the body to use. The other kind, called *non-heme iron*, is also needed for growth and development, and is present in eggs, dried beans and peas, and grains. Table 5 shows some common sources of non-heme iron.

Iron absorption can be helped by some things such as vitamin C, but may also be inhibited by other substances such as tea, antacids, and some additives put in food as preservatives or flavors. If your child has particular trouble getting enough iron, you may need to look into some of these inhibitors and enhancers for additional ideas. Table 6 shows some common enhancer and inhibitor foods.

Some clinics, physicians, and other people recommend giving high doses of vitamins to help children with Down syndrome to function better, but there have never been any studies that proved any value to the treatments. Often special vitamin preparations are expensive, or are given instead of other medical attention. Chapter 15 discusses alternative therapies in detail. Remember, a well balanced diet will most likely meet your child's nutritional needs.

When There Is a Problem

There are a few children with feeding problems that are not simply behavioral or related to their developmental progress. They may continue to have trouble getting enough calories to grow, or be unable or unwilling to eat anything but liquids or a few additional foods. They may very frequently have problems with choking or gagging while eating. These kinds of problems may be a lit-

Table 6: Enhancer and inhibitor foods.

ENHANCER FOODS
Enhancer foods are foods that can enhance the availability of non-heme iron.

- ✓ Meat, fish or poultry *(MFP factor)*
- ✓ Ascorbic acid *(vitamin C)*
- ✓ Some foods high in ascorbic acid *(vitamin C)*

Portion	mg. vitamin C
Orange, 1 medium	66
Orange juice, 1/2 cup	55
Broccoli, cooked, 1/2 cup	55
Cantaloupe, 1/4	45
Strawberries, 1/2 cup	44
Strained infant juice, 4.2 oz	42
Grapefruit juice, 1/2 cup	42
Spinach, cooked, 1/2 cup	25
Tomato juice, 1/2 cup	20

INHIBITOR FOODS
Inhibitor foods are foods that can decrease the availability of non-heme iron.

- ✓ Tea *(tannic acid)*
- ✓ Sequestering additives *(such as EDTA, which is used in fats and soft drinks to clarify and prevent rancidity)*
- ✓ Antacids
- ✓ Egg yolk *(phosvitin)*, unless a food containing vitamin C is eaten at the same time

tle more common in children with Down syndrome, and may be signals that your child needs to be looked at by a specialist in feeding issues. Your local physician is a good place to start, and should be able to refer you to specialists if that becomes necessary.

Constipation

Constipation is a common problem in babies and children with Down syndrome. Your child is constipated if she has hard, infrequent stools that are difficult for her to pass. The large bowel functions to store stool and absorb water from the stool; consequently, the longer it stores stool, the harder the stool becomes and the more difficult to pass. Less frequent bowel movements alone are not a sign of constipation if the stools are soft and easy to pass; this may just be your child's particular pattern. If, however, her stools are both infrequent (less than once in two days) and hard, your child may be constipated.

Constipation may result from a variety of causes—hypotonia, lack of exercise, inappropriate diet, and inability to establish a routine bowel pattern. If left untreated, constipation can lead to a condition called *stool hoarding* or *encopresis*. In these conditions, the lower bowel fills with hard stool that is not moving. This is called an *impacted bowel*, and can result in an enlarged colon.

There are several dietary treatments to ease your child's constipation. First, increasing fluid intake and the amount of roughage in the diet may be useful. Roughage is food substances that absorb water in the gut and help keep the stool moist. Adding bran, which is the fiber hull of grains and is high in roughage, to your child's cereal, or to other baked goods such as muffins or pancakes, may prove helpful. Other sources of roughage include many vegetables such as green beans, peas or corn. Prunes and prune juice contain natural laxatives, and are frequently effective. If your child's constipation persists or becomes painful, consult your pediatrician. The medical treatment of constipation is discussed in Chapter 9.

Nutrition Resources

A number of federal and state programs are aimed at improving the nutrition of infants and children, Most state and local health departments have nutritionists on staff who can provide a variety of services, including nutrition education, consultation on nutrition problems, and information about services that are available. Nutrition screening, counseling, education, follow-up, and referral are provided in many community clinics that serve children with special health care needs. These clinics may be associated with WIC (Women, Infants, and Children), Maternal and Child Health, and other state and federal programs. Services may also be available through early intervention programs that serve children from birth to age 3.

The federal Special Supplemental Food Program for Women, Infants, and Children (WIC) provides specific food supplements to infants and children who are at nutritional risk, including children with special needs. Families must also qualify within specified income guidelines. This program provides baby formula or foods for the breastfeeding mother. As the baby grows, additional foods high in required nutrients are provided, including eggs, cheese, cereals, and juices. Types of formulas, quantities of food, and the method of providing the food vary from state to state. Many states give vouchers that can be redeemed at the grocery store for the specific foods; other states give the food out directly. Usually the WIC program will provide some health monitoring, as well as information about nutrition. More information about WIC is available through your child's doctor, or local office of human services.

Conclusion

Nutrition and growth are often serious concerns of parents of children with Down syndrome. Because of the differences in the feeding, eating, and growth of patterns children with Down syndrome, they need careful monitoring. Problems can be treated, and most children grow up healthy. Your child's doctor and a nutritionist can help you ensure your child's diet is healthy and tailored to her individual needs.

References

Bennett, F.C., et al. "Vitamin and Mineral Supplements in Down's Syndrome." *Pediatrics,* Vol. 72, 1983, 707.

Bjorksten, et al. "Zinc and Immune Function in Down's Syndrome." *Acta Paediatrica Scandinavia,* Vol. 69, 1980, 183.

Cronk, C.E. "Growth of Children with Down Syndrome." *Pediatrics,* Vol. 61, 1978, 564.

Francheschi, C., et al. "Oral Zinc Supplementation in Down's Syndrome: Restoration of Thymic Endocrine Activity and Some Immune Defects." *Journal of Mental Deficiencies Research,* Vol. 32, 1988, 169.

Palmer, S. "Influence of Vitamin A Nuture on the Immune Response: Findings in Children with Down Syndrome." *International Journal of Vitamin and Nutrition Resources,* Vol. 48, 1980, 189.

Pipes, P. and Holm, V.A. "Food and Children with Down Syndrome." *Journal of American Dietetic Association,* Vol. 77, 1980, 277–281.

Pipes, P., "Nutritional Aspects," in Pueschel, S.M. and Pueschel, J.K., *Biomedical Concerns in Persons with Down Syndrome* (Baltimore: Paul H. Brooks, 1992), 39–46.

Schapiro, M.B. and Rapaport, S.I. "Basal Metabolic Rate in Healthy Down Syndrome Adults." *Journal of Mental Deficiencies Research,* Vol. 33, 1989, 211.

18 | Planning for Health Care in Adulthood

Marta Little, M.D. and
David Leshtz, M.A.

Introduction

People with Down syndrome are living longer today than ever before. Their life expectancy has increased dramatically over the last 50 years. During the 1940s only a few children with Down syndrome lived to adulthood, with only 50 percent surviving to their first birthday and only 40 percent surviving to age five. Heart defects, for which there were no effective treatment, were the leading cause of the high childhood mortality. Today, the majority of children with Down syndrome can be expected to become adults. Medical care and community living have led to increased lifespans that are still on the rise.

In the past, many children with Down syndrome died at an early age from the effects of congenital heart disease. Today, almost all heart defects are repaired surgically, and these children survive into adulthood. However, improved life expectancy is not only the result of timely surgical treatment of congenital heart disease, but also reflects changing attitudes toward children with Down syndrome in general. In the past, children with Down syndrome were frequently institutionalized, and medical services and educational opportunities were lacking or substandard. Today it is clear that children who receive appropriate health services and educational opportunities enjoy a longer and more meaningful life and contribute to society.

Because in the past few people with Down syndrome survived into adulthood, services for adults did not exist. As the number of people with Down syndrome who live full lives increases, there is a greater need for long-term planning, including planning for adult health care. This chapter discusses the challenges that adults with Down syndrome and their families face in managing health care and in dealing with the health care system. It will also address the special health concerns of adults with Down syndrome.

Self-Advocacy

You have raised your Down syndrome child much as you would raise any child. By the time your child reaches young adulthood, you will have experienced the triumphs, frustrations, joys, and sorrows that all parents experience with their children. You will have learned that children with Down syndrome are far more similar to other children than they are different. You will know that your child, despite having some special characteristics, is "normal" in most ways. You will know that your child with Down syndrome is a person, his own person.

For health care, you will have tried to instill good habits in your child. All parents want their children to learn to brush their teeth regularly, to get enough exercise, to eat as nutritiously as possible. With your child, you may have had to work harder to make sure that these habits are learned. Parents also need to be aware of the health problems their child is more likely to face, such as obesity, thyroid disorders, joint problems, and heart defects. One of the most important things that you can do for your child with Down syndrome is to help him learn the skills to manage his own health care. Teaching a child to take personal responsibility for his own health is the best way to help that child stay healthy as an adult.

Many parents find it very hard to help their child become more responsible for their own health care. One reason may be that these parents still struggle with low expectations and negative predictions for their child. Although great strides have been made in recognizing the abilities of people with Down syndrome, attitudes based on old stereotypes will not go away. Even the best efforts of well-informed and determined parents can be hurt by people who think their child is unable to learn, unable to become a more mature adult, or unlikely to gain the skills and confidence needed to live and work independently.

Another difficulty for parents may be their own attitudes about the medical profession. Many people were conditioned as children to give doctors their unquestioning respect. The common image of a doctor for many of us was that of a stern, busy man with framed degrees on the wall. The medical profession has changed a lot, but old fears or discomforts may remain. It is difficult to teach a child to be assertive and ask questions of a doctor if we ourselves feel intimidated.

To make things even more complicated, parents sometimes encounter a medical professional who does not see beyond the diagnosis of Down syndrome. We now know that Down syndrome results from a chromosomal abnormality, but is *not* itself a disease. Unfortunately, some physicians may have the same mind-set that much of society has. A doctor or nurse, like anyone else, may need encouragement to view your son or daughter as a multi-faceted person, not simply "a Downs."

Starting early to overcome these difficulties will give your child a good chance of being able to manage his own health care as an adult. Managing one's own health care is a skill, like crossing the street, handling money, or acting appropriately in social situations. The sooner your child gains experience and practice, the more likely he will add health care management to the list of important activities he can do on his own.

There are several ways you can help your child move along the road to independent health care. The most important early step is to give your child, even at a very young age, opportunities to make decisions.

- Offer your child a choice of clothes in the morning.
- Encourage him to choose the breakfast cereal he prefers.
- Let your child decide which direction you will go for a walk together.
- Have him pick a toothbrush in the color he likes best.

Getting used to making small decisions will prepare your child to make bigger, more important decisions as he grows older. All children gain confidence from making decisions. Although it may be hard at times, you will contribute to your child's self-esteem by taking his decisions seriously.

There are many ways you can help an older child become more independent in managing his health care. The suggestions below are adapted from *Speak Up for Health,* produced by Minnesota's PACER Center:

- An older child might be responsible for calling to make his own doctor's or dentist's appointments. It is a good idea to rehearse the call with your child before the actual call is made, and to notify the doctor's staff ahead of time.
- Have your child take part in his health care. Make your child increasingly responsible for keeping a calendar of health care appointments as well as social activities.
- When your child is an adult, how will he travel to appointments with a doctor or dentist? Introduce your child to the various transportation options available in your community by using them together.
- Be familiar with your health insurance policy. Learn when or whether your child will no longer be eligible for coverage under your policy. Learn

about the various options that are available to your child for health care coverage, and then talk with your child about these options. Ask other parents, local disability organizations, your employer, and local and state insurance agencies.

Learning to Manage Health Care

Expressing pain or discomfort is the first health care skill any child needs to learn. Communicating "where it hurts" requires practice by your child, and patience by you. Your child will be able to provide more accurate information if he has learned and regularly uses the correct names for body parts. Help him learn them.

Your words and behavior before going to a doctor may influence your child's attitude about medical care. Threatening your child ("If you keep doing that, you will have to go to the doctor!") is unwise. Try a plan of positive reinforcement, where he is rewarded for cooperation with such things as stickers, a movie, or a family meal at a local restaurant. In addition, taking your child to the doctor every time he expresses a mild complaint may teach him to use medical problems for attention-seeking. If possible, take your child with you to some of your own medical appointments. Let him know that visits to the doctor are a regular part of life for everyone, and are not to be feared.

If your child is very resistant or panic-stricken, there are some things that can help. First, ask your doctor to balance the need for a treatment or procedure to happen immediately with your child's fear. Perhaps, the treatment can be delayed until your child is calmer. Second, it sometimes helps to give your child choice during treatment. For example, if your child needs a shot, but does not want it, giving him the choice of which arm to have it in may give him some sense of control and help him stay calm.

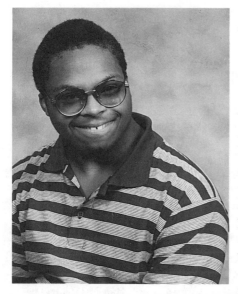

It is important to model correct behavior for your child, whether at the doctor's office, the grocery store, or the park. When your child visits the doctor, do not automatically answer the doctor's questions for him. Prompt your child to answer to the best of his ability. If your child will not answer directly, try to involve him in the discussion as much as possible.

You may also need to model correct behavior for your child's doctor, to make sure that your child is treated with respect and dignity. Avoid talking about your child as if he were not in the room. Maintain eye contact with your child when talking with him, and show that you expect the same from the doctor. Treating your child as part of "the team" will demonstrate to medical personnel that you expect your child to become an active participant in his health care.

Over time, gradually withdraw from the interaction between the doctor and your child. You will, of course, continue to give additional information to health care professionals and help them understand your child's needs. However, the less you act as an intermediary or interpreter, the more likely your child will develop the ability to speak for himself.

Most pediatricians will follow your lead, and will treat your child with courtesy and consideration. You will know you have a good one if he or she treats your child in the same way he or she would treat any child of the same age. If you believe that your child is not being treated respectfully, find another doctor! In addition, most doctors will appreciate your suggestions and knowledge about your child. If your child cannot identify letters, for example, an eye specialist will find it useful to know what kinds of symbols would be more appropriate.

All children have a right to privacy, and all children need to develop physical modesty in a healthy manner. Parents and doctors who respect a child's privacy and modesty help lay the groundwork for good social skills, self-esteem, and positive sexual attitudes as an adult. You may need to help your child's doctor become sensitive to these issues. Removal of clothing is obviously necessary in a doctor's office, for example, but extended periods of nakedness are not necessary. Doctors should be encouraged to limit the number of people present during an examination. Your adult son or daughter should receive the same courtesy and consideration as you would expect from your doctor.

You, or your child, can bring a friend or advocate with you to health care appointments. The presence of a friend or neighbor or relative may boost your confidence and provide objectivity in a confusing or emotional situation.

The issue of privacy is just one example of the need for children with Down syndrome to learn how to assert their feelings. Encouraging your child to express his opinions will help him protect himself as an adult. Your child will receive better medical care if he understands that he has rights as a patient and as a human being. Every state and many counties have chapters of The Arc (formerly known as the Association for Retarded Citizens). Each state also has an office of Protection and Advocacy Services. You or your child can call either of these organizations if you feel your child is not getting good treatment, or if you are uncertain of the rights you and your child have as patients. More information about these two organizations is included in the resource section at the end of this chapter.

Health Care Resources

In many cases, a team of professionals is involved in the health care of children and adults with Down syndrome. Often the most efficient and effective way to arrange access to the health care system will be through a trusted family doctor (your *primary care physician*), who can provide basic care and who will coordinate referrals to other health care professionals (such as a pediatric cardiologist for heart problems). This can prevent you from feeling as though you are being shuffled from one specialist to another without direction. If you and your adult child identify one person to be in charge of health care coordination, your child will know where to turn, and will be more likely to achieve independence and confidence in the patient-doctor relationship. Optimally, the primary care physician should:

- be personally interested in your child;
- be comfortable communicating directly with your child;
- be familiar with specific health concerns of people with Down syndrome; and
- be capable of coordinating referrals to community resources and other health care professionals.

Some physicians may have little or no experience caring for an adult with Down syndrome, especially because until recently so few people with Down syndrome have grown up to live full lives in the community. It may be helpful to provide your doctor with a copy of the *Down Syndrome Preventative Medicine Checklist* listed among the resources at the end of this chapter. In most areas of the United States there are also regional clinics specializing in the care of individuals with Down syndrome or other developmental disabilities. These centers may be a useful resource to your physician and your family; they are listed in the resource section of Chapter 19.

Health Care Goals

The goals of health care for adults with Down syndrome are, as for anyone, to maintain good health and to promptly recognize and treat medical problems that develop. Attention to these goals is especially important, however, since certain medical conditions mentioned in this book occur more frequently in people with Down syndrome. These conditions can lead to other health problems and impair development if they are not promptly recognized and treated. Your child's physician can talk with you about the appropriate frequency of check-ups for preventive care and health maintenance. An annual check-up is a good rule of thumb, but depending upon your child's age and any health problems, check-ups may be necessary more or less often than this. Routine dental care is also recommended every 6 to 12 months (dental care is discussed in detail in Chapter 12).

Ideally, you and your child's physician will talk with him about such health-related issues as alcohol, smoking, substance abuse, sexual activity (and AIDS), and family stresses, and provide counseling as needed. Blood pressure and weight should be routinely monitored, and dietary counseling should be recommended if your child is overweight.

Surveys of young adults with Down syndrome suggest that the most common health complaints involve the skin, the teeth and gums, and the joints, so these areas may require particular attention during a physical exam. The medical issues are the same for children and adults; refer to the chapters where they are discussed. For women, periodic breast exams, pelvic exams, and Pap smears are recommended. It is generally recommended that women have a baseline mammogram between the ages of 35 and 40, then every one to two years thereafter. For men, periodic testicular and prostate exams are recommended. Some of these recommendations are being reviewed and revised, but remember, people with Down syndrome should receive the same medical attention and treatment as anyone else.

Immunizations will need to be kept current. Your child should receive a tetanus-diphtheria booster at least every ten years. Vaccination for influenza in the fall of each year is also appropriate for many adults, including those with Down syndrome. Vaccination for pneumonia (Pneumovax) is generally recommended after age 65 and may be advisable at an earlier age for many adults with Down syndrome. People with Down syndrome are more likely to have immune problems with each of these kinds of infections than other people, so it is more important that they receive regular vaccinations to improve their defenses.

People with Down syndrome develop vision impairments, hearing impairments, and thyroid dysfunction more often than other people. Identifying and treating these conditions early can often prevent more serious deterioration, and with it the loss of important life skills. Eye exams by an ophthalmologist and blood tests to check thyroid function are recommended at regular intervals. Auditory testing should be performed about every 5 to 10 years after school age, but may be needed more often if there are repeated ear infections or indications of hearing loss. During the school years, it is likely your child's school will conduct regular screening. Concerns with the ears are discussed in detail in Chapter 8.

Special Concerns in Adults with Down Syndrome

This section reviews the health issues of special concern to adults with Down syndrome.

Cardiac Concerns

Congenital heart defects are found in approximately 40 percent or more of babies with Down syndrome, and a thorough cardiac evaluation is necessary for every child early in infancy. Surgical correction of these heart defects is often performed during infancy or early childhood, and is responsible for the significantly improved survival of children with Down syndrome. In adolescence and adulthood, there may be late complications that result from the heart defect and surgical correction. In children and adults with heart defects and those who have had corrective surgery, blood flow within the heart is never entirely normal. Turbulence in the flow can leave these people prone to developing *endocarditis*, an infection of heart tissues and of artificial heart valves or conduits. To protect against the development of endocarditis, antibiotics should be administered prior to dental care and prior to certain surgical procedures. Cardiac problems and treatment are discussed in detail in Chapter 3.

If surgical correction of the heart defect requires the placement of an artificial heart valve, regular use of anticoagulant medications that inhibit blood clotting may be necessary. Disturbances of cardiac rhythm may also be seen in adult life as a late complication of congenital heart defects and surgical correction. Your doctor will talk with you and your adult child if vigorous exercise needs to be limited due to concern about exercise-induced heart rhythm disturbances. People with Down syndrome who did not have heart defects at birth are also prone to developing dilation (*mitral valve prolapse*) or leaks of heart valves (*aortic insufficiency*). A special study known as a *cardiac echo*, in which sound waves are used to produce an image of the heart, is useful in assessing the size and function of the heart chambers and valves, and is recommended during early adulthood.

Thyroid Concerns

People with Down syndrome appear to be unusually prone to thyroid disorders. Thyroid disorders may develop at any age. Underactive thyroid (*hypothyroidism*) is the most common problem. In adults, the signs and symptoms of hypothyroidism include slowed speech, hoarse voice, dry skin, constipation, apathy, and fatigue. Because symptoms may be subtle at first, yearly blood tests to assess thyroid function are

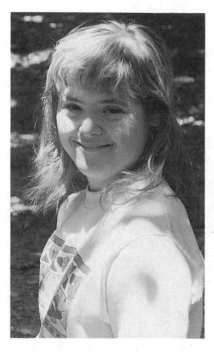

recommended. Hypothyroidism is treated with thyroid hormone replacement, and this replacement results in substantial improvement. All symptoms caused by hypothyroidism should disappear with thyroid replacement therapy as long as daily replacement therapy is maintained.

Overactive thyroid (*hyperthyroidism*) and inflammation of the thyroid (*thyroiditis*) also occur. The signs and symptoms of hyperthyroidism are nervousness, irritability, poor sleep, tremor, weight loss, and frequent stools. There are several different therapies available to block the release or effect of excessive thyroid hormone, and the response to therapy is generally very good. Thyroid problems are discussed in detail in Chapter 5.

Musculoskeletal Concerns

Due to low muscle tone and lax ligaments, people with Down syndrome have an increased risk of developing joint problems with age. The same type of problems—flat feet, hip dislocation, and knee cap problems—become more common and can have a great impact on daily life. It is important to respond promptly to any new problem that appears and to continue to monitor existing problems.

Psychiatric Concerns

Overall, the prevalence of psychiatric disorders in people with Down syndrome is less than that in people with mental retardation due to other causes. It is also not different from the prevalence of psychiatric disorders due to organic causes in the normal population. Nevertheless, adults with Down syndrome may be particularly vulnerable to depression. The symptoms of depression include withdrawal, disinterest, and inactivity, often accompanied by a deterioration in social skills and intellectual functioning. Depression is treatable with counseling; sometimes antidepressant medications may be helpful.

Many people, including medical professionals, mistakenly believe that a diagnosis of Down syndrome is sufficient to explain a wide range of behaviors. No one should assume that a child or adult "acts that way because he has mental retardation or Down syndrome." While mental illness is not especially common in people with Down syndrome, it does occur. It is a possibility that you should be aware of, particularly if you are concerned about unusual moods or behavior in your child.

Alzheimer's Disease

For aging adults with Down syndrome (ages 40 to 70), the greatest neurological concern is Alzheimer's disease. In this disease, there is progressive degeneration and loss of nerve cells in the brain. When Alzheimer's disease develops, there is a gradual deterioration of memory, social interaction, language, and life skills. A person's gait may become slow and clumsy, and some affected people develop seizures. This is a progressive disease for which there is currently no effective treatment to stop or reverse the symptoms.

It is very important not to prematurely attribute new symptoms or problems in older adults with Down syndrome to Alzheimer's disease. When a person develops new symptoms—memory loss, for example—a thorough evaluation for other treatable conditions that could cause the symptoms should be carried out. For example, when an adult with Down syndrome who normally revels in social interaction becomes less talkative and socially withdrawn, a thorough medical evaluation, including an assessment of thyroid function, is necessary. The possibility of depression should also be considered. Alzheimer's disease is discussed in detail in Chapter 14.

Summary

Changing attitudes and advances in medical care have resulted in increased length and better quality of life for people with Down syndrome. In preparing your child for adult life, you will want to lay the foundations for independent living and self-care as much as possible. In the area of health care, this means instilling good health habits, fostering your child's sense of responsibility for his own health care, and building his confidence in dealing with the health care system.

Choosing an interested family doctor or other primary care physician as the main provider of your child's health care is important. Attention to certain health problems that occur with greater frequency in people with Down syndrome, especially treatable conditions that can impair function such as visual impairment, hearing loss, thyroid dysfunction, orthopedic problems, and depression, is important.

As greater numbers of children with Down syndrome reach adulthood, there will be new challenges. You may find that some parts of the health care system are behind the times in attitudes toward and expectations for your child with Down syndrome. You may find health insurance companies uncooperative as you work to provide for your child's health. Nevertheless, the dramatic changes in attitudes and expectations over the last 50 years suggest that you can be optimistic about meeting these challenges, and about your ability to prepare your child with Down syndrome to lead a long, productive, and healthy life.

Resources

The Arc, P.O. Box 1047, Arlington, TX 76004; 800/433–5255.

Connections, the Newsletter of the National Center for Youth with Disabilities, University of Minnesota, 420 Delaware St. SE, Box 721, Minneapolis, MN 55455. A good source of information on disability issues that affect young people with disabilities.

Disability Rag, 1962 Roanoke, Louisville, KY 40201. One of the best advocacy magazines, it looks at disability issues from a consumer viewpoint, and has a strong civil rights emphasis.

Down Syndrome Preventative Medicine Checklist, available from the National Down Syndrome Congress, 1605 Chantilly Drive, Suite 250, Atlanta, GA 30324–3269; 800/232–1555.

Exceptional Parent Magazine, P.O. Box 3000, Denville, NJ 07834–9919; 800/247–8080.

National Association of Protection and Advocacy Systems, 900 Second Street NE, Suite 211, Washington, DC 20002. Can provide you with information about your state P&A office, and also your state planning council for developmental disabilities and your state university affiliated program(s) that serve people with disabilities.

National Council on Independent Living, 211 Wilson Boulevard, Suite 405, Arlington, VA 22201; 703/525–3406 (voice); 703–525–3407 (TTY). The independent living movement stresses self-advocacy, peer mentoring, and independence. Many communities have Independent Living Centers that your child can tap to acquire the skills and self-confidence needed to live more independently.

National Information Center for Children and Youth with Disabilities (NICHCY), P.O. Box 1492, Washington, D.C. 20013–1492; 202/884–8200, 800/695–0285. A clearinghouse of information resources for parents of children with disabilities. It can provide information about both national and local agencies and organizations.

PACER Center, 4826 Chicago Avenue South, Minneapolis, MN 55417. An excellent source of information on a variety of disability issues, including education, vocational services, and advocacy.

The People First Handbook describes the People First philosophy; it is available from People First of Washington, P.O. Box 381, Tacoma, WA 98401. People First is an advocacy organization established by people with disabilities; many states have chapters.

World Institute on Disability, 510 Sixteenth Street, Oakland, CA 94612–1502. Can provide information on independent living programs, self-advocacy, and other consumer-driven approaches to dealing with disability issues.

19 | Resources for "Resilient" Families

Susan Schoon Eberly, M.A.

Introduction

When you first learned that your child has Down syndrome, you may have felt a little panicky. You were probably prepared to deal with the responsibilities of a new baby. No doubt you had done some thinking about how you would balance looking after your new arrival with meeting the everyday needs of the rest of your family. But when you learned that your baby has Down syndrome, you may have worried that you would not know how to care for her. You may have wondered how the other people in your family would feel about the baby. And you may have worried about what the future holds for all of you.

This chapter gives you information about some resources that can help you answer these questions. First, it describes the characteristics of strong, or *resilient,* families. Then it details a range of resources—support groups, government programs and offices, and publications—that will be useful during your child's infant, preschool, school-age, and young adult years.

What Makes a "Resilient" Family

In the last few years, a lot of research has been done to learn more about families that do well, even when the going is tough. Chances are you know some families that have fallen apart when confronted with ongoing stress—the loss of a job, chronic illness, the birth of a child with disabilities. You prob-

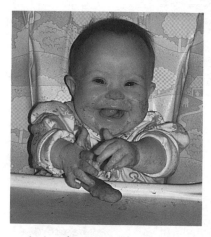

ably also know families that are "resilient"—families that have grown stronger and more loving even though faced with hard times. How can you help your family to be one of these "resilient" families?

By studying a wide range of families, researchers in psychology and sociology have learned that the most important characteristic of resilient families is their commitment to *family*. These families recognize the benefits of working together. They understand how difficult it would be to cope without the love and support of family members. They talk with pride about how important their family is to them, and about how pulling together to deal with their concerns has made them all closer and more appreciative of each other.

Within strong, supportive families, the roles of the different generations are clearly defined. The parents are in charge, and they work as a team to deal with problems and make decisions. They show their love and respect for each of their children, while encouraging their growth and increasing independence. Children feel secure in the stability of the love of their parents and siblings.

Sometimes these roles are disrupted if one parent becomes too involved with the child who has the disability. This can threaten the stability of the family. If the child is encouraged to be too dependent, overinvolvement can slow the development of that child.

The stability of the family can also be disturbed when many different service providers—doctors, therapists, educators, social workers—become part of the family's life. Too much "intervention" can upset the way a family functions.

When family roles and routines are shaken up, family members may have the feeling that "outsiders have taken over our lives!" In other cases, families can become locked into dependency upon service providers.

In resilient families, parents protect family privacy. They are assertive in deciding what roles professionals will—and will not—play. These families typically have a businesslike relationship with professionals, rather than becoming their "friends." They keep family routines intact, and set priorities for family activities. Of course, the family itself is the best judge of what constitutes an effective relationship with professionals— very businesslike for some families and more informal and relaxed for others.

Research also shows that strong families communicate well, both the good news and the bad. Members of these families know it is OK to talk freely about how they feel—whether it is joy over a brother's accomplishments, concern about a mother's hectic schedule, grief about a new baby's disability, or fear about a father's illness. Conflicts are talked about with understanding and respect. All of the members of the family know that they "have permission" to be honest about how they feel. Sometimes, individual or family counselling can help to build good communication in families.

Another characteristic of resilient families is that although they are close-knit, they do not have an isolated, us-against-the-world perspective. Instead, they know how to reach out to a network of friends, relatives, service providers, parent groups, and others. They get, and give, support, in much the way that Emily Perl Kingsley describes in her preface to this book. The "family support networks" that these families are part of may be formal or informal. They provide the family with:

- emotional support;
- a way to test out ideas by discussing them with other more experienced families;

- access to a wide range of valuable information—about child development, Down syndrome, community services and programs, and so forth; and
- a channel through which they can share what they have learned and provide support to other families.

Family support groups come in as many different varieties as families themselves. Some groups focus primarily on young families; others are made up of families whose children are nearly grown. It is important to recognize that groups will evolve as the needs of their members evolve. If the first group you make contact with does not feel quite right for you, look into other groups.

Recently, computers have begun to play a role in parent support. Through the many different online computer services, parents can "talk" with other parents from around the country and around the world with other parents. They can exchange electronic mail (E-Mail) and participate in real-time conferences much like a parent support group meeting. For many this is the preferred way to reach out. Almost all of the online computer services—CompuServe, America Online, Genie, and Prodigy—have groups that focus on Down syndrome or disabilities. In addition, the Internet, a worldwide network of computer systems offers a support group devoted specifically to Down syndrome.

Encouraged and informed by a range of personal and community supports, resilient families are better prepared to take an active role in meeting the needs of *all* family members. Resilient families do not wait passively for information or services to come their way. They seek them out. If appropriate services do not exist, these families will work to create them. If none of the family support groups they talk with seem to right for them, they look for kindred souls and start a group of their own.

Resilient families find a way to balance the needs of their child with Down syndrome with her non-disability related needs, and with the needs of other family members. They are secure enough to be flexible—they adjust, adapt, and laugh a lot. Parents find ways to make time—for themselves, and also for their children. Their child's Down syndrome is not allowed to become the central, driving reality for the family.

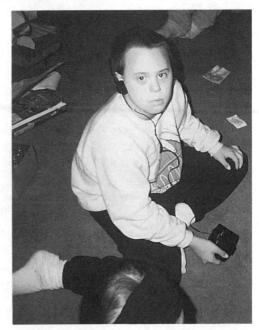

Finally, resilient families look for and build on the positive aspects of the situation. When asked what the birth of a child with Down syndrome has meant in their lives, members of these families will often talk about how it has made them more accepting of individual differences and more aware of what is really important in life. Brothers and sisters of a child with Down syndrome say they have learned a lot about caring. Priorities, these resilient families report, have changed—and changed for the better.

If you would like to learn more about resilient families, a good place to start is an article called "Family Resilience to the Challenge of a Child's Disability," by Joan M. Patterson. This article, was published in the September 1991 issue of *Pediatric Annals*, and contains an excellent bibliography that will guide you to further information. The librarian at your local library can help you get a copy of this article, and of the other information resources mentioned at the end of this chapter.

Local Resources for Your Family

There are many resources you can tap as you work to make your family one of these "resilient" families. You can, for starters, find out about parent support groups in your community. Talk to your family doctor or pediatrician, a member of your local school's special education department, or the staff of the local office of your state's department of human services to find out about such groups in your community. Talking with other families will provide you with both information and emotional support.

If you do not know of any local parent groups, you may be able to get help from the National Down Syndrome Congress or the National Down Syndrome Society. Both of these organizations maintain lists of support groups and contact people.

This contact with other parents, families, and family support groups may begin as early as when your child is still in the hospital nursery. In the introduction to this book, Dr. Allen Crocker draws upon his own long experience with (and obvious respect and affection for) families in discussing how to work most effectively with the medical staff you will encounter as you supervise the health care of your child. Part of this will involve keeping good records of your child's care. This may be something of a job, but it will create one of the most valuable resources you can have in making important decisions about your child's care.

In most health care settings, you will work with professionals to create a care plan for your child. What this plan is called will vary from agency to agency; it may be an "ISP," or *individual service plan*, and "IFSP," or *individual family service plan*, or an "IEP," or *individual education plan*. This plan outlines in writing the care your child receives, the goals of this care, and the outcomes. The care plan is a tool that you can use to plan, monitor, and evaluate your child's care. As your child begins to be involved in a broader range of community services, such as school, this plan can be used to coordinate services from a variety of sources.

Your state has a number of government organizations that can provide you with useful information about Down syndrome, parent support groups, and local programs. These organizations include:

- Your state *developmental disabilities planning council.* This organization, located in every state capital, advocates with and for people with disabilities and their families. Your local department of human services office can tell you how to contact this council. You can get information from the DD Council about how to contact the other state organizations and advocacy groups listed on the pages that follow.

- Your state *University Affiliated Program (UAP).* Each state has at least one UAP. These federally-funded programs provide treatment, research, training, and information services for individuals with developmental disabilities and their families. For information about your state's UAP, contact their national office:

  American Association of University Affiliated Programs
  8630 Fenton Street, Suite 410
  Silver Spring, MD 20910
  Phone: 301–588–8252

- Your state *Protection and Advocacy Services (P&A)* organization. You can find out about your legal rights and the rights of your child from your state P&A office, which is located in your state capital.

Local Resources: Advocacy Groups and Parent Centers

Advocacy groups are another excellent source of information. You can contact the national office of any of the organizations listed below to learn about chapters in your area, and to learn what specific services they provide for families.

The ARC/USA
2501 Avenue J
Arlington, Texas 76005
Phone 871–640–0204

March of Dimes
1275 Mamaroneck Avenue
White Plains, NY 10605
Phone 914–428–7100

National Down Syndrome Congress
1605 Chantilly Drive
Suite 250
Atlanta, GA 30324–3269
Phone 800–232–6372

National Down Syndrome Society
141 Fifth Avenue
New York, NY 10010
Phone 800–221–4602

National Easter Seal Society
1600 Stout Street, Suite 1420
Denver, CO 80202
Phone 303–573–0264

If your community does not have an active advocacy or parents' support group, you may want to talk with other parents about creating one.

Most states have special resource centers for families with children who have disabilities. These are often called parent centers, and you can use them to find local services, family support groups, disability-specific information, and a range of other valuable resources. You can learn about the parent center in your state by contacting your Technical Assistance for Parent Programs (TAPP) Regional Center:

Midwest Region: PACER Center
4826 Chicago Avenue South
Minneapolis, Minnesota 55417
612/827–2966

Northeast Region: Parent Information Center
151A Manchester Street
P.O. Box 1422
Concord, New Hampshire 03302
603/224–6299

South Region: ARC of Georgia
1851 Ram Runway, Suite 104
College Park, Georgia 30337
404/761–3510

West Region: Washington State PAVE
6316 South 12th Street
Tacoma, Washington 98465
206/565–2266

National Office: TAPP Project
Federation for Children with Special Needs
95 Berkeley Street, Suite 104
Boston, Massachusetts 02116
617/482–2915

Resources for Early Intervention—From Birth to Age Three

The first three years of your child's life are crucial—at no other time will your child's development be as fast, or as complex. For this reason, *early intervention services*—services to promote optimal physical, mental, emotional, and social development—are provided to youngsters up to the age of three. These services can have a life-long impact on your child's development.

Many states have recently begun to offer early intervention services that are part of a program created by the Federal Individuals with Disabilities Education Act (IDEA). Part H of the IDEA directs services to children who have, or are at risk for, disabilities, and to their families. It calls for family members and service providers to work as a team in order to help each child develop to the fullest. Participating in this program can give you access to:

- Infant education;
- Medical intervention;
- Occupational therapy;
- Parent education/training;
- Physical therapy; and
- Speech/communication therapy.

You may be contacted by your state's IDEA Part H early intervention program through its "Child Find" activities. If you are not, talk with your local human service office to learn if this early intervention program is available in your area.

Under IDEA Part H, families and professionals work together to prepare an Individual Family Service Plan (IFSP). This plan spells out in detail what services the child and family will use, how services will be provided, and what outcomes are desired.

A good, carefully thought-out IFSP is a planning tool that will connect you with the best, most appropriate services for your child and your family. It will highlight the importance of your role in your child's development, because *you* are the single most important person in your child's life. As a parent, you will always be there for your child, while other "care providers"—doctors, therapists, and teachers—will play only a temporary role. Because of your love, knowledge, and commitment to your child, you are your child's most important resource.

Resources for the Preschool Child, Ages Three to Five

Research shows that children with Down syndrome learn best by watching and imitating other children, and this is the strongest argument for encouraging your child's involvement with other children from an early age. In many states, your child will be eligible for *preschool* services from the ages of three to five. The IDEA guarantees your child a *free, appropriate public education*, provided in the *least restrictive, age-appropriate environment*. Your state Protection and Advocacy Services office can provide you with information about your child's rights under this law, and the education services available in your state. Other sources of information include your local school's department of special education, and your state department of education's branch of special education.

Another good source of information about education issues and about advocacy groups in your state is:

National Information Center for Children and Youth with
    Disabilities
P.O. Box 1492
Washington, D.C. 20013–1492
800/695–0285

When your child begins preschool, you will again be part of a team that will design a plan to guide the services your child will use. This plan is called the Individualized Education Program, or IEP. Another parent who has "been through the system" can be a really good source of information for you as you prepare to design this plan. It is also a good idea to have an experienced parent accompany you to IEP meetings with school staff.

The IEP process begins with an assessment of your child. If you disagree with the results of the assessment, you may request another. You want to be sure that you start the IEP process with an accurate assessment of your child's abilities because this assessment will guide many crucial decisions about placement and programming. Once again, this is a time when you need to remember that you are the most important "expert" when it comes to deciding what will be included in your child's IEP. Do not hesitate to bring experienced parents or other experts with you to IEP meetings. Take time before the meetings to gather information from teachers, other parents, and service providers. Be clear in your own mind about your goals. Write them down, and bring this list with you to the meeting. Make sure that the IEP is appropriate for your child. The services your child uses should be based on the individual strengths and needs of your child, not on what the school can most easily provide.

Resources for the Elementary and Secondary School Child—Ages Five to Twenty-Two

Your child has the right to attend your neighborhood school, and to be in classes with non-disabled students. The issue of integration—also called *mainstreaming* or *full inclusion*—is very important. A child learns to get along in the real world, with a variety of people in a variety of settings, through experience—ongoing, regular, all-day experience. A segregated or "self-contained" classroom, in which all students have disabilities, is not the best overall learning environment for any child. It simply cannot provide experience in getting along with all kinds of people, disabled and non-disabled.

For inclusive education to work, however, your child's needs must be known, and supporting services must be provided in the classroom. If your child is placed in a regular classroom, but not given the resources necessary to learn, it is not "full inclusion." If the placement does not work out well, it is not your child's fault. The IEP is the best tool to ensure that the school and the teacher have all the supports they need to help your child to succeed.

Your child's IEP is an important tool, one that you can use to guide your child's education throughout grade school and high school. If you feel your child needs a segregated or "special ed" setting for some classes, then be sure that the IEP includes mainstreaming into non-segregated classes whenever appropriate—for music, art, physical education, lunch, recess, creative writing, and so forth. The IEP should also include a full range of extracurricular activities—band, chorus, sports, 4–H, drama.

As your youngster approaches junior high, the IEP should begin to include *vocational*—employment—objectives. A generation ago, adults with Down syndrome almost always lived in institutions and worked—if they worked at all—in segregated "workshops." Today, many people with Down syndrome live far more independent lives. They have jobs and live in their own homes or apartments. You can work with friends, local human services programs, and local employers to design the system of supports your young adult with Down syndrome needs to live as independently as possible. But for this to happen, planning for adult life needs to begin in late grade school or early junior high.

Often, a teenager with Down syndrome can work in part-time jobs in the community, sometimes with the assistance of a job coach. Your child may want to experience a variety of different jobs to learn what work is most satisfying and what skills are needed. Equally important, as your teenager learns about the world of work, employers in the community will be learning about this young adult's potential as an employee. Training and actual employment during the teenage years may be formally arranged through the school, or informally set up by you.

In the final two years of high school, your child's IEP should include a *transition plan* to guide her transition from school to adult life. Sometimes your state office of vocational rehabilitation services will be involved. At other times, the student and the parents may work with school staff, members of the community, and service providers to create appropriate post-secondary education, work, and living arrangements. If your community has no programs for independent or supported living and employment, you may need to work with other members of your community to create them. Beginning to plan for your child's options as an adult while your child is still a youngster will give you time to learn, organize, and act.

I know of a young woman with Down syndrome who lives in a midwestern community of about 45,000. She has a signifi-

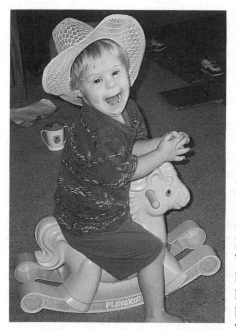

cant level of mental re-tardation, and cannot read or do arithmetic. Nonetheless, she lives in her own apartment in a "regular" apartment house (she is the only resident with a disability). Her independent living counselor (provided by the state human services agency) lives nearby, and is on hand if problems arise. Once a week, the two meet to plan meals and go shopping. Once a month they pay bills together. This young woman has two part-time jobs—she stocks shelves at a discount store, and cleans a neighborhood clothing store. At first, she was supervised by a job coach. Today, her job coach is contacted only when she needs to learn new skills. She attends church with her family each Sunday, and is the member of a bowling league. She uses the city bus for transportation.

All this happened because of careful planning and preparation that started when she was a freshman in high school. The team that made this possible included the young woman herself, her family, school staff, local business people, and her local human services department office. It takes a concerted effort, but with similar forethought and planning, you can create an outcome that will be as appropriate and fulfilling for your child.

As you prepare for your child's transition into the adult world, you may want to talk with the local offices of your state's department of human services, public health, education, human rights, and vocational rehabilitation services. You may also want to introduce your child to consumer advocacy groups like the Centers for Independent Living or People First. These groups can help your child learn to advocate for herself, and some also offer assistance with living skills. To learn if either group has local chapters in your area, contact:

People First International
P.O. Box 12642
Salem, OR 97309
503/378–5143

Centers for Independent Living
National Council on Independent Living
3233 Wesleyan, Suite 100
Houston, TX 77027
713/960–9961

People with disabilities make up the membership of these two highly effective self-advocacy groups.

Other sources of information on options for living and working are advocacy groups like The Arc and Easter Seals, whose addresses were given earlier.

Conclusion

You can tap a wide range of resources as you work to keep yourself mentally, emotionally, and physically healthy; to help your family stay strong and resilient; and to encourage your child with Down syndrome to develop to her fullest. Use these resources to learn and to grow, and in the process you can take pride in the way that you yourself *become* a resource— for your child, your family, your community, and yourself.

Resources

Each of the publications listed below is useful in itself, and also provides a bibliography of additional resources that you can use to locate more detailed information.

_____. *Pocket Guide to Federal Help for Individuals with Disabilities.* Washington, DC: U.S. Department of Education, Clearinghouse on Disability Information. (Request Publication #249–950/0086, Superintendent of Documents, U.S. Government Printing Office, Washington, DC, 20402, 1989.

Anderson, Winifred, et al. *Negotiating the Special Education Maze: A Guide for Parents and Teachers* (Bethesda, MD: Woodbine House, 1990).

Children's Health Issues. A newsletter that provides excellent information about health care issues, policies, and programs. It is published by the Center for Children with Chronic Illness and Disability, Box 721, University of Minnesota, 420 Delaware Street S.E., Minneapolis, MN 55455.

Exceptional Parent. A magazine for parents that deals with a wide range of disability issues. It is an excellent source of information. 1995 subscription rates are $24 a year; for further information, contact *Exceptional Parent Magazine*, P.O. Box 3000, Denville, NJ 07834–9919, or call 1–800–247–8080.

Geralis, Elaine, ed. *Children with Cerebral Palsy: A Parents' Guide* (Bethesda, MD: Woodbine House, 1991). Although its focus is children with cerebral palsy, this book provides excellent information for all families that include children with disabilities.

Healy, Alfred, M.D. and J.A. Beck. *Improving Health Care for Children with Chronic Conditions: Guidelines for Families.* Produced at the Iowa University Affiliated Program, this publication is available from Campus Stores, 208 GSB, University of Iowa, Iowa City, IA 52242.

Patterson, J.M. "Family Resilience and the Challenge of a Child's Disability." *Pediatric Annals,* Vol. 20, No. 9, 1992, 491–500.

Pueschel, Siegfried M. *The Young Person with Down Syndrome: Transition from Adolescence to Adulthood* (Baltimore: Paul H. Brookes, 1988).

Stray-Gundersen, Karen, ed. *Babies with Down Syndrome: A New Parent's Guide* (Bethesda, MD: Woodbine House, 1986).

Tingey, Carol, ed. *Down Syndrome: A Resource Handbook. (Boston: Little, Brown & Company, 1988).*

Down Syndrome Clinics

Alabama

University of Alabama at
Birmingham
331 Sparks Center
1720 7th Avenue South
Birmingham, AL 35294–0017
205/975–2380
Contact: Dr. Ditza Zachor

Arizona

Family and Community Medicine
Dept.
University of Arizona
Family Practice Office
1450 N. Cherry Avenue
Tucson, AZ 85719
602/626–6186
Contact: Dr. Tamsen L. Bassford

California

Dr. Milton L. Kolchins
5400 Balboa Blvd., Suite 105
Encino, CA 91316
818/789–0347

Children's Hospital Medical
Center of Northern California
747 52nd Street
Oakland, CA 94609
415/428–3351
Contact: Dr. Richard Umansky

University of California at San
Francisco
400 Parnassus, ACC Building
2nd Floor, Room A226
San Francisco, CA 94143
415/476–4988
Contact: Dr. Lucy Crain

Georgia

Department of Genetics
Emory University School of
Medicine
2040 Ridgewood Drive
Atlanta, GA 30322
404/727–5731
Contact: Dr. R. Dwain Blackston
Dr. P. Fanning

Department of Pediatrics
Medical College of Georgia
BG-121
Augusta, GA 30912
706/721–2809
Contact: Dr. Bonnie Salbert

Illinois

KaRabida Children's Hospital and
Research Center
E. 65th at Lake Michigan
Chicago, IL 60649
312/363–6700
Contact: Dr. Nancy Roizen

UAP Family Clinic M/C 626
University of Illinois
1640 West Roosevelt Road
Chicago, IL 60608–6902
312/413–1871
Contact: Dr. Ann Cutler
            Dennis McGuire

Lutheran General Children's
    Hospital
Subspecialty Outpatient Center
1255 N. Milwaukee Avenue
Glenview, IL 60025
708/318–2980
Contact: Dr. Nancy Keck

Lutheran General Adult Down
    Syndrome Clinic
Department of Family Practice
1775 Ballard Road
Park Ridge, IL 60068
708/318–2878
Contact: Dr. Brian Chicoine

Indiana

Ann Whitehill Down Syndrome Pro-
    gram
James Whitcomb Riley Hospital for
    Children
702 Barnhill Drive, Room 1601
Indiana University Medical Center
Indianapolis, IN 46223
317/274–4842
Contact: Dr. Marilyn J. Bull

Riley Hospital for Children
Room 1601
702 Barnhill Drive
Indianapolis, IN 46223
Contact: Candace Zickler, CPNP

Iowa

Division of Developmental
    Disabilities
University of Iowa Hospital & Clinic
Iowa City, IA 52242
319/353–6460
Contact: Dr. Don Van Dyke

Louisiana

LSU Medical
1542 Tulane Avenue
New Orleans, LA 70112
504/568–4850
Contact: Dr. Thomas E. Elkins

Maryland

Kennedy Institute Down Syndrome
    Clinic
707 N. Broadway
Baltimore, MD 21205
410/550–9420
410/550–8839 Clinic Coord.
Contact: Dr. George Capone

Massachusetts

Down Syndrome Program
Children's Hospital
300 Longwood Avenue
Boston, MA 02115
617/735 6509
Contact: Dr. Allen Crocker

Michigan

University of Michigan Medical
Center
Department of Obstetrics &
Gynecology
MPB D2202
Ann Arbor, MI 48109–0718
313/763–6670
Contact: Dr. Elisabeth H. Quint

Minnesota

Group Health, Inc.
6845 Lee Avenue North
Brooklyn Center, MN 55429
Contact: Dr. J. Margaret Horrobin

Developmental and Rehabilitative
Services
Minneapolis Children's Medical
Center
2525 Chicago Avenue S.
Minneapolis, MN 55404
612/863–6593
Contact: Dr. Kim McConnell

University of Minnesota
Department of Educational
Psychology
Burton Hill, Room 255
178 Pillsbury Drive, SE
Minneapolis, MN 55455
612/624–5241
Contact: John E. Rynders, Ph.D.

Missouri

Children's Mercy Hospital
2401 Gillham Road
Kansas City, MO 64108
816/234–3290
Contact: Dr. David Harris

Down Syndrome Medical Clinic
Children's Hospital
Washington University Medical
Center
400 S. Kingshighway Blvd.
St. Louis, MO 63110
314/454–6095
Contact: Dr. Arnold Strauss

New Hampshire

Down Syndrome Program
Clinical Genetics & Child
Development Center
Dartmouth Medical School
Hanover, NH 03756
603/646–7884
Contact: Dr. W. Carl Cooley

New Jersey

D.D.C. #60
Morristown Memorial Hospital
100 Madison Avenue
Morristown, NJ 07962–1956
201/971–4095
Contact: Dr. Theodore A. Kastner

UMDNJ-Robert Wood Johnson
    Medical School
Dept. of Family Medicine (Rm 284C)
1 Robert Wood Johnson Place
New Brunswick, NJ 08903
908/937–7662
Contact: Dr. Robert C. Like

Department of Family Medicine
New Jersey Medical School
Med. Science Bldg., B-636
185 South Orange Avenue
Newark, NJ 07013
201/982–6481
Contact: Dr. Caryl J. Heaton

New York

Genesee Developmental Unit
224 Alexander Avenue
Rochester, NY 14607
716/263–5237
Contact: Dr. Nancy Lanphear

Institute for Basic Research
    in Developmental Disabilities
1050 Forest Hill Road
Staten Island, NY 10314

718/494–0600
Contact: Dr. Krystyna Wisniewski

Down Syndrome Interdisciplinary
    Clinic
Mental Retardation Institute
Cedarwood Hall
New York Medical College
Valhall, NY 10595
914/347–4514
Contact: Dr. Taesun Chung

North Dakota

Children's Hospital
MeritCare Down Syndrome Service
737 Broadway
Fargo, ND 58102
701/234–2568
Contact: Dr. Guy Carter

Down Syndrome Outpatient Service
Coordinated Treatment Center
St. Luke's Hospitals-Meritcare
720 4th Street, N
Fargo, ND 58122
701/234–5737
800/443–4779
Contact: Dr. Gerald T. Atwood

Ohio

Blick Clinic for Developmental
    Disabilities
640 W. Market Street
Akron, OH 44303
216/762–5425
Contact: Dr. Jane Holan

Cincinnati Center for Developmental Disorders
University of Cincinnati
Pavilion Building
Elland and Bethesda Avenues
Cincinnati, OH 45229
513/559–4691
Contact: Dr. Bonnie Patterson

ARC/Baker International
Resource Center for Down
Syndrome
Keith Bldg., Suite 514
1621 Euclid Avenue
Cleveland, OH 44115
216/621–5858
Contact: Rebecca J. Hoffman, R.N.

Down Syndrome Clinic
Rainbow Babies and Children's
Hospital
2074 Abington Road
Cleveland, OH 44106
216/844–1517
Contact: Dr. Joanne Mortimer

Children's Hospital
700 Children's Drive
Columbus, OH 54304
614/461–2663
Contact: Dr. Annemarie Sommers

Down Syndrome Clinic
Department of Pediatrics
Medical College of Ohio
Health Center

Box 10008
Toledo, OH 43699
419/381–3831
Contact: Dr. Eileen Quinn

Pennsylvania

Dr. Gertrude A. Barber Center
136 East Avenue
Erie, PA 16507
814/459–4211
Contact: Dr. Joseph Barber

Department of Pediatrics
PA State University
College of Medicine
Hershey, PA 17033
Contact: Dr. Roger Ladda

Department of Genetics
Milton S. Hershey Medical Center
Division of Genetics
Box 850
Hershey, PA 17033
717/531–8414
Contact: Maria Mascari, Ph.D.

Down Syndrome of Center of
Western Pennsylvania
Children's Hospital of Pittsburgh
One Children's Place
3705 Fifth Avenue
Pittsburgh, PA 15213–2583
412/692–7693 or 5560/6546
Contact: Dr. William I. Cohen
Nancy Murray, MS

Rhode Island

Child Development Center
Rhode Island Hospital
593 Eddy Street
Providence, RI 02902
401/277–5071
Contact: Dr. Siegfried M. Pueschel

Texas

Down Syndrome Clinic
Children's Medical Center of Dallas
4th Floor-Genetics
1935 Motor Street
Dallas, TX 75235
Contact: Dr. Golder Wilson

Santa Rosa Medical Center
Box 7330, Station A
San Antonio, TX 78285
512/228–2386
Contact: Dr. Robert J. Clayton

University Family Health Center-
Southeast
3819 S. Gevers
San Antonio, TX 78223
210/531–5500
Contact: Sue Doty, M.D., Ph.D.

Virginia

Children's Hospital of the Kings
Daughter
Eastern Virginia Medical School
601 Children's Lane
Norfolk, VA 23507

804/628–7473
Contact: Dr. Thomas Montgomery

Dr. Patricia Hunt
7834 Forest Avenue
Richmond, VA 23225
804/272–8197

Wisconsin

Waisman Center Down Syndrome
Clinic
1500 Highland
Madison, WI 53705
608/263–7335
Contact: Dr. Renata Laxova

St. Michael Family Care Center
2400 W. Willard Avenue
Milwaukee, WI 53209
414/527–8191
Contact: Dr. David Smith

Argentina

Hospital Aleman
Caallia Correo 41310
1118 Pueyrredon 1640
Buenos Aries, Argentina
Contact: Dr. Rafael Durlach

Australia

Health Promotion Clinic for the
Developmentally
Disabled, Clinic 5
Royal North Shore Hospital and
Area Health Service

Pacific Highway
St. Leonard's 2065
New South Wales, Australia
02/438/7688
Contact: Dr. Helen Beange

Brazil

Pediatrician/ Public Health
Rua Dr. Louis County, 159–Pinhei-
ros
Sao Paulo-SP-Brazil-05436–030
55/011 282/8130
Contact: Dr. Jose Torres Assuncao

Canada

Down Syndrome Clinic
North York General Hospital
4001 Leslie Street
Toronto, Ontario, Canada
416/756–6000

Montreal Children's Hospital
2300 Tupper Avenue (#A331)
Montreal, Quebec H3H 1P3
Canada
1/514–934–4324 or 4475
Contact: Dr. Jean-Francois Lemay

Surrey Place Centre
University of Toronto
2 Surrey Place
Toronto, Ontario M5S 2C2
Canada
416/925–5141
416/923–8476
Contact: Dr. John Lovering

Japan

University of Tokyo
Department of Maternal and Child
Health
7–3–1, Hongo, Bunkyo
Tokyo, 113 Japan
Contact: Dr. Makoto Higurashi

Spain

Centre Medic Down
Valencia, 231, 4o 4a
08007 Barcelon, Spain
930215–7699
Contact: Dr. Augustin Seres-San-
tamaria

Fundacion Sindrome de Down de
Canabria
Universidad de Santander
Santander, Spain
34–42–338800
Contact: Dr. Jesus Florez

Sweden

Department of Clinical Genetics
Children's Hospital
University of Uppsala
751 85 Uppsala
Sweden
46–18 554025
Contact: Goran Anneren, PhD.

Index

About the Editors

Don C. Van Dyke, M.D.

Don C. Van Dyke, M.D., is Associate Professor of Pediatrics at the University Hospital School in the Division of Developmental Disabilities, Department of Pediatrics, University of Iowa Hospitals and Clinics, where he works in a number of programs for individuals with developmental disabilities, including Down syndrome. For the past ten years, he has conducted research and provided direct clinical care and clinical management for individuals with Down syndrome.

Philip Mattheis, M.D.

Philip Mattheis, M.D., is a developmental pediatrician who received most of his training at the University of Iowa at Iowa City. He works at the University of Montana, in Missoula, at the Rural Institute on Disabilities. Down Syndrome and other disabilities that affect thinking, learning, and speaking are his primary interests in clinic and research. He is the father of three children, and his youngest child has Down syndrome (whom he credits with providing the rest of his training in developmental disabilities).

Susan Schoon Eberly, M.A.

For the past decade, Susan Schoon Eberly, M.A., has worked at the University of Iowa Hospitals and Schools as an editor and then as publications supervisor in the Division of Developmental Disabilities, which is also Iowa's University Affiliated Program. Her work as a writer and editor of materials for children, families, and professionals reflects her personal experience with the ways in which a child's disability can affect a family.

Janet K. Williams, M.A., Ph.D.

Janet K. Williams, M.A., Ph.D., is an Assistant Professor of Nursing at the University of Iowa and a member of the University's Down syndrome clinic team. She provides genetic counseling to families of individuals with Down syndrome who attend these clinics at various sites across the state of Iowa.